AF601254

Advanced Practice in Nursing

Under the Auspices of the International Council of Nurses (ICN)

Series Editor

Christophe Debout, GIP-IFITS
Health Chair Sciences- Po Paris/IDS UMR Inserm 1145
Paris, France

April Kapu • Jackie Rowles
Jennifer Manning • Mavis N Schorn
Editors

A Global View on Clinical Autonomy for Advanced Practice Nurses

Enhancing Decision-Making, Leadership, and Collaborative Care

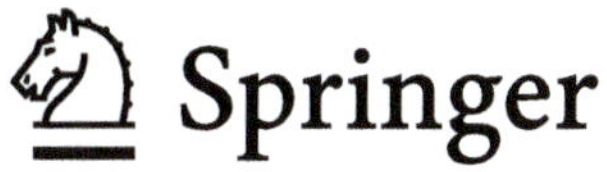

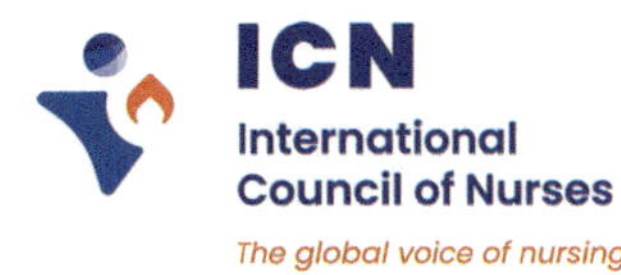

Editors
April Kapu
School of Nursing
Vanderbilt University
Nashville, TN, USA

Jennifer Manning
School of Nursing
Louisiana State University Health Science
New Orleans, LA, USA

Jackie Rowles
School of Nurse Anesthesia
Harris College and Nursing
and Health Sciences
Texas Christian University
Fort Worth, TX, USA

Mavis N Schorn
Vanderbilt University School of Nursing
Vanderbilt University
Nashville, TN, USA

ISSN 2511-3917 ISSN 2511-3925 (electronic)
Advanced Practice in Nursing
ISBN 978-3-032-21457-7 ISBN 978-3-032-21458-4 (eBook)
https://doi.org/10.1007/978-3-032-21458-4

This Springer imprint is published by the registered company Springer Nature Switzerland AG
The registered company address is: Gewerbestrasse 11, 6330 Cham, Switzerland

Preface

This volume advances a conversation that has been waiting to be written. Clinical autonomy, rooted in centuries of philosophical thought and refined through modern bioethics, is often discussed in the abstract. Here, we examine clinical autonomy in practice, centered on Advanced Practice Nurses (APNs), and follow its implications through ethics, regulation, payment, organizational design, and measurement, and ultimately, outcomes for people and communities. Our contributors, from healthcare clinics and educational universities to ministries of health and influential boards, trace how autonomy becomes care through increased access, safer decisions, and more equitable reach.

This is the first book to treat APN clinical autonomy as a global, practice-oriented construct. It builds on prior syntheses and empirical studies that conceptualized APN clinical autonomy in practice and began to specify how it is supported, constrained, and measured [24, 25]. It is both synthesis and blueprint, and deliberately a beginning. We invite readers to test, adapt, and refine what follows so that autonomy is consistently understood, responsibly exercised, reliably measured, and transparently accountable, wherever people, families, and communities seek care.

Nashville, TN, USA — April Kapu
Fort Worth, TX, USA — Jackie Rowles
New Orleans, LA, USA — Jennifer Manning
Nashville, TN, USA — Mavis N Schorn

Introduction

Why Clinical Autonomy Matters

Clinical autonomy sits at the center of safe, equitable, person-centered care. Properly understood, it is neither isolation nor unilateral independence; it is the earned capacity to exercise professional judgment within clear standards, ethical duties, and collaborative systems. In practice, autonomy enables clinicians to act decisively on behalf of people receiving care, reason through complexity, consult judiciously, and be accountable for outcomes. Its stakes are universal, but they are most visible where access is constrained and the healthcare workforce is stretched [1–5]. Recent scholarship frames APN clinical autonomy as a dynamic, practice-embedded construct with clear organizational determinants and person-facing consequences [24], and empirical evidence indicates it increases with accumulating clinical experience and is reinforced by supportive organizational culture [25].

For clarity, in this volume, autonomy refers to accountable clinical decision-making authority exercised within a regulated scope of practice, professional standards, and collaborative care systems. We intentionally avoid describing APN practice as fully "independent," because advanced practice nursing is enacted in interprofessional environments with defined consultation, referral, and escalation pathways. Autonomy is, therefore, best understood as practiced self-governance and responsibility, not isolation.

This book places clinical autonomy for advanced practice nurses (APNs) at the forefront of a global, practice-oriented conversation. ICN guidance underscores that "APN" is not a single, uniform role internationally; across its 2020 and 2021 publications, ICN describes advanced practice nursing roles that include clinical nurse specialists (CNSs), nurse practitioners (NPs), and nurse anesthetists [26, 27].

However, advanced practice roles are organized and titled differently across countries and regions, and some advanced clinical roles are not uniformly classified as APN roles across global frameworks. Accordingly, this volume uses "advanced practice nursing" as an umbrella term that collectively refers to nurse anesthetists, nurse-midwives, clinical nurse specialists, and nurse practitioners in settings where these roles are regulated, graduate-prepared, and authorized for advanced scope and responsibilities. Throughout the book, we therefore attend carefully to role distinctions, titles, and country context rather than assuming a single global role model.

When APNs are both regulated and supported to practice to the full range of their education and training, they measurably contribute to timely access, quality outcomes, prevention, continuity, and experience of care, particularly in primary care, chronic disease management, maternal health, mental health, and rural settings [1–5, 12–14, 21]. The aim of this book is not merely to defend the concept but to demonstrate how autonomy—embedded within standards, ethics, and interprofessional collaboration—becomes a system-level lever for health improvement of populations.

ICN Anchor for Advanced Practice Nursing Role Development

The International Council of Nurses Guidelines on Advanced Practice Nursing 2020 emphasize that advanced practice nursing development requires educational preparation beyond that of a generalist nurse, role-specific competencies and standards, and clear mechanisms for regulation and credentialing to support role clarity and accountability across settings [26]. ICN also notes that the breadth and depth of autonomy associated with the APN often arises across an extensive range of community-based services, including primary healthcare, ambulatory services, and out-of-hospital settings, and that autonomy may evolve over time as advanced practice nursing gains recognition [26]. Across contexts, ICN emphasizes that the APN is fundamentally a nursing role built on nursing principles and enacted through collaboration, including consultation and referral when appropriate [26].

The Philosophical Roots of Autonomy and Their Clinical Relevance

The term autonomy, from autos (self) and nomos (rule), originated in ancient Greece as self-governance of city-states, later evolving into a personal attribute of self-governance central to moral agency and rights. Kant's view frames autonomy as self-legislation through reasonable freedom from controlling influences and the capacity to bind oneself to moral law, while Aristotelian traditions emphasize rational desire, deliberation, and moral responsibility. These perspectives converge on a practical insight that matters in the clinical setting: autonomy requires the capacity to understand, deliberate, and own one's reasons for action [22, 23].

Modern bioethics adapted these ideas into the principle of respect for autonomy, shaping informed consent, decisional capacity, and freedom from coercion or undue influence. In clinical practice, this means autonomy has both negative obligations, such as avoiding controlling and unnecessary constraints, and positive obligations, such as fostering capacity for informed and voluntary decision-making [6–11].

From Patient Autonomy to Professional Autonomy

- **Person autonomy:** Contemporary standards require informed consent grounded in adequate disclosure, comprehension, voluntariness, and decision-making capacity. The Belmont Report and the Declaration of Helsinki formalize these principles, and practical guidance is reinforced by clinical and legal frameworks (e.g., capacity assessment in primary care and privacy protections for access to information). Respect for autonomy has moved care from paternalism toward shared decision-making models that align treatments with the person's values [7–11].
- **Professional autonomy:** Nurses, physicians, and other healthcare providers require autonomy to exercise expert judgment in real time within ethical codes and regulatory scope. Professional autonomy is not absolute; it is accountable to evidence, standards, resource stewardship, and the person's right to self-determination. The ICN Code of Ethics emphasizes professional responsibility for evidence-informed practice, advocacy, cultural safety, and collaboration, while acknowledging that autonomous practice is inseparable from accountability for outcomes [2]. In nursing, autonomy includes authority and accountability for practice and extends to decisions about practice environments, including policies and operations [1–5].

Clinical autonomy for APNs bridges these domains. It presumes deep respect for person-centered self-determination while enabling advanced nursing judgment to deliver safe, effective, equitable care.

Defining Clinical Autonomy for APNs

We use clinical autonomy to mean the capacity and authority of APNs to make and enact accountable clinical decisions within regulated scope, professional standards, and ethical obligations. This framing aligns with ICN guidance that APN practice is grounded in graduate education and defined competencies, with autonomy and accountability shaped by country-specific regulation, credentialing, and scope-of-practice policies [26]. Clinical autonomy in APN practice is characterized by:

- Eliciting and interpreting person-centered narratives and clinical data; formulating differential diagnoses; ordering and interpreting tests; initiating and adjusting treatments; and evaluating outcomes.
- Exercising judgment while engaging in timely consultation and referral when care needs exceed scope or competency.
- Being accountable for decisions, including documentation, communication, safety, quality, and stewardship of resources.

This autonomy is developmental. Early practice is bounded by supervision and collaborative oversight; with advanced education, specialization, mentoring, and a track record of outcomes, the circle of discretion expands. Mature practice is characterized by interdependence, including the ability to act decisively and consult judiciously in service of people and populations [1–3, 21]. These components align with an empirically derived definition of clinical autonomy as self-determination, including competence, relatedness, and autonomy, paired with the authority to complete full episodes of evidence-based care (diagnosis, prescribing, referrals, discharge) within enabling regulation and organizational culture [24, 25].

What Clinical Autonomy Is Not

- **Not absolute independence:** Comparative evidence cautions against equating autonomy with independence [24, 25]. "Independent" implies self-sufficiency detached from interprofessional team-based care. Nursing autonomy is both autonomous and collaborative, with structured pathways for consultation and referral [1–3].
- **Not competition with physicians:** APN autonomy complements, rather than displaces, medical practice. Mature systems delineate scopes clearly, coordinate care, and realize gains in access, continuity, and person-centered experience [4, 5, 12–14, 21].
- **Not unregulated discretion:** Clinical autonomy is exercised within codified scope, ethical codes, standards, and outcome accountability. It grows with competency and demonstrated safety [1–3, 6].

Ethical Grounding: Autonomy Alongside Beneficence, Nonmaleficence, and Justice

The four-principles approach, which includes respect for autonomy, beneficence, nonmaleficence, and justice, offers a practical framework for clinical judgment. Autonomy is often "first among equals" in liberal-individualist contexts, but not absolute; its limits are negotiated when beneficence or justice present compelling counterclaims (e.g., coercive measures justified only under severe risk and impaired capacity). In nursing, ethical codes embed this balance: respect person-centered self-determination, prevent harm, promote well-being, and steward fair use of resources [2, 6, 16–18].

Relational Autonomy and Shared Decision-Making

Autonomy is personal and relational. People make choices within family, cultural, and social contexts. Respecting autonomy includes respecting how people wish to decide, including family involvement, provided influence is not coercive. APNs foster autonomy by building capacity through clear explanations, teach-back, deliberate support, and time to consider options. APNs' strengths in communication, education, and continuity make them well-positioned to operationalize relational autonomy in practice [1–3, 16–18]. In addition, field studies of APNs illustrate this relational dimension in practice, described as "living it," through communication, capacity building, and continuity that enable informed and voluntary decisions [24, 25].

Why APN Clinical Autonomy Matters for Access, Quality, and Equity

When APNs practice with clear authority, people experience:

- **Faster access and continuity:** APNs expand primary care panels, reduce wait times, and stabilize services in rural and underserved settings [4, 5, 21]. Synthesis across settings directly associates APN autonomy with improved patient flow and reduced waits [24].
- **Strong performance on prevention and chronic disease:** Emphasis on education, lifestyle support, and evidence-based care improves adherence and control in conditions such as diabetes, hypertension, COPD, and depression [11, 16–18, 21].
- **Person-centered communication and shared decision-making:** People report high satisfaction with APN-led care, citing time for questions, comprehensible explanations, and a sense of partnership [11, 16–18].
- **System efficiency:** Appropriate test ordering, timely follow-up, avoidance of avoidable emergency department visits and admissions, and improved transitions reduce fragmentation [4, 5, 12–14, 21].
- **Workforce resilience:** Meaningful autonomy correlates with professional satisfaction and retention; conversely, ambiguous scope and unnecessary constraints contribute to moral distress and attrition [1–3, 12–14, 21, 24, 25].

These outcomes are not attributable to autonomy alone, but to autonomy embedded in coherent structures: competency-based education, enabling regulation, aligned payment, supportive organizational policies, and outcome measurement [1–5, 21].

Early Examples of APN Autonomy Driving Access

These illustrative vignettes preview the detailed cases explored later in the book. They are composites grounded in documented patterns from healthcare systems with robust APN roles.

- **Rural primary care continuity:** In a remote district clinic facing months-long wait times for care, a newly credentialed APN is granted authority for diagnosis, prescribing within formulary, and chronic disease management protocols. Within six months, median time-to-appointment decreased from 28 to 7 days; hypertension control rates improved, supported by standardized education and follow-up plans. The APN coordinated teleconsultation with regional specialists for complex cases, illustrating interdependence rather than isolation [4, 5, 11, 16–18, 21].

- **Community mental health access:** In a safety-net setting, an APN with mental health specialization led an integrated program for depression and anxiety. With standing screening protocols, brief interventions, and prescriptive authority, time-to-first-treatment decreased from weeks to days. Shared decision-making and clear consent processes increased adherence and reduced acute, urgent, and emergency care visits [8–11, 16–18].
- **Maternal health in underserved areas:** A midwifery APN model with prescriptive authority for prenatal and postpartum care standardized risk assessment, managed routine cases autonomously, and co-managed high-risk pregnancies with obstetrics. Prenatal visit adherence increased, and postpartum complications decreased through proactive follow-up and education. Formal escalation pathways for referral were used when needed to ensure comprehensive and safe care [1–5, 16–18].
- **Urban safety-net diabetes program:** At a large clinic facing high HbA1c levels and poor follow-up adherence among uninsured and underinsured people, APNs led a protocolized care pathway that combined prescriptive authority, point-of-care testing, and shared decision-making tools. They coordinated social supports, medication access programs, and group education to address barriers beyond the clinic. Outcomes included improved glycemic control, fewer emergency visits for hyperglycemic crises, and higher person-reported understanding of self-management. People attributed improvements to rapid treatment adjustments, care personalization, continuity with the care team, and informed consent practices [10, 11, 16–18, 21].
- **Telehealth-enabled chronic care in dispersed regions:** In dispersed communities, people with COPD and heart failure experienced delays in medication titration and preventable hospital admissions. APNs, practicing with authority to order diagnostics, adjust evidence-based therapies, and initiate advance care planning, used remote monitoring to guide care. Clear escalation criteria and virtual consultation pathways with physicians and pharmacists were codified. As a result, time to therapy optimization decreased, readmissions fell, engagement in care plans improved, and documentation of preferences demonstrated active participation [8–11, 16–18, 21].

Regulatory and Economic Determinants: From Principle to Practice

Policy architecture determines whether APN autonomy is implemented diligently or constrained.

- **Scope-of-practice clarity:** Statutory authority for diagnosis, ordering, and prescribing, aligned with education and certification, enables APN judgment at the point of care [33–36]. Ambiguity invites institutional barriers, such as unnecessary co-signature rules, that delay decisions and dilute accountability [1–5, 21].

- **Collaboration requirements:** Requirements that make consultation a resource rather than gatekeeping improve timeliness without compromising safety. During public health emergencies, streamlined collaboration, paired with escalation and documentation standards, showed safe, scalable pathways for expanded APN authority [4, 5]. Evidence from Ireland illustrates how national policy reforms (e.g., removal of collaborative practice requirements) can be blunted by local governance practices, underscoring the need to align regulation with organizational implementation [24, 25].
- **Payment recognition:** Direct billing privileges and inclusion in value-based arrangements allow APNs to manage panels and invest in prevention. Where payment requires physician intermediation regardless of service, APN-led access improvement is curtailed. Aligning incentives with outcomes (e.g., chronic disease control and readmission reduction) recognizes and rewards APN strengths [4, 5, 21].
- **Organizational governance:** Credentialing, privileging, standing orders, and decision support translate legal scope into daily practice. Effective governance includes explicit criteria for legally permitted actions and mandatory consultation; peer case review focused on learning; and access to guidelines, order sets, and documentation templates supporting consent and capacity assessment [1–3, 10, 11, 16–18].
- **Ethical and legal compliance as enablers:** Informed consent frameworks, capacity assessments, and privacy protections clarify roles and protect people receiving care and clinicians. These processes structure transparent, person-centered decision-making aligned with autonomy and accountability [7–11].

Measuring Clinical Autonomy and Its Impact

Validated instruments can complement outcome portfolios. The Dempster Practice Behaviors Scale (DPBS) assesses professional autonomy behaviors, while the Advanced Nursing Practice Clinical Autonomy Impact Scale (ANPCAIS) captures actual clinical autonomy in practice. In national data, ANPCAIS demonstrated good reliability and sensitivity to NP experience [25]. Lockwood's review also noted the scarcity of APN-specific autonomy measures and called for continued psychometric development [24]. A practical measurement portfolio links autonomy to outcomes and should be used for improvement:

- **Structure and process indicators:** Degree of discretion in assessment, diagnosis, prescribing, and follow-up within defined scope; consultation and referral timeliness; consent and capacity documentation completeness; privacy rights in practice [8–11].
- **Outcome indicators:** Safety (adverse events and escalation), quality (guideline adherence and disease control), access (wait times and panel size), experience

(understanding, involvement, and satisfaction), and equity (reach and results in underserved groups) [4, 5, 11, 16–18, 21].
- **Professional environment:** Clinician-reported autonomy, decision latitude, moral distress, and intention to stay [1–3, 12–14].
- **Learning and governance:** Case reviews on decision quality and escalation; rapid-cycle improvements that refine protocols and documentation [6, 10, 11, 16–18].

Ethical Nuances in Application: Capacity, Coercion, Culture

Although autonomy is discussed here in the context of APN-led practice, APNs, as well as other clinicians, must guard against coercion and undue influence. Ethical guidance requires distinguishing supportive family involvement from manipulative pressure and ensuring voluntariness in decisions, especially in high-stakes or vulnerable contexts [6–8]. The Declaration of Helsinki and the Belmont Report underscore that valid consent depends on freedom from controlling influences and adequate understanding. Consent processes should therefore include strategies to identify and mitigate overt threats, excessive inducements, or subtle pressures while maintaining space for people to voice their preferences [7, 8]. When influence crosses into control, consent is invalid and must be re-established with protections in place [6–8].

Relational autonomy and cultural humility are essential to ethical practice. Many people prefer family-inclusive deliberation; ethically sound care respects this preference while centering the person's voice and values and using communication practices that foster understanding and voluntariness [11, 22, 23]. Nursing frameworks emphasize person-centered care, caring science, and cultural safety as the ethical context in which autonomy is realized. Clinicians build trusting relationships, surface what matters to the person, and attend to power, identity, and context, particularly where historical or structural inequities shape clinical encounters [1–3, 16–18]. The ICN Code of Ethics and renewed ICN definitions explicitly position nurses' autonomous and accountable decision-making within collaborative practice and regulation, highlighting that professional autonomy is exercised in partnership with people, families, and communities to protect dignity, rights, and equity [1–3].

Practical Guidance: Making APN Autonomy Work Day-to-Day

- **Policymakers:** Align scope with preparation; authorize prescriptive rights; enable direct billing and value-based participation; require performance reporting on access, quality, and equity [4, 5, 21].
- **Health system leaders:** Privilege APNs to full legal scope; remove unnecessary co-signatures; standardize consultation thresholds; invest in consent and capacity tools and privacy workflows [6–11, 16–18]. Implementation strategies that

explicitly support self-determination needs, including competence, relatedness, and autonomy, appear to strengthen APN clinical autonomy and its impact [25].

- **Educators:** Embed consent, capacity, shared decision-making, and documentation excellence in curricula and continuing education; use simulation and case review for complex scenarios such as health literacy, family engagement, and limited capacity [6, 10–11, 16–18].
- **APNs:** Exercise judgment within scope; consult early for complexity; make consent a conversation; document reasoning and follow-up; track outcomes for improvement [8–11, 16–18, 21].

First of Its Kind and a Deliberate Beginning

This is the first comprehensive volume to center APN clinical autonomy as a global, practice-oriented construct, connecting philosophical roots, bioethics, legal frameworks, regulation, payment, organizational governance, measurement, and real-world cases. It is intentionally a starting point, a blueprint for iterative refinement toward a globally accepted, locally adaptable framework. We anticipate debate and welcome improvement. The trajectory is clear: people and communities benefit when APNs are prepared, authorized, and supported to exercise clinical judgment and practice autonomously.

The textbook contains five main sections, with chapters authored by internationally recognized experts in the field of advanced practice. The sections are as follows:

- **Part I: APN Roles Globally**
  Maps titles, scopes, and educational pathways; identifies how culture and system design shape autonomy.
- **Part II: Regulation and Levels of Authority**
  Reviews legislation, licensure, prescriptive rights, and collaboration and supervision requirements; analyzes the implications of reforms and emergency waivers.
- **Part III: Benefits of Autonomous Practice**
  Synthesizes evidence on access, quality, safety, person-centered experience, and efficiency; includes case studies from varied health systems.
- **Part IV: Global Variations and Challenges**
  Examines barriers (e.g., payment misalignment, professional opposition, legal ambiguity) and enabling strategies.
- **Part V: Enhancing APN Clinical Autonomy in Low-Resource Settings**
  Offers practical approaches for education, mentorship, regulation, governance, and measurement suitable for constrained environments.
- **Conclusion: The Path Forward**
  Proposes elements of a globally accepted framework: standardized definitions, competency-based education, enabling regulation, aligned payment, robust measurement, and interprofessional partnership.

Through these writings, it is clear that a globally accepted, locally adaptable framework would include standardized definitions linking person and professional autonomy; competency-based education in consent, capacity, shared decision-making, and documentation; enabling regulation; aligned payment; robust measurement tied to improvement; and interprofessional partnership anchored in respect and clarity [1–6, 11, 16–18, 21]. We invite readers to apply, test, and refine the tools and principles offered here, moving from localized exemplars to shared architecture, and from aspiration to sustainable, equitable impact.

References

1. International Council of Nurses. Renewing the definitions of 'nursing' and 'a nurse': Final project report. Geneva: ICN; 2025. Available from: https://www.icn.ch/
2. International Council of Nurses. The ICN code of ethics for nurses. Geneva: ICN; 2021. Available from: https://www.icn.ch/system/files/2023-06/ICN_Code-of-Ethics_EN_Web.pdf
3. International Council of Nurses. Nursing definitions (current and archival). Geneva: ICN; 2002. Available from: https://www.icn.ch/resources/nursing-definitions
4. World Health Organization. Global strategic directions for nursing and midwifery 2021–2025. Geneva: WHO; 2021. Available from: https://www.who.int/publications/i/item/9789240033863
5. World Health Organization. State of the world's nursing 2025: investing in education, jobs and leadership. 2025. https://www.who.int/publications/i/item/9789240110236
6. Beauchamp TL, Childress JF. Principles of biomedical ethics. 8th ed. New York: Oxford University Press; 2019.
7. World Medical Association. Declaration of Helsinki – ethical principles for medical research involving human subjects. Ferney-Voltaire: WMA; 2013 (rev). Available from: https://www.wma.net/policies-post/wma-declaration-of-helsinki-ethical-principles-for-medical-research-involving-human-subjects/
8. U.S. Department of Health and Human Services, Office for Human Research Protections. The Belmont Report. Washington (DC): HHS; 1979. Available from: https://www.hhs.gov/ohrp/regulations-and-policy/belmont-report/index.html
9. U.S. Department of Health and Human Services. HIPAA for individuals: your rights under HIPAA. Washington (DC): HHS; 2024. Available from: https://www.hhs.gov/hipaa/for-individuals/index.html
10. American Academy of Family Physicians. Evaluating medical decision-making capacity in practice. Am Fam Physician. 2018;98(1):40–6.
11. Elwyn G, Frosch DL, Thomson R, Joseph-Williams N, Lloyd A, Kinnersley P, et al. Shared decision making: a model for clinical practice. BMJ. 2012;344:e245.
12. Aiken LH, Clarke SP, Sloane DM, Sochalski J, Silber JH. Hospital nurse staffing and patient mortality, nurse burnout, and job dissatisfaction. JAMA. 2002;288(16):1987–93.
13. McHugh MD, Aiken LH, Sloane DM, Windsor C, Douglas C, Yates P. Effects of nurse-to-patient ratio legislation on staffing and patient outcomes. Lancet. 2021;397(10288):1905–13.
14. Aiken LH, Sloane D, Griffiths P, Rafferty AM, Bruyneel L, McHugh M, et al. Nursing skill mix in European hospitals: cross-sectional study. BMJ Qual Saf. 2017;26(7):559–68.
15. All-Party Parliamentary Group on Global Health. Triple Impact: how developing nursing will improve health, promote gender equality and support economic growth. London: APPG; 2016. Available from: https://www.appg-globalhealth.org.uk/
16. McCormack B, McCance T, Bulley C, Brown D, McMillan A, Martin S. Fundamentals of person centred healthcare practice. 2nd ed. Hoboken: Wiley-Blackwell; 2021.
17. Watson J. Nursing: the philosophy and science of caring. Boulder: University Press of Colorado; 2008.

18. Ramsden I. Cultural safety and nursing education in Aotearoa and Te Waipounamu [dissertation]. Wellington: Victoria University of Wellington; 2002.
19. OECD. Health at a glance 2023: OECD indicators. Paris: OECD Publishing; 2023. Available from: https://www.oecd.org/health/
20. International Labour Organization. Nursing Personnel Convention, 1977 (No. 149) and Recommendation (No. 157). Geneva: ILO; 1977. Available from: https://www.ilo.org/
21. National Academies of Sciences, Engineering, and Medicine. The future of nursing 2020–2030: charting a path to achieve health equity. Washington (DC): National Academies Press; 2021.
22. Stanford Encyclopedia of Philosophy. Personal autonomy. 2018. Available from: https://plato.stanford.edu/entries/personal-autonomy/
23. Oxford Bibliographies. Autonomy. Available from: https://www.oxfordbibliographies.com/abstract/document/obo-9780195396577/obo-9780195396577-0167.xml
24. Lockwood EB, Lehwaldt D, Sweeney MR, Matthews A. An exploration of the levels of clinical autonomy of advanced nurse practitioners: a narrative literature review. Int J Nurs Pract. 2022;28(1):e12978. doi:10.1111/ijn.12978. https://pubmed.ncbi.nlm.nih.gov/38651183/
25. Lockwood EB, Schober M. Factors influencing the impact of nurse practitioners' clinical autonomy; a self-determining perspective. Int Nurs Rev. 2024;71(2):375–395. 10.1111/inr.12948. https://onlinelibrary.wiley.com/doi/10.1111/inr.12948
26. International Council of Nurses (ICN). Guidelines on advanced practice nursing 2020. Geneva, Switzerland: International Council of Nurses; 2020. Available at: https://www.icn.ch/sites/default/files/2023-04/ICN_APN%20Report_EN.pdf
27. International Council of Nurses. Guidelines on advanced practice nursing: nurse anesthetists. 2021. https://www.icn.ch/resources/publications-and-reports/guidelines-advanced-practice-nursing-nurse-anesthetists-2021

Contents

Clinical Autonomy for Nurse Practitioners

Nilufeur McKay and April Kapu

The global health-care environment is one of converging pressures: accelerating population aging, a rising burden of chronic disease and comorbidities, persistent access to care gaps, and significant workforce shortages. Within this context, nurse practitioners (NPs), advanced practice nurses with master's or doctoral preparation, deliver comprehensive care anchored in diagnostic acumen, pharmacotherapeutics, and a preventive, person-centered approach. The International Council of Nurses (ICN) defines advanced practice nursing (APN) as practice grounded in expert knowledge, complex decision making, and advanced clinical competencies shaped by the practice context; a master's degree is recommended for entry [1]. For NPs, clinical autonomy links this competence to impact: where law, regulation, and organizational policy enable autonomous practice within governance systems and collaborative care models, NPs can reduce delays, streamline care, and extend access, particularly in underserved communities, while supporting informed choice, continuity, and shared decision making. This chapter synthesizes the international evidence and experience, mapping the relationship between autonomy and outcomes, and offering policy and practice insights to advance NP roles globally.

N. McKay (✉)
School of Nursing and Midwifery, Edith Cowan University, Perth, WA, Australia
e-mail: n.mckay@ecu.edu.au

A. Kapu
School of Nursing, Vanderbilt University, Nashville, TN, USA

A. Kapu et al. (eds.), *A Global View on Clinical Autonomy for Advanced Practice Nurses*, Advanced Practice in Nursing,
https://doi.org/10.1007/978-3-032-21458-4_1

Historical Evolution of Nurse Practitioners Across World Health Organization (WHO) Regions

The NP role did not globalize in a uniform manner; rather, it evolved through locally specific responses to access gaps, professional leadership, and regulatory opportunity. Across settings, NP role development has been driven by community health needs and the goal of strengthening person-centered primary care, particularly for populations experiencing barriers to timely services. Because NP's roles and regulatory models vary widely, this section highlights selected country exemplars across WHO regions to illustrate common pathways and policy levers rather than providing a comprehensive review of every jurisdiction.

Region of the Americas

The United States launched the first NP program in 1965 at the University of Colorado, responding to primary care shortages amplified by Medicare and Medicaid expansions. Early growth was consolidated via professional standard-setting, national board certification, and incremental state-level reforms. Over time, NP practice diffused from pediatrics and family practice into adult–gerontology, psychiatric–mental health, women's health, and specialty services. Today, state laws range from full to restricted practice, with a clear trend toward what is defined as Full Practice Authority (FPA). States with FPA demonstrate larger NP workforces in primary care and more NP-led practices in underserved areas [2, 3].

Canada's trajectory broadly parallels the United States but with provincial regulation. Provinces established Primary Health Care NP programs and, in some jurisdictions, acute, pediatric, and neonatal pathways; NPs now practice across community, emergency, rural/remote, and long-term care [4].

Across Latin America and the Caribbean, APN's/NP's roles are emergent. The Pan American Health Organization (PAHO) has advocated since 2013 for expanding nursing in primary care [5]. Chile, in 2022, educated its first cohort of oncology NPs via an academic–service partnership to expand cancer services—an exemplar of specialty-first role development within national priorities [6]. Jamaica, with a history of advanced roles, approved prescriptive authority for APNs in 2023 under defined public-sector conditions, illustrating stepwise policy reform [7].

Europe

In the United Kingdom, advanced nurse practitioners emerged in the late 1980s as general practice confronted workforce pressures. Autonomous prescribing expanded for nurses completing approved programs, although the "nurse practitioner" title lacks uniform national protection and education remains heterogeneous, leading to variation in role clarity [8, 9]. The Republic of Ireland adopted a more tightly coupled model: graduate education tied to accredited Advanced Practice posts and autonomous prescribing within scope, underpinned by revalidation—producing clear accountability and durable role integration [10].

The Netherlands redesignated NPs as "verpleegkundig specialist" (nurse specialist), built dual master's-level programs (somatic and mental health), and codified authority for defined medical acts, including autonomous prescribing. National evaluations reported safe care and high patient satisfaction, consolidating autonomous authority [11]. Finland aligned diverse master's-level curricula with a national APN competence framework to harmonize outcomes and support role clarity as services shift toward primary/community care [12].

Africa

The African Region faces profound primary care shortages and a dual burden of infectious and noncommunicable diseases. International bodies identify NPs as strategic for universal health coverage; early adopters and pilot programs demonstrate both promise and the critical need for harmonized education pathways, prescriptive frameworks, and role regulation to avoid ad hoc integration [13]. Currently, three countries in Africa have adopted the nurse practitioner role, and in those countries, further policy and regulations are needed to promote an autonomous role [14].

Eastern Mediterranean

Several countries are exploring APN roles to bolster primary care and chronic disease services. Oman has piloted NP roles and is among the few Arab countries authorizing nurse prescribing under defined conditions. Across the region, role development hinges on foundational legislation, title protection, prescriptive frameworks, and accredited graduate education [15].

South-East Asia and Western Pacific

In both regions, trajectories are diverse. Singapore established a structured Master of Nursing pathway with title protection and standardized clinical training, integrating NPs into acute and mental health services [16]. Japan has progressed advanced nursing certifications and selective expansions of task autonomy, though autonomous prescribing is limited. Australia legislated NP title protection early, with nationally consistent standards and endorsement; NPs practice autonomously across acute, primary, rural/remote, and specialty settings. Removal of federal "collaborative arrangement" requirements for Medicare and Prescribing Benefits Scheme (PBS) access in 2024 exemplifies regulatory streamlining to support access. In 2025, the Australian Federal Government passed a legislation for authorized nurse prescribers to meet the needs of primary care, residential aged care and remote communities. Nurse prescribers will be required to undertake accredited nurse prescriber courses and practice under the guidance of an NP or medical practitioner. This change provides a pathway for nurses interested in pursuing the more autonomous role of an NP [17–19]. New Zealand likewise embeds NPs with protected title, master's preparation, and autonomous prescribing within scope and similar to the United Kingdom authorizes a role of the nurse prescriber. Nurse prescribers have designated medication formularies based on their specialty and population of practice [20].

Workforce Considerations Across Regions

Global Distribution and Shortages

The WHO estimates roughly 28–29 million nurses worldwide, with a projected shortfall of approximately 5 million by 2030, concentrated in the African, Eastern Mediterranean, and South-East Asian regions and parts of Latin America [21]. Maldistribution is stark: most nurses work in countries serving a minority of the global population. In this context, advanced nursing roles represent a capacity multiplier where scopes and financing enable practice. Workforce policy is therefore also a people-centered equity issue: aligning education, regulation, and financing helps to ensure individuals, families, and communities, especially in rural and underserved areas, can access timely, appropriate care and participate in decisions about their treatment.

Demand Drivers

Population aging and increasing comorbidities raise demand for the expansion of primary care; persistent physician shortage, especially in rural areas, amplify access gaps; and evidence demonstrating NP quality and cost-effectiveness strengthens the policy rationale for expanded roles [3, 8, 9, 21]. Where regulation enables clinical autonomy and payment recognizes NP services, NP workforces grow more rapidly and distribute more equitably.

Scalability and Growth

The United States reports rapid growth in NP employment and outsized growth projections relative to other health professions, with the majority of NPs practicing in primary care [2]. Australia counts thousands of endorsed NPs across states and territories, with notable impact in rural/remote and priority populations; consistent national standards support mobility [17–19]. The Netherlands and the Republic of Ireland have increased nurse specialist/NP posts across general practice, emergency, and mental health, anchored by legal scopes and prescribing [10, 11]. In low- and middle-income countries (LMICs), growth remains limited, constrained by regulatory ambiguity, financing, and limited graduate education capacity [13, 18].

Education and Training

ICN recommends graduate-level preparation (minimum master's), nationally accredited programs, and credentialing aligned to scope and context [1]. High-performing systems share competency-based curricula mapped to scope; substantial supervised clinical practice; structured preceptorship and evaluation; and established pathways for certification, licensure, and endorsement. The content of nurse practitioner graduate degrees shares similarities with a focus on advanced pathophysiology, physical assessment, pharmacology, and research methods to drive health system level changes.

Selected Country Models

United States

Bachelor of Science Nursing-to-Master of Science Nursing/Doctor of Nursing Practice (DNP) pathways aligned to population foci (family, adult–gerontology, pediatrics, neonatal, women's health, psychiatric–mental health), through certified accrediting bodies (Commission on Collegiate Nursing Education [CCNE]/ Accreditation Commission for Education in Nursing [ACEN]) and national board certification preceding state NP licensure [2].

Canada

Provincial regulation and certification govern master's/post-master's NP programs (e.g., primary health care; some provinces: acute care/pediatric/neonatal), with strong community and rural/remote presence [4].

Australia

Endorsement requires completion of a Nursing and Midwifery Board of Australia (NMBA)-approved NP master's, demonstration of advanced practice competence, and 5000 advanced practice hours. Programs are accredited by the Australian Nursing and Midwifery Accreditation Council; endorsement confers title protection and autonomous prescribing within scope [17, 23, 24].

United Kingdom and Republic of Ireland

The UK supports MSc-level advanced practice and autonomous prescribing for qualified nurse prescribers, but NP title protection and standardized preparation are incomplete [8, 9]. The Republic of Ireland links graduate education to accredited posts and autonomous prescribing with revalidation, ensuring alignment of education, scope, and accountability [10].

The Netherlands and Finland

The Netherlands' dual master's programs (somatic, mental health) prepare nurse specialists registered in a dedicated registry, with legal authority for defined medical tasks and autonomous prescribing [11]. Finland's national competence framework harmonizes master's-level APN outcomes across institutions [12].

Singapore and Chile

Singapore's Master of Nursing pathway includes rigorous admission standards, structured clinical training, and title protection [15]. Chile's master's-level oncology NP program, launched in 2022 via academic–service partnership, targets urgent specialty gaps with simulation-enhanced training [6].

Educational Alignment with Clinical Autonomy

Where graduate competencies map directly to legal scopes, prescribing authority, and reimbursement, NPs practice autonomously, and employers can design services confidently. Inconsistent standards or lack of title protection impede clarity for health-care teams and the public.

Impact of Optimal Clinical Autonomy in Practice Quality and Safety

Quality and Safety

Decades of trials and observational studies demonstrate that NP-led care produces outcomes comparable to physician-led care across primary and specialty ambulatory settings. The Cochrane review by Laurant et al. found equivalence in patient outcomes and process measures with high patient satisfaction in primary care [22]. Large syntheses (Newhouse et al.; Stanik-Hutt et al.) report similar or better results for chronic disease control, preventive care, and patient experience [25, 26]. Specialty-focused and acute/ED reviews show equal or better performance on throughput, length of stay, and clinical quality [25, 26].

Access and Equity

Jurisdictions granting FPA see more NPs working in primary care and a greater likelihood of NP-managed clinics without on-site physicians, particularly in rural and underserved areas. Kuo et al. documented larger increases in patients seen by NPs in less restrictive states [27]. Xue et al.'s systematic review links expanded scopes with improved access indicators and greater NP deployment [3]. Natural experiments exploiting staggered FPA adoption show increased primary care access without adverse health effects [28].

Cost and Utilization

Economic evaluations conclude NP care is cost-effective: similar or lower costs per episode, reductions in emergency visits and hospitalizations in select models, and favorable cost–utility in primary and specialized ambulatory settings [29]. Hospital studies and integrated care models show equal or reduced length of stay under NP-inclusive teams [25, 26, 29].

System Exemplars

In the Netherlands, codified authority for nurse specialists to perform medical acts and prescribe has been accompanied by positive safety and satisfaction outcomes and clear interprofessional role delineation [11]. The Republic of Ireland's model streamlines emergency and primary care pathways through autonomous prescribing tied to accredited posts [10]. Australia's nationally regulated, autonomous NP practice improves timeliness and continuity across rural/remote clinics, urgent care, and mental health; recent federal policy changes further reduce administrative barriers to access [17–19].

Impact of Clinical Autonomy on Patient Care

- **Access:** Clinical autonomy, including prescribing authority, correlates with increased NP supply in primary care, higher rates of NP-led clinics, and improved access in rural/underserved settings [3, 27, 28]. During the COVID-19 emergency, temporary relaxation of restrictions enabled rapid NP-led expansion of telehealth, testing, and vaccination, underscoring the latent capacity unlocked by autonomy.
- **Outcomes:** Across chronic disease management, preventive services, and specialty ambulatory care, quality of care persists regardless of physician supervision mandates, indicating that additional mandated supervision does not improve clinical results when graduate education and certification are rigorous [22, 25, 26].
- **Utilization and Cost:** Clinical autonomy is associated with increased use of timely primary care and reduced utilization of costly downstream services for ambulatory care–related conditions; economic reviews consistently find NP models cost-effective [28, 29].
- **Workforce:** Enabling autonomy strengthens recruitment and retention into advanced practice, while restrictive collaborative/supervisory requirements depress NP supply and employer demand—particularly in clinics serving underserved communities [3, 27, 30].

Levers to Augment Autonomy to Impact Outcomes

Autonomy is necessary but insufficient on its own. Clear team norms, consultation pathways, and shared governance support continuity and shared decision making and help prevent fragmented care that can otherwise shift coordination burdens onto patients and families. Quality and sustainability depend on resourcing (diagnostics, IT, pharmacy access), team norms (consultation pathways, shared governance), and payment parity. Supportive practice environments—preceptorship, peer networks, manageable panels—mitigate burnout and sustain quality, especially in rural clinics [16, 18].

Regulation and Levels of Authority Regulatory Models

Regulatory frameworks should enable timely access to care while maintaining public protection through clear accountability, quality assurance, and interprofessional safeguards that sustain public trust. Jurisdictions span a spectrum from full, autonomous practice and prescribing within scope (e.g., Australia; many U.S. states; Republic of Ireland; The Netherlands) to reduced or restricted models requiring collaboration or supervision. Prescriptive authority ranges from autonomous to supplementary/protocol-limited, sometimes with formulary constraints [8–11, 16, 21].

Exemplars

- **The Netherlands**. Competency-based legal authority for nurse specialists to perform defined medical acts and prescribe, supported by a dedicated registry and accredited master's programs [11].
- **Republic of Ireland.** Graduate preparation integrated with accredited advanced practice posts and autonomous prescribing, with five-year revalidation—producing clarity and accountability [10].
- **Australia.** National title protection and endorsement linked to standards for practice and accredited programs; autonomous prescribing within scope; policy updates reduce administrative barriers to funding/subsidies [17–19, 23, 24].
- **United States**. State-by-state patchwork persists; Full Practice Authority states demonstrate stronger NP primary care presence and improved access indicators [2, 3, 27].
- **Jamaica.** Cabinet-approved prescriptive rights for APNs under defined conditions in public institutions represent incremental reform aligned to service needs [7].

Policy Levers

Effective autonomy constructs combine: (1) clear scope and title protection; (2) accredited graduate education aligned to scope; (3) equitable reimbursement; (4) outcomes tracking and data; and (5) public and interprofessional engagement to reduce role ambiguity [1, 11, 16, 19–21].

Perspectives on Nurse Practitioner Care Patients

Patients consistently report high satisfaction with NP care, citing communication quality, shared decision making, and holistic focus. Trials and observational studies show equal or higher satisfaction relative to physician-led primary care with comparable clinical outcomes [22, 25, 26].

Health-Care Team Members

Physicians collaborating with NPs report more favorable views of NP competence, prescribing, contributions to access, and workload than those with limited exposure [28]. Nurses and administrators often emphasize NPs' impact on throughput, quality, and cost containment in primary care, emergency/urgent care, long-term care, residential aged care, and transitions [11, 16]. Team success improves with role clarity, reliable consultation pathways, and aligned incentives. Ensuring health-care organizations and leaders understand the NP role supports effective collaboration and appropriate use of NP competencies. Clear role delineation, consultation pathways, and fit-for-purpose prescribing policies reduce duplication and delays; so, patients are not caught between professional boundaries and experience coordinated, timely care.

Conclusion

The global story of nurse practitioners is one of pragmatic innovation refined by evidence. Where graduate education, regulation, and practice environments align to support clinical autonomy, NPs deliver care that is safe, effective, and cost-efficient—expanding primary care capacity, improving access in underserved communities, and advancing health system performance. Comparative analyses show that autonomy, especially prescribing authority, is associated with increased access and NP workforce, quality outcome equivalence to physician-led care, and favorable cost profiles. Priorities for the next phase include (1) advancing title protection and standardized competence frameworks while preserving contextual flexibility; (2) scaling equitable reimbursement and data-driven workforce planning; (3) expanding high-quality NP education via academic–service partnerships; and (4) investing in interprofessional practice environments that sustain autonomy and mitigate burnout. These steps will position NPs to contribute fully to global health and universal health-care coverage.

Appendices 1 and 2 provide selected, illustrative examples of NP and NP-equivalent regulatory and education models across WHO regions and are not intended to be exhaustive.

Acknowledgments We thank colleagues across NP programs, regulatory bodies, and clinical services whose insights informed this synthesis.

Appendices

Appendix 1: Regulatory Status and Autonomy (Selected Countries by WHO Region)

WHO Region	Country	NP or NP-equivalent APN title protection	Prescriptive authority	Practice authority	Collaboration/ supervision requirement	Primary regulator (nursing; other key bodies)	Notes
Americas	United States	Yes (APRN/NP; varies by state)	Autonomous within scope (FPA states); collaborative–supplementary (restricted states)	Full/reduced/ restricted (state dependent)	None specified (FPA states)/ required by law (restricted states)	State boards of nursing; boards of medicine (varies)	FPA linked to greater NP primary care presence [2, 3, 27]
Americas	Canada	Yes (provincial/ territorial)	Autonomous within scope or collaborative–supplementary (province dependent)	Full/reduced (province dependent)	Required by law or employer/setting (varies)	Provincial/territorial nursing regulators; ministries (varies)	PHC and specialty NP streams [4]
Americas	Chile	Program-level (e.g., oncology NP)	Protocol based (specialty settings)	Restricted (employer/ setting-defined)	Protocol based	Nursing bodies/ universities; Ministry of Health	Master's oncology NP [6]
Americas	Jamaica	Emerging	Collaborative–supplementary (public sector; conditions apply)	Reduced	Required by employer/setting	Nursing council; Ministry of Health and wellness	2023 cabinet approval [7]
Europe	United Kingdom	Partial	Autonomous within scope (qualified nurse prescribers)	Reduced (employer-defined advanced practice)	Required by employer/setting	NMC (prescribing); employers/ credentialing bodies	Advanced practice widespread; title not uniformly protected [8, 9]
Europe	Republic of Ireland	Yes (ANP)	Autonomous within scope	Full (within accredited posts)	Required by employer/setting (accredited post model)	NMBI; health service employers	Revalidation strengthens accountability [10]

Europe	The Netherlands	Yes (nurse specialist)	Autonomous within scope	Full (for defined medical acts)	None specified (within legal task framework)	Nursing regulator/ registry; Ministry of Health (legal acts framework)	Competency-based legal tasks [11]
Europe	Finland	Emerging	Limited formulary–restricted (expanding)	Reduced	Required by employer/setting	National bodies; universities	National APN competence framework [12]
Africa	South Africa (example)	Emerging/role dependent	Protocol based (PHC)	Restricted	Required by law and/or protocol	SANC; Department of Health	Role clarity varies; formal NP title limited [13]
EMR	Oman (example)	Emerging	Limited formulary–restricted (preset medications)	Restricted	Required by law/ employer	National nursing council; Ministry of Health	Early-stage APN policies [15]
SEARO	India	Program level (NP critical care)	Limited formulary–restricted (state/institution dependent)	Restricted	Required by employer/setting	Indian nursing council; state bodies	Postgraduate residency model
WPRO	Australia	Yes	Autonomous within scope	Full	None specified (within scope/ endorsement)	NMBA/AHPRA; funders/payers	National standards and endorsement; funding reforms [17–19, 23, 24]
WPRO	New Zealand	Yes	Autonomous within scope	Full	None specified	Nursing Council of New Zealand	Mature role across primary and aged care [20]
WPRO	Singapore	Yes	Autonomous within scope (defined services)	Reduced	Required by employer/setting	Singapore nursing board; service governance	Structured master of nursing pathway [16]
WPRO	Japan	Emerging (certification models)	None/limited formulary–restricted (nonautonomous)	Restricted	Protocol based/ required by employer	National bodies	Incremental expansion; limited autonomous prescribing

- WHO: World Health Organization
- NP: Nurse practitioner
- FPA: Full Practice Authority
- PHC: Primary health care
- APRN: Advanced Practice Registered Nurse (United States)
- MOHW: Ministry of Health & Wellness
- NMC: Nursing and Midwifery Council (United Kingdom)
- ANP: Advanced Nurse Practitioner (Republic of Ireland)
- NMBI: Nursing and Midwifery Board of Ireland
- APN: Advanced practice nursing
- SANC: South African Nursing Council
- Dept Health: Department of Health
- EMR: Eastern Mediterranean Region (WHO)
- SEARO: WHO South-East Asia Region
- WPRO: WHO Western Pacific Region.
- NMBA: Nursing and Midwifery Board of Australia
- AHPRA: Australian Health Practitioner Regulation Agency
- NZ: New Zealand

Appendix 2: Education and Training Mapped to Autonomy (Selected Countries)

Country	Entry qualification	Degree/ program	Accreditation/ approval	Clinical preparation	Certification/ licensure	Link to autonomy
United States	RN + BSN	MSN/DNP (population foci)	CCNE/ACEN; state boards of nursing	Extensive supervised clinical hours	National certification; state NP/APRN licensure	State scope-of-practice determines full vs. reduced/ restricted practice authority and prescribing authority [3]
Canada	RN + BSN	Master's/ post-master's NP	Provincial/ territorial approval; universities	Supervised clinical placements	Provincial/territorial certification/licensure	Provincial/territorial frameworks enable autonomous prescribing and practice within scope [4]
Australia	RN + BSN + advanced practice experience (plus specified postgraduate study as required)	Master's (NP)	ANMAC (program accreditation); NMBA (endorsement)	Advanced practice portfolio + supervised clinical hours	AHPRA NP endorsement	National title protection and endorsement support autonomous practice and prescribing within scope [23, 24]
United Kingdom	RN + experience	MSc advanced practice + prescribing	Universities; NMC (prescribing annotation)	Supervised practice aligned to role	RN registration + NMC prescriber annotation	Autonomy varies by employer governance and service model; prescribing authority is within scope for credentialed nurse prescribers [8, 9]
Republic of Ireland	RN + experience	MSc advanced practice + prescribing	NMBI (posts and prescribing); employers (accredited posts)	Competency-based practice in accredited posts	Registration as ANP + prescriber	Autonomous prescribing and practice authority operate within accredited posts and defined scope [10]

(continued)

Country	Entry qualification	Degree/ program	Accreditation/ approval	Clinical preparation	Certification/ licensure	Link to autonomy
The Netherlands	RN + experience	Master's (nurse specialist)	National accreditation; nurse specialist register	Competency-based clinical practice	Nurse specialist registration	Legal authority supports autonomous performance of defined medical acts and prescribing within scope [11]
Finland	RN + experience	Master's (APN)	Universities; national competence framework	Clinical practicum	RN licensure + advanced role recognition (as applicable)	Competence framework supports role clarity and expansion of scope within governance arrangements [12]
Singapore	RN + experience	Master of nursing (NP)	Singapore nursing board	Structured clinical residency	Registration/title protection	Autonomous practice and prescribing operate within defined services, scope, and organizational governance [16]
Chile	RN + experience	Master's (oncology NP)	Universities; academic–service partnership	Simulation + specialty immersion	Institutional credentialing	Role autonomy is defined within oncology pathways and organizational protocols [6]

- RN: Registered nurse
- BSN: Bachelor of Science in Nursing
- MSN: Master of Science in Nursing
- DNP: Doctor of Nursing Practice
- CCNE: Commission on Collegiate Nursing Education
- ACEN: Accreditation Commission for Education in Nursing
- ANMAC: Australian Nursing and Midwifery Accreditation Council
- NMBA: Nursing and Midwifery Board of Australia
- AHPRA: Australian Health Practitioner Regulation Agency
- NMC: Nursing and Midwifery Council (United Kingdom)
- ANP: Advanced Nurse Practitioner (Ireland)
- APN: Advanced practice nursing
- NP: Nurse practitioner
- MSc: Master of Science

References

1. International Council of Nurses. Guidelines on advanced practice nursing. Geneva: ICN; 2020. Available from: https://www.icn.ch/system/files/documents/2020-04/ICN_APN%20 Report_EN_WEB.pdf
2. U.S. Bureau of Labor Statistics. Occupational Employment and Wages: Nurse Practitioners, May 2022. Washington (DC): BLS; 2023. Available from: https://www.bls.gov/oes/current/ oes291171.htm
3. Xue Y, Ye Z, Brewer C, Spetz J. Impact of state nurse practitioner scope-of-practice regulation on health care delivery: systematic review. Med Care Res Rev. 2016;73(2):197–230.
4. Canadian Nurses Association. Nurse Practitioners. Ottawa: CNA; 2022. Available from: https://www.cna-aiic.ca
5. Pan American Health Organization. Expanding roles of nurses in primary health care. Washington: PAHO; 2013. Available from: https://www.paho.org
6. University of Miami. First Nurse Practitioners Educated in Chile. Coral Gables (FL): University of Miami News; 2022. Available from: https://news.miami.edu/sonhs/stories/2022/10/first-nurse-practitioners-educated-in-chile.html
7. Ministry of Health & Wellness, Jamaica. Cabinet gives approval for Prescriptive Rights for Advanced Practice Registered Nurses [press release]. Kingston: MOHW; 2023 Nov 21. Available from: https://www.moh.gov.jm
8. Royal College of Nursing. Advanced level nursing practice: introduction. London: RCN; 2018. Available from: https://www.rcn.org.uk
9. World Health Organization Regional Office for Europe. Nurse prescribing across Europe: current status and future prospects. Copenhagen: WHO Europe; 2019. Available from: https://www.euro.who.int
10. Nursing and Midwifery Board of Ireland. Guidance for nurse and midwife prescribing. Dublin: NMBI; 2020. Available from: https://www.nmbi.ie
11. World Health Organization Regional Office for Europe. Advancing nursing roles in primary care: The Netherlands – delivering safe, good-quality care leading to high patient satisfaction. Copenhagen: WHO Europe; 2019. Available from: https://www.who.int/europe/publications
12. Jokiniemi K, Meretoja R, Kotila J. Advanced practice nursing in Finland: a national competence framework. J Adv Nurs. 2020;76(1):220–30.

13. Pulcini J, Jelic M, Gul R, Loke AY. The global shortage of health workers – the case for nurse practitioners. Int Nurs Rev. 2020;67(3):323–31.
14. Gray DC, Rogers M, Miller MK. Advanced practice nursing initiatives in Africa, moving towards the nurse practitioner role: experiences from the field. Int Nurs Rev. 2024;71(2):205–10.
15. Al-Ameri A, Al-Rawajfah O, Al-Awamreh K, Al-Maaitah R. Advanced practice nursing roles in Arab countries in the Eastern Mediterranean region: a scoping review. J Nurs Manag. 2023;31(8):2900–11.
16. National University of Singapore. Master of nursing: admission requirements. Singapore: NUS; 2025. Available from: https://medicine.nus.edu.sg/nursing/education/graduate/master-of-nursing/
17. Nursing and Midwifery Board of Australia. Nurse practitioner standards for practice. Melbourne: NMBA; 2021. Available from: https://www.nursingmidwiferyboard.gov.au/Nursing.aspx
18. Australian Government Department of Health and Aged Care. Nurse practitioner workforce plan. Canberra: DoHAC; 2022. Available from: https://www.health.gov.au
19. Australian College of Nurse Practitioners. Changes to improve access to Medicare funding and PBS subsidies for NP care – effective 1 November 2024 [press release]. Canberra: ACNP; 2024. Available from: https://www.acnp.org.au
20. Snell H, Budge C, Courtenay M. A survey of nurses prescribing in diabetes care: practices, barriers and facilitators in New Zealand and the United Kingdom. J Clin Nurs. 2022;31(15–16):2331–43.
21. World Health Organization. State of the world's nursing 2020: investing in education, jobs and leadership. Geneva: WHO; 2020. Available from: https://www.who.int/publications/i/item/9789240003279
22. Laurant M, van der Biezen M, Wijers N, Watananirun K, Kontopantelis E, van Vught AJ. Nurses as substitutes for doctors in primary care. Cochrane Database Syst Rev. 2018;7:CD001271.
23. Australian Nursing and Midwifery Accreditation Council. Nurse practitioner accreditation standards. Canberra: ANMAC; 2015. Available from: https://www.anmac.org.au
24. Nursing and Midwifery Board of Australia. Approved programs of study – nurse practitioner. Melbourne: NMBA; 2025. Available from: https://www.nursingmidwiferyboard.gov.au/Accreditation/Approved-programs-of-study.aspx
25. Newhouse RP, Stanik-Hutt J, White KM, Johantgen M, Bass EB, Zangaro G, et al. Advanced practice nurse outcomes 1990–2008: a systematic review. Nurs Econ. 2011;29(5):230–50.
26. Stanik-Hutt J, Newhouse RP, White KM, Johantgen M, Bass EB, Zangaro G, et al. The quality and effectiveness of care provided by nurse practitioners. Nurs Outlook. 2013;61(6):400–15.e13.
27. Kuo YF, Loresto FL Jr, Rounds LR, Goodwin JS. States with the least restrictive regulations experienced the largest increase in patients seen by nurse practitioners. Health Aff (Millwood). 2013;32(7):1236–43.
28. Traczynski J, Udalova V. Nurse practitioner independence, health care utilization, and health outcomes. J Health Econ. 2018;58:90–109.
29. Martin-Misener R, Harbman P, Donald F, Reid K, Kilpatrick K, Carter N, et al. Cost-effectiveness of nurse practitioners in primary and specialised ambulatory care: systematic review. BMJ Open. 2015;5:e007167.
30. Donelan K, DesRoches CM, Dittus RS, Buerhaus P. Perspectives of physicians and nurse practitioners on primary care practice. Health Aff (Millwood). 2013;32(11):1942–8.

Clinical Autonomy in Midwifery

Pandora Hardtman, Yvonne Delphine Nsaba Uwera,
Karen Feltham Johnson, Deveree Stewart,
and Joeri Vermeulen

Clinical Autonomy in Midwifery

The clinical evolution of Midwives and Nurse-Midwives across the World Health Organization (WHO) regions is as varied as the scope of practice of Midwives themselves. At its core, the word "midwife" has commonly been accepted to mean "with woman," and globally, this concept remains central to the implementation of autonomous midwifery models of care. The practice of midwifery is arguably the oldest of the accepted advanced practice specialties, with historical and anthropological evidence documenting its presence across continents and civilizations. Wholistic midwifery care—encompassing physical, emotional, and spiritual dimensions—can be traced through both secular and religious texts, as well as in early art and oral traditions. From ancient depictions of birth attendants in Egyptian hieroglyphics to midwifery's integral role in indigenous birthing rituals across Africa, Asia, and the Americas, the midwife has long held a central place in community health and well-being. Anthropologists and global health scholars have noted that

P. Hardtman (✉)
Progressive Journeys LLC, Atlanta, GA, USA

Y. D. N. Uwera
University of Rwanda, Kigali, Rwanda

K. F. Johnson
D'Youville University, New York, NY, USA
e-mail: felthamk@dyc.edu

D. Stewart
University of the West Indies School of Nursing, Kingston, Jamaica

J. Vermeulen
Vrije Universiteit Brussel (VUB), University of Luxembourg, Esch-sur- Alzette, Grand Duchy of Luxembourg, Brussels, Belgium
e-mail: Joeri.vermeulen@ehb.be

A. Kapu et al. (eds.), *A Global View on Clinical Autonomy for Advanced Practice Nurses*, Advanced Practice in Nursing,
https://doi.org/10.1007/978-3-032-21458-4_2

midwives historically acted not only as birth attendants but also as healers, educators, and spiritual guides [18, 32]. This deep cultural embeddedness, alongside the addition of midwifery practice to the United Nations Educational, Scientific, and Cultural Organization's (UNESCO's) list of intangible cultural heritage, affirms midwifery's longevity and adaptability, even as its scope and regulatory frameworks have evolved over time [37, 79].

Today, midwives have various titles, education preparation, scope of practice, and regulation across the globe. The International Confederation of Midwives (ICM) states "A midwife is a person who has successfully completed a midwifery education programme based on the ICM Essential Competencies for Midwifery Practice and the framework of the ICM Global Standards for Midwifery Education, recognized in the country where it is located; who has acquired the requisite qualifications to be registered and/or legally licensed to practice midwifery and use the title 'midwife,' and who demonstrates competency in the scope of practice of the midwife" [38].

In many countries, this definition reflects a distinct professional cadre regulated through independent midwifery legislation and regulatory authorities. However, in other jurisdictions, maternity care is delivered primarily by professionals educated and regulated as nurses, including nurse-midwives and maternity nurses whose scope of practice includes pregnancy, birth, and postpartum care. In these contexts, maternity care falls within the regulated scope of nursing practice and is governed by nursing regulatory bodies. Recognizing both models is important for conceptual clarity: while the ICM definition describes the international standard for the midwifery profession, maternity nursing remains a legitimate and regulated domain of nursing practice in many health systems. These differences in professional regulation reflect historical, legal, and workforce development pathways across countries and should be considered when interpreting maternity workforce roles and competencies. Emerging evidence also suggests that regulatory and conceptual conflation of midwifery and nursing may influence professional identity formation and workforce sustainability; studies have found that diminished professional identity and unclear professional boundaries can negatively affect the recruitment and retention of midwives globally [56] This chapter therefore uses the term "midwife" in alignment with the ICM definition while acknowledging that maternity care globally is delivered through multiple professional and regulatory pathways.

People who are educated as both nurses and midwives are referred to as *nurse-midwives* and will be the primary focus. The emerging title *advanced practice midwife* is yet another title that is not consistent globally. The variations in titles and regulation regarding midwives make clarity of the role difficult. For example, there are nurses in some areas of the world who are educated as maternity nurses and are referred to as midwives; however, they have not been educated and trained in accordance with the ICM definition. This group is critical to the perinatal workforce and performs a legitimate scope of nursing practice; however, the term *nurse-midwife* subsumes the competencies necessary to be a fully qualified and regulated nurse and a midwife. The credentials and regulation are quite varied for midwives within and between counties. Our focus will be primarily on nurse-midwives unless specified otherwise.

The International Council of Nurses (ICN) defines an Advanced Practice Nurse (APN) as a registered nurse who has acquired expert knowledge, complex decision-making skills, and clinical competencies for expanded practice, typically holding a master's degree or higher [30]. While the ICN does not specifically define the role of an Advanced Practice Midwife, its APN framework—emphasizing autonomy, advanced clinical judgment, and leadership—has influenced how advanced midwifery roles are conceptualized, particularly in countries where nursing and midwifery are regulated under the same body. In parallel, the International Confederation of Midwives (ICM) outlines a scope for midwives that may include expanded or specialist competencies such as prescribing, performing ultrasounds, managing emergencies, or leading public health initiatives. These extended roles often mirror those of advanced practice nurses and are shaped by country-specific regulations, health system needs, and educational frameworks. Thus, while the title "Advanced Practice Midwife" is not universally defined, it generally refers to midwives who have received postgraduate education and who function with a high level of clinical autonomy, contributing significantly to leadership, education, and direct care within their scope of practice.

The midwifery workforce is essential to meeting the sexual and reproductive health needs of women, adolescents, newborns, and their families in multiple national and global strategic plans, which emphasizes investment in the midwifery workforce as one of the key pathways for accelerating progress toward ending preventable maternal mortality and morbidity. Investment in the midwifery workforce has been shown to yield significant returns in terms of improved health and social outcomes [51]. For example, a recent study concluded that universal coverage of midwife-delivered interventions would reduce mortality rates by two-thirds. [50]. In the third State of the World's Midwifery Report 2021, four major priorities for action were highlighted: strengthening midwifery leadership and governance; building on progress in midwifery education and training; midwife-led improvements for sexual, reproductive, maternal, and newborn health and rights (SRMNH) service delivery, and improved workforce planning, management, regulation and working environment [81]. Since that time, several regional reports have also been launched including East, Central and Southern Africa, Arab, Caribbean, and Asia Pacific, all of which indicate that autonomy of practice in midwifery will be essential to attain the full range of sexual reproductive health needs of women.

In May 2021, member states of the World Health Organization (WHO) fully endorsed the policy priorities of the new WHO Global Strategic Direction for Nursing and Midwifery (SDNM). During the World Health Assembly 2025, this SDNM was used as a pivotal document to guide nursing and APN practice, and the document was re-ratified. The SDNM highlighted specific policy priorities that included: strengthening leadership; improving education and training; better jobs (creating jobs, recruiting, retaining), and service delivery (ensuring decent working conditions, better regulation).

Clinical autonomy in midwifery is a cornerstone of effective, responsive, and high-quality health-care delivery. When health systems recognize that midwives as independent or collaborative, providers are capable of making timely, evidence-based decisions within their scope of practice—they enhance both provider performance and patient outcomes [79]. This recognition not only empowers these professionals but also translates into measurable improvements in continuity of care, treatment adherence, and overall client satisfaction [63].

This chapter will provide a snapshot of the historical evolution of clinical autonomy in nurse-midwifery practice in a few select regions. An introduction to cross-regional workforce considerations and how clinical autonomy and levels of authority impact the quality of midwifery care will be provided. Drawing from global examples and perspectives of midwives themselves, we seek to illuminate the role of nurse-midwifery.

Africa

Historical Evolution

Across the African continent, especially in Sub-Saharan Africa, the evolution of Midwifery professions replicates a multifaceted interaction of traditional practices, colonial influences, and postcolonial developments. Specifically, midwifery was rooted in indigenous practices where the practices were deeply embedded into the cultural fabric of several communities' local perspective, and the role of midwives had a significant cultural and community importance (Sharif, 2023). Midwives' role in Africa has progressed significantly throughout the decades, formed by various cultural, social, and political influences that reflect the various contexts of the continent.

In many African cultures, childbirth has traditionally been a community event, with experienced older women serving as midwives. This cultural backdrop shapes the community expectations and practices of midwives that often passed traditional roles to the formal health context [52]. The arrival of colonial rule in the nineteenth and twentieth centuries marked a turning point. Colonial administrations following norms in their countries of origin sought, or forced, replacement of traditional birthing practices with biomedical models, labeling traditional midwifery as unsafe or unscientific. European-style nurse-midwife training schools were established, primarily to serve colonial elites, often excluding local knowledge and subordinating African midwives within racialized and gendered hierarchies. This era initiated a systemic devaluation of traditional care and a fragmentation of midwives' authority, which remains as a barrier today.

Following independence movements across Africa in the mid-twentieth century, many governments recognized the strategic importance of midwives in reducing maternal and infant mortalities. Ministries of health launched national training programs, though often under nursing umbrellas, which may have limited midwifery's professional autonomy. International initiatives such as the Safe Motherhood

Initiative of the 1980s and the WHO's Making Pregnancy Safer strategy in the early 2000s helped re-center midwives as critical frontline health workers.

Unceasing tension between traditional practices and modern health-care standards led to a varied acceptance of midwives, especially when social confidence in health-care settings was low. This dynamic cultural scenario was further complicated by undefined scopes of practice and lack of recognition of the profession by the national health systems [81].

In East Africa, particularly in countries like Kenya, political variations after independence led to the formalization of the nursing profession and a more structured role for national nurses within the health system. Kimani and Gatimu [35] highlight the establishment of regulatory frameworks and training programs that sought to professionalize nursing and midwifery. While midwives are often referred as the backbone of the maternal health system in various environments, midwives still deal with social perceptions that often favor obstetrical high-tech practices, and midwives are often considered as "doctors' helpers" rather than autonomous practitioners [33].

The global health discourse emphasizes the need for qualified midwives, and while many reforms and efforts to integrate the midwifery profession have been implemented, there still remain many challenges that need to be addressed [80]. In 16 African countries, only about 56% had expected governance structures for nursing and midwifery practice in place. Even fewer had functioning governance instruments like clear scopes of practice, ethical codes, strategic plans, and schemes of service. The absence of these frameworks curtails professional autonomy, as providers lack official guidance and legal legitimacy to practice fully and confidently.

Broader issues, such as inadequate training, financial constraints, employment and retention, limited resources, and bureaucratic challenges, continue to hinder the effective integration of the nursing and midwifery professions into the health system in many African countries [39]. The lack of adequate training, support, and recognition often leaves these professionals to feel undervalued and overloaded, which further complicates their role in maternal care [80].

The historical evolution of the midwifery profession across many African countries demonstrates a complex interaction of cultural, social, and political influences that have shaped their practices and roles in healthcare. As health-care models continue to evolve, recognizing the contributions of nurses and midwives is crucial to promoting equitable health systems [56].

Workforce Considerations

In Africa, nurses and midwives face a multitude of challenges that prevent their effectiveness and professional development. The continent is marked by a shortage of health professionals especially in rural and hard to reach areas and humanitarian settings, with a nurse/midwife-population relationship that remains critically low compared to global standards [64]. Issues such as inadequate training, unemployment, low job satisfaction, limited access to continuous professional development, and systemic barriers within health structures exacerbate this shortage ([10]). Several African nations have adopted innovative strategies to improve the competence, image, and capacities of their midwifery workforce, but investment in sustainable health system recognition is quasi nonexistent.

Among the major challenges faced by nurses and midwives in Africa, especially Sub-Saharan Africa, is the nonrecognition of both professions by the health system. This leads to inadequate distribution of the workforce resulting in nurses and midwives often operating without the latest knowledge or skills necessary for effective practice and provision of quality health-care services [43]. In addition, the work environment for nurses and midwives in Africa is often characterized by a high workload and lack of support in the health system, contributing to exhaustion and job dissatisfaction [44]. This challenge is amplified during public health crises, as seen during the COVID-19 pandemic, when health professionals faced unprecedented pressure [49]. Midwives in Africa often remain marginalized in health sectors, which leads to insufficient representation in decision-making processes [48].

Impact of Optimal Clinical Autonomy in Practice

Research has demonstrated that greater clinical autonomy significantly reduces occupational stress and burnout, factors closely tied to workforce retention and care quality [34]. For instance, in Ethiopia and Rwanda, nurses have been trained to independently manage noncommunicable diseases (NCDs) at the primary health-care level, filling critical gaps in access and efficiency [53].

Despite these promising models, clinical autonomy remains inconsistently granted across African nations, often hindered by outdated regulatory frameworks and entrenched hierarchical norms. In many countries, nursing and midwifery scopes of practice remain limited by regulation that fails to reflect modern educational advancements or the evolving complexity of frontline care roles [53]. Power dynamics within health systems—particularly physician-dominated cultures—can create resistance to nurse-led decision-making, while ambiguous policies and fear of litigation discourage autonomous practice even when competence exists.

Midwives in Malawi, for example, have cited limited leadership opportunities, institutional inertia, and weak accountability structures as key constraints on their clinical decision-making capacity [16]. Additionally, the lack of legal protections and clear role definitions further erodes confidence and curtails the exercise of autonomy in complex clinical scenarios.

To advance clinical autonomy in a sustainable manner, health systems must modernize regulatory frameworks, invest in advanced practice education, clarify professional roles, and ensure legal protection for independent practice. Such reforms not only uplift nursing and midwifery professionals but also strengthen the entire health system through more equitable, accessible, and person-centered care.

Regulation and Levels of Authority

The regulation of nurses and midwives across Africa plays a vital role in defining clinical autonomy, shaping professional recognition, and safeguarding public health. As frontline providers in diverse settings—including remote, underserved communities—midwives often serve as the first, and sometimes only, point of contact within the health system. Their ability to act autonomously, however, is deeply influenced by the strength and clarity of regulatory systems, which vary significantly across the continent.

In many countries, professional regulation is managed by Nursing and Midwifery Councils or Orders, which oversee education standards, licensure, and scope of practice. Where these systems are robust, midwives are more likely to have clearly defined roles and pathways for continuous professional development (CPD). Yet, disparities in the structure and enforcement of these frameworks continue to impede autonomy in practice, and in some countries, functional Councils do not exist or are in their infancy. A debate is also ongoing regarding whether nursing and midwifery should separate out into separate councils to better serve the specific needs of the professions.

South Africa is widely recognized for having one of the most advanced nursing and midwifery regulatory systems on the continent. The South African Nursing Council (SANC) provides a comprehensive classification of nursing cadres, and midwives practicing at the primary care level are authorized to prescribe essential medications, reflecting an expanded scope of practice. Nonetheless, the full integration of advanced practice nurses and midwives into leadership and health governance structures remains an ongoing challenge.

In East Africa, Kenya and Rwanda have developed well-structured regulatory frameworks. Kenya's Nursing Council oversees a tiered licensure system aligned with educational levels, promoting greater professional accountability. Rwanda's National Council of Nurses and Midwives has also established strong mechanisms for licensure renewal and continual professional development. However, both countries still face limitations in operationalizing fully autonomous scopes of practice, particularly in institutional settings.

In West Africa, Ghana has made notable strides, including the introduction of a graduate diploma in midwifery and revisions to job descriptions that enhance midwives' clinical and professional independence. These efforts have been recognized by the WHO Regional Office for Africa as promising for scaling midwifery autonomy. However, many francophone countries in the region continue to struggle with inconsistent education standards, limited regulatory capacity, and weak enforcement of licensure requirements.

Amid these challenges, several exemplary models across the continent demonstrate what expanded midwifery autonomy can look like in practice. The Edna Adan Maternity Hospital in Somaliland, founded by nurse-midwife Edna Adan Ismail, serves as both a referral center and a midwifery training institution. Run by midwives and dedicated to cultivating future leaders, the hospital exemplifies a context in which midwifery leadership, education, and clinical practice are fully integrated and respected.

Collectively, these examples reveal both the diversity and unevenness of midwifery regulation in Africa. Where regulation is strong, clear, and backed by political will, midwives can practice with greater clinical independence, ultimately improving health outcomes for women and newborns. Scaling these successes will require sustained investment in regulatory infrastructure, harmonized education standards, and continued advocacy for the professional autonomy of midwives as essential to achieving universal health coverage.

While global momentum continues to champion the role of qualified midwives in achieving universal health coverage, the path toward meaningful professional autonomy in Sub-Saharan Africa remains obstructed by deeply entrenched systemic barriers. The absence or weakness of formal governance structures undermines clarity in scope and accountability, while persistent educational limitations leave practitioners underprepared to exercise independent clinical judgment. Compounding this are leadership gaps that restrict advocacy, representation, and daily operational constraints—ranging from resource scarcity to inconsistent quality assurance practices—that further inhibit autonomous decision-making at the point-of-care. Despite regional and international reform efforts, these interlinked deficits in regulation, education, leadership, and institutional support continue to constrain the full realization of autonomy for the region's nursing and midwifery workforce. Addressing these challenges is not only critical for improving health system performance but also for empowering the professions to deliver the respectful, rights-based care that communities across the continent deserve.

Americas

Historical Evolution

Historically, midwifery in the United States (USA) and Canada was rooted in community-based care. As described in *Varney's Midwifery (7th ed., Ch. 2),* European-trained immigrant midwives as well as African American "granny midwives" in the South played essential roles in maternal and newborn care. As medicine became increasingly professionalized in the late nineteenth and twentieth centuries, these community midwives became increasingly marginalized [9].

U.S. Midwifery

The formalization of nurse-midwifery education in the USA began in response to poor maternal and infant outcomes in underserved areas. Mary Breckinridge's establishment in 1925 of the Frontier Nursing Service in Kentucky significantly influenced the path of midwifery in the USA bringing trained nurse-midwives to remote communities [8]. In 1932, the first U.S. nurse-midwifery education program opened at the Maternity Center Association in New York City. The founding of the American College of Nurse-Midwives (ACNM) in 1955 further standardized education, certification, and practice [5]. Currently, there are three recognized midwifery education routes in the USA: 1) a Certified Nurse-Midwife (CNM) is a registered nurse with an advanced practice education in midwifery that includes the Core Competencies for Basic Midwifery Practice in a program accredited by the Accreditation Commission for Midwifery Education (ACME), a graduate degree, and has passed the American Midwifery Certification Board (AMCB) national exam [41]. The CNM credential is recognized and can be licensed in all fifty states of the USA. A Certified Midwife (CM) does not have a nursing degree but has completed science and health courses along with requirements to complete an ACME accredited graduate degree in midwifery, and has passed the national AMCB exam [9]. The CM is recognized may be licensed in thirteen states with the same scope and prescriptive authority as CNMs. CNM and CM scope of practice includes gynecologic and primary care across the lifespan and gender spectrum in addition to antepartum, intrapartum, postpartum, and care of the newborn in the first 28 days of life.

The Certified Professional Midwife (CPM) credential is issued by the North American Registry of Midwives (NARM) and is designed specifically for practice in community settings such as homes and birth centers. CPMs often complete their education through programs accredited by the Midwifery Education Accreditation Council (MEAC), although NARM also allows competency-based entry through its Portfolio Evaluation Process. This structure reflects the CPM model's emphasis on competency demonstration, intensive supervised clinical experience in out-of-hospital environments, and verification of skills by qualified preceptors [41].

CPMs are licensed or regulated in many U.S. states, though the specific legislation, regulatory mechanisms, and permitted scope of practice vary widely. Their training focuses on physiologic birth, autonomous practice, and early identification of conditions requiring consultation or referral—elements that distinguish CPM education from the hospital-based training of Certified Nurse-Midwives or Certified Midwives [9] The combined use of MEAC-accredited curricula and NARM's competency examinations ensures that CPM certification includes both didactic education and apprenticeship-based clinical training tailored to community birth settings [9, 41].

Canadian Midwifery

Canadian midwives complete an undergraduate degree in midwifery. Midwives are not APNs in Canada but rather enter the profession through a direct-entry program. Canadian midwives are trained through a single, standardized model. Midwifery education is regulated at the provincial or territorial level with each jurisdiction overseeing licensure, practice standards, and continuing education requirements. Candidates pass a national exam [12].

Historically, Indigenous midwives have held a distinct traditional role within Indigenous, First Nations, Inuit, and Métis communities, which included all aspects of the health of women and their families throughout the lifecycle. The colonial systems took away much of the independent practice of Indigenous midwifery; however, despite this, practice has continued and today, Indigenous midwives are represented by the National Aboriginal Council of Midwives (NACM), officially formed in 2008. NACM and Canadian Association of Midwives (CAM) work in partnership to represent the profession of midwifery in Canada. Together, these two foundations, alongside research, evidence-based guidelines and clinical practice, have helped to develop and solidify the current Canadian midwifery model of care [12].

In contrast, French settlers imported midwives under the order of the King of France, and later, in the twentieth century, nurse-midwives were recruited—often from the UK—to practice in remote communities where physicians were unavailable. Despite marginalization, some nursing schools offered postgraduate certificates in midwifery to support outpost settings. A grassroots movement, born out of social activism and the struggle for women's rights, resulted in the development of a parallel midwifery practice in Canada [61]. It was only after a loud consumer movement increased demand for midwives during the 1970s–1980s, and visible poor perinatal outcomes triggered coroner inquests, that midwifery regulation was first enacted in Ontario in 1994. Since that time, the vast majority of provinces and territories have regulated and funded midwifery [45, 61].

In Central and South America, midwifery is practiced across much of the region; however, its organization does not align with the advanced practice nursing (APN) framework common in North America. In several countries, midwifery exists as a stand-alone profession—such as the *matronas* in Chile—while in others it is situated within nursing, as in the obstetric nurse model in Brazil [19, 36]. Education for these roles is generally offered at the undergraduate level and does not consistently provide the level of clinical autonomy or graduate-level preparation associated with midwifery in North America. Although expanded nursing and midwifery roles, including advanced practice nursing, are being discussed and promoted by regional organizations, widespread formalization through legislation, regulation, and standardized graduate-level education remains limited in Latin America. [84].

Workforce Considerations

Across the Americas, the midwifery workforce is shaped by regional differences, education models, regulation, and health-care system integration with results being a significant impact on accessibility to maternal and newborn care. In the USA, midwifery is integrated into an advanced practice model but faces inconsistencies in scope and regulation across states. CNMs and CMs attend roughly 10% of vaginal births, though geographic distribution varies widely [5]. CNMs are disproportionately located in urban areas, while many rural and underserved communities face a shortage of maternity providers. The uneven access contributes to persistent disparities in maternal outcomes, particularly among Black, Indigenous, and low-income populations. CMs are licensed in only thirteen states—despite equivalent training and AMCB certification, they, therefore, have limited impact on workforce gaps. Although CNMs provide high-quality, cost-effective care with fewer interventions [63], workforce growth is constrained by limited and expensive midwifery education programs, lack of federal investment, and state-level practice barriers. CPMs primarily attend out-of-hospital births with varying integration into health systems, resulting in inconsistent workforce utilization.

In Canada, provincial regulation results in differing workforce availability, with stronger midwifery programs in Ontario and British Columbia [12]. Canadian midwives attend approximately 11–12% of all births with significant differences in provinces where midwives are better integrated into the health-care system (such as British Columbia and Ontario). Data on birth attendance in British Columbia includes both midwife-involved (29.2%) to midwife-led births (15.4%). Data regarding births attended by indigenous midwives is imprecise. The National Council of Indigenous Midwives (NCIM) advocates for and supports the expansion and restoration of Indigenous midwifery supporting reproductive justice, sovereignty, and culturally safe care [47]. In communities such as Nunavik (northern Quebec), indigenous midwives may attend a majority of local births.

Midwifery in Mexico has a long history rooted in Indigenous practice. With the arrival of the Spanish colonizers in the sixteenth century came the push for institutionalization of obstetric care and Western medicine. The shift to move away from traditional community birth to hospitals expanded after the Mexican Revolution (1910–1920) with efforts to modernize healthcare. Midwives were excluded from this model—especially in urban areas [65].

Central and South America present fragmented models with varying levels of recognition and autonomy for midwives. In Brazil, obstetric nurses—registered nurses with additional midwifery training—provide maternity care within public hospitals functioning under the supervision of physicians [19].

Education and Training

U.S. education and training pathways to midwifery certification and licensure include a minimum of a postbaccalaureate masters degrees—as is the case with CNMs and CMs—and high school completion with a nondegree apprenticeship model in CPM education. Nurse-Midwife education requires a nursing degree and license as a registered nurse for program entry. Nurse-Midwife education programs are primarily housed within schools of nursing in universities. There are forty-six nurse-midwifery education programs in the USA accredited by the Accreditation Commission for Midwifery Education (ACME) as of July 2025. Of these forty-six, fourteen require a Doctor of Nursing Practice (DNP) for graduation reflecting a trend by some nursing schools to offer only a DNP for APN entry to practice. The DNP requires a minimum of 1000 postbaccalaureate clinical hours [4]. Nurse-midwifery (and midwifery) education programs generally adhere to a competency-based model in which students demonstrate proficiency in the core competencies of clinical practice including primary care; reproductive and sexual health; preconception, antepartum, intrapartum and postpartum; care of the newborn for the first 28 days of life; and professional issues. Clinical experience in these programs will exceed 700 hours [2]. Some financial assistance exists for nurse-midwifery and midwifery education programs—including Federal Financial Aid, Nurse Faculty Loan Programs, and loan repayment programs in which graduates working in underserved areas are eligible for loan repayment (such as the Indian Health Service). Student midwives compete with medical students and other APN specialties for clinical experiences; thus, student midwives may face the necessity for short-term relocation to satisfy the clinical practicum requirements. Education debt influences workforce trends as newly graduated midwives seek higher-paying positions to maximize salary and pay off student-loan debt making higher-salary practices more appealing.

Some ACME accredited programs in the USA combine online didactic education with in-person clinical practice mentored by a qualified preceptor. This model may allow students to remain in their home communities during their education and training. This route is especially valuable in rural and underserved areas and for students with home and work responsibilities pursuing advanced practice opportunities.

Impact of Optimal Clinical Autonomy in Practice

States where CNMs and CMs practice autonomously without physician oversight consistently demonstrate better maternal outcomes, higher workforce density, and more midwife-attended births than states with restrictions to practice [69]. For example, in Washington State where CNMs have full practice authority including prescriptive privileges, midwives attend approximately 12% of births with low intervention rates for people who have low-risk pregnancies [83]. In Alabama, a restrictive state without clinical autonomy and one of the highest maternal mortality rates in the USA, more than half of the counties lack maternal care providers and less than 2% of births are attended by midwives [82].

Caribbean

Historical Evolution

The Caribbean region, spanning island nations from the Bahamas to Trinidad and Tobago, as well as Guyana and Suriname in South America, is home to about 16 million people. While populations and living standards vary, most countries are classified as upper middle-income by the World Bank.

Midwifery in the Caribbean has been shaped by indigenous traditions and colonial influences from the British, Dutch, French, and Americans. During the transatlantic slave trade, the need for improved birth outcomes led to the emergence of trained midwives as vital contributors to the local economy. In the English-speaking Caribbean, midwifery remains closely tied to the British model and is typically viewed as a pathway within nursing linked to career progression and reimbursement structures rather than an as an independent profession a recent development.

During the pre-emancipation period in the early 1800s, efforts were being made in the Caribbean to improve the medical conditions of enslaved populations. These efforts were often driven not by humanitarian concerns but by economic motives, as the health and reproductive capacity of enslaved people was crucial to plantation profitability [6, 67].

On each estate, there existed rudimentary health-care facilities, such as estate hospitals or "Yaws Huts," named after a common tropical infection. Within this structure, an older enslaved woman—often over the age of 50—was designated as the "Grandy." According to Orlando Patterson in Sociology of Slavery, the Grandy played a central role in maternal care. She was responsible for the well-being of pregnant women throughout their pregnancy and supervised both infants and young children on the estate. However, contrary to popular belief, the Grandy did not typically oversee the actual birth of babies [17].

As Patterson further elaborates, about 2 weeks prior to giving birth, enslaved women were transferred to the care of a "Nana," a traditional midwife who operated independently, often from her own establishment. The "Nana" functioned as a midwife and was central to the birthing process among enslaved populations [57] According to Verderse and Turnbull [70], the Nana—or Traditional Birth Attendant (TBA)—was typically an older, postmenopausal woman who had herself given birth to at least one child. Deeply embedded in her community, she often extended her services to nearby villages. Her domain was childbirth, a sphere in which she commanded significant authority and influence. Her practices were rooted in a blend of experience, mysticism, and cultural ritual, often reinforced through traditional ceremonies and spiritual beliefs.

Nana's authority lay squarely in the domain of childbirth, where she exercised both medical and spiritual influence. Her methods combined practical knowledge with mystical and ritual practices, often involving herbs, roots, and ceremonial rites. She acted as a healer and herbalist, preparing remedies to ease pregnancy discomfort, induce labor or abortion, and treat gynecological ailments such as dysmenorrhea. Although she lacked formal medical training and legal recognition, she was highly respected, known for her patience, calm demeanor, and the intimate, continuous care that she provided.

Thus, even in the absence of institutional medical systems, enslaved communities created and sustained complex networks of maternal and child healthcare. Figures like the Grandy and the Nana were not only caregivers but also custodians of cultural and spiritual traditions, maintaining the health of their communities under oppressive and inhumane conditions.

Despite lacking formal registration or legal recognition, the Nana held a position of considerable respect and trust within the community. Her demeanor was typically calm and patient, providing both emotional and physical support to women throughout the childbirth process. Known by various titles across different cultural contexts, the Nana's presence extended beyond maternity care into broader aspects of communal and familial life, making her a vital figure in both health and social structure. The Nana was the precursor to the visioning of today's modern midwife.

By the late nineteenth century, formal midwifery training had begun to take shape in the Caribbean under colonial influence. In Jamaica, the establishment of the Victoria Jubilee Lying-in Hospital in 1891 marked a turning point in structured maternal healthcare. The hospital introduced a midwifery training program for "respectable women of good character and strong constitution," offering instruction that led to a certificate in midwifery [28]. This program represented the transition from informal apprenticeship models of birth assistance to standardized, institutionalized education for midwives.

Workforce Availability

The English-speaking Caribbean has recorded increasing enrollments in nursing and midwifery programs over the last decade, reflecting a growing recognition of the importance of these professions to health system strengthening. Despite this progress, the region continues to face significant challenges in ensuring the availability of qualified midwives across health-care institutions. Geographical, informational, attitudinal, and financial barriers continue to restrict the distribution and retention of midwives, particularly in rural and underserved areas [23].

Caribbean Community's (CARICOM's) Human Resource Development 2030 Strategy outlines a vision for a Seamless HRD System that includes prior learning recognition, multiple entry and exit points, open and distance learning, and structured continuous professional development (CPD) pathways [13]. These measures are particularly relevant to nursing and midwifery education, often with rigid structures that limit workforce expansion and recognition of prior competencies. Expanding access through more flexible educational approaches could significantly improve workforce availability.

Regulatory infrastructures across the Caribbean vary significantly, yet the Caribbean Community (CARICOM) has undertaken important efforts to standardize health professional education. A major advancement has been the recognition of the Caribbean Regional Midwives Association (CRMA) as an affiliate of the CARICOM Regional Nursing Body (RNB). This affiliation has provided midwifery with a formal voice in regional policy discussions where it previously lacked representation. CARICOM has also established a regional licensing examination for nursing and continues to advance the development of a harmonized nursing curriculum. Importantly, the RNB now acknowledges CRMA as the official body representing midwifery, ensuring that the profession contributes directly to shaping the regional midwifery agenda.

There is ongoing movement toward establishing a regional harmonized midwifery entrance examination, modeled after the existing regional nursing exam. Regulation in nursing and midwifery is a cornerstone of public protection, ensuring that only competent, qualified, and safe professionals provide care. These frameworks define professional roles and responsibilities and act as benchmarks for maintaining high standards of practice. In the Caribbean, regulation is widely supported, as it helps secure consistent and reliable health services across communities.

However, the scope and strength of regulatory structures differ considerably. Countries such as Jamaica, Trinidad and Tobago, The Bahamas, Guyana, St. Lucia, and Barbados have formal nursing regulations in place, while midwifery-specific regulation remains uneven. Among these, Jamaica is notable for having a more comprehensive framework for midwifery education and practice.

At the same time, workforce shortages extend beyond education and training. Recruitment, retention, and workplace conditions play an equally important role. CARICOM has highlighted the urgent need for governments to prioritize investments in the health workforce, as shortages of nurses and midwives are reaching critical levels [14]. The Pan American Health Organization (PAHO) projects a deficit of 600,000 to 2 million health workers across the Americas by 2030 if current trends continue [54]. Although some Caribbean states exceed the WHO threshold of 44.5 health workers per 10,000 population, inequities remain, with smaller states and rural communities experiencing acute shortages [54].

Addressing these challenges requires comprehensive action. Continuous professional development, workplace wellness initiatives, and effective leadership and governance structures are essential for retention [23]. Governments must also prioritize remuneration, career advancement opportunities, and succession planning to sustain the workforce. Regional collaboration, including the development of specialist pools of midwives who can work across countries, could strengthen health system resilience in smaller island states [13].

Ultimately, workforce availability is not solely a matter of training numbers but of creating a supportive ecosystem that enables midwives to enter, remain, and advance within the profession. Coordinated investment and implementation of CARICOM's workforce protection strategies will be critical to building a sustainable and equitable midwifery workforce for the region.

Europe

Historical Evolution

Across Europe, the role of midwives has evolved from informal, superstitious practices to a formalized and regulated profession. As countries transitioned from rural, community-based care to hospital-centric systems, midwives' roles expanded and contracted, often depending on local medical and political landscapes.

The nineteenth century was a critical period for the professionalization and legal recognition of midwifery across Europe. The century saw significant reforms in the legal status of midwifery. Midwives were increasingly recognized as medical professionals, and certification systems were introduced to regulate the profession. In countries like France and Germany, midwifery schools with formal curricula were established, combining both theoretical and practical training. Midwifery began to be more structured, and professional associations emerged to advocate for midwives' rights, set professional standards, and improve working conditions, including better pay and benefits. In the Czech Republic, midwifery had long been regulated with exams starting as early as the sixteenth century. However, it was in the nineteenth century that the profession was formalized with the establishment of specialized midwifery schools and improved training systems. This trend also spread to other countries such as Poland and Hungary, where midwifery education was made more comprehensive, laying the foundation for a more professionalized approach to childbirth [46].

One of the most significant shifts of the twentieth century was the move from home births to hospital births. In most other Western European countries, there has been an important shift in midwifery care after World War II, when childbirth moved from home to hospital. The reason for this shift was the introduction of a compulsory health and disablement insurance scheme, which specified that births in hospital and all specialist medical care would be reimbursed by health insurance, regardless of whether they were complicated or uncomplicated [22]. The rise of obstetrics as a medical specialty led to physicians taking a more central role in childbirth, and midwives increasingly found their role confined to assisting obstetricians in the hospital setting. This transition marked a decline in the autonomy of midwives, as physicians began to oversee and manage most births, including those that were previously within the domain of midwives. The twentieth century witnessed the widespread medicalization of childbirth, with significant shifts in the role of midwives within the health-care system. The role of midwives became increasingly institutionalized, with midwives working under the supervision of obstetricians and within hospital settings in ante-, intra- and postpartum settings. The twentieth century marked a shift to medicalized childbirth, and today, midwifery continues to balance between medical practice and holistic care, with an ongoing focus on professionalization, autonomy, and the health of women and children. In Belgium, the transition from home births to hospital births accelerated after World War II, especially as health insurance systems began to prioritize hospital care. Although midwives were still recognized as medical practitioners under legislation such as the Royal Decree of 1967, their roles in the birthing process were limited, and obstetricians took over much of the responsibility [73]. After the end of the Austro-Hungarian period, midwifery in Bosnia and Herzegovina became more formalized, with midwifery schools being established to train practitioners. However, by the late twentieth century, midwives' roles had become increasingly restricted, and their focus shifted to specific areas of maternal and neonatal care. The trend toward medicalization and the involvement of obstetricians in all births further reduced the midwifery role in birth management [46]. The twentieth century saw the establishment of many national and international professional organizations for midwives, including the International Confederation of Midwives (ICM). These organizations played crucial roles in standardizing training, advocating for improved working conditions, and promoting continuing education. The ICM also represented midwives at the global level, advancing professional standards and promoting the role of midwives in healthcare [3].

The last two decades have been especially important for midwifery, as midwives have gained independence and many new competences [46]. In the twenty-first century, midwifery continued to evolve, with a focus on autonomy, professional development, and the role of midwives in advocating for women's reproductive rights. Midwifery has been increasingly recognized as a distinct profession independent from nursing in many European countries, with legislation that defines midwives' roles and competencies. Countries such as France, Belgium, Poland, and the Czech Republic have passed laws granting midwives more autonomy, including the right to prescribe medication and perform ultrasounds in certain contexts. These legal advancements signify a growing recognition of midwifery as a valuable and independent health-care profession. While hospital births remained dominant, there has been a resurgence of interest in home births and midwife-led models of care, particularly in countries like the Netherlands and the United Kingdom. This shift is partly a response to the medicalization of childbirth and a desire for more personalized, holistic care during pregnancy and childbirth. Some women seek more autonomy in their birth choices, preferring the continuity of care that a midwife can provide.

Workforce Considerations

There are significant differences in the number of midwives across European countries, both in absolute numbers and when measured per population. Western European countries generally have higher densities of midwives compared to Eastern European countries, and there are notable variations even within regions of the same country. Key differences include (1) Large variations: There is a 3.5–4.5-fold difference in the density of nurses and midwives between the highest and lowest regions in Europe. For example, Denmark has a much higher nursing and midwifery density than Bulgaria, and these differences are even more pronounced at the regional level within countries [77]. (2) Regional patterns: Densely populated regions, such as capitals and major cities, tend to have higher physician densities, while the density of nurses and midwives is often higher in less populated areas [77]. These disparities have remained largely unchanged over the past decade, underscoring the persistent regional imbalances in access to midwifery care. In Germany, for example, a shortage of midwives has resulted in understaffed hospitals and even the closure of birth units, despite rising birth rates. (3) Trends over time: From 2000 to 2018, the average number of midwives per 100,000 population in European OECD countries increased by 14%. However, the increase was more pronounced in Western Europe compared to Eastern Europe [21]. (4) Western versus. Eastern Europe: The number of health-care professionals, including midwives, per 100 hospital beds is significantly higher in Western European countries than in Eastern European countries [21]. (5) Policy and planning challenges: The absence of a central register for midwives further complicates workforce planning [77]. While most high-income European countries have strong educational and regulatory frameworks for midwives, the lack of midwife leaders at the national level often hinders effective policy development [50]. Current workforce planning models for physicians may not be directly applicable to midwifery due to differences in service delivery and health-care systems, indicating a need for new, tailored approaches [60]. Economic evaluations suggest that midwifery-led care is generally cost-effective, but comprehensive studies to guide workforce investment and planning are lacking [11].

Education and Training

In the last decade, midwifery education in all European countries has moved into higher education institutions (*WHO European Region. Strengthening the skills of future midwives*, 2024). Within the World Health Organization (WHO) European Region, which spans 53 Member States across Europe and Central Asia, midwifery education varies significantly due to differences in health-care systems, cultural contexts, and available resources (*WHO European Region. Strengthening the skills of future midwives*, 2024). A study on the education levels at which midwives complete their training in EU countries found that, in most countries, midwifery training culminates in either a bachelor's or master's degree [58]. In majority of countries, midwives can pursue postgraduate education, such as a Master's or Doctorate in midwifery or related disciplines [75]. A growth in midwifery research has been observed across Europe, with many midwives in various countries engaging in research and advancing their studies through postgraduate degrees [66].

The Bologna Declaration and EU Directive 2005/36/EC played a key role in the aforementioned changes in midwifery education across Europe [25]. The European Union established minimum standards for midwifery education and practice through Directive 2005/36/EC, supporting the recognition of professional qualifications across member states. This directive outlines the required duration and content for midwifery training, with Annex V specifying the professional activities and scope of midwifery practice. According to this directive, midwives must possess a thorough understanding of obstetrics, gynecology, professional ethics, and relevant legislation, along with knowledge in areas such as anatomy, physiology, pharmacology, and neonatal care. Clinical training in licensed health-care facilities is essential for midwifery students to gain the practical experience necessary to provide prenatal care, attend births, and offer postnatal care [74]. To ensure a harmonized approach to midwifery education across the EU, the European Midwives Association conducted surveys in 2014 and 2016 to assess the implementation of Annex V. The surveys found that most member countries had integrated the directive into their national regulations. However, challenges remain in acquiring certain competencies, such as managing breech births and assessing perineal trauma.

A recent European Commission's study [24] aimed to evaluate the implementation of Directive 2005/36/EC and identify gaps and areas for improvement in midwifery training. This study, which includes consultations with professional organizations and national authorities, may inform potential updates to the directive [24]. The proposed updates to Directive 2005/36/EC focus on incorporating contemporary health-care needs into midwifery education. These updates include integrating perinatal mental health, respectful care for women with special needs, evidence-based practices, leadership, and digital technologies. By aligning midwifery training with modern health-care demands and facilitating the mobility of midwives across the EU, the European Commission aims to enhance the quality of maternity care and ensure midwives are equipped to meet diverse health-care challenges across member states.

Clinical Autonomy

Midwives' autonomy in Europe varies significantly by country, but it may be limited in some regions despite progress in education and professional recognition. While midwives are increasingly recognized as key health-care professionals, their ability to practice independently and influence maternity care policy is often constrained. In Europe, the current state of midwifery autonomy is shaped by significant advancements in education and professionalization, alongside ongoing challenges in clinical practice and regulation. Midwifery education is embedded in higher education institutions in Europe, offering opportunities for postgraduate study and research. However, despite these advancements, progress in education has not always translated into greater autonomy in clinical practice or leadership roles [26, 75]. In some countries, midwives are undervalued and underutilized, with their roles in decision-making and policy development not fully realized [26, 71, 75]. There are notable regional differences in the levels of autonomy. For instance, in Belgium, midwives in Brussels report higher autonomy compared to those in Wallonia, and primary care midwives generally experience more autonomy than those working in hospitals ([72]. In Italy, midwives are gaining increasing autonomy in discharging women after physiological childbirth, although this responsibility is still shared with obstetrician [62].

To enhance midwives' autonomy, several recommendations are proposed: prioritizing midwife-led continuity of care, fostering interprofessional collaboration, tailoring continuous professional development, increasing public awareness of midwives' roles, and advocating for supportive policy changes. Addressing the lack of recognized authority is crucial, as it underpins many of the other challenges and is essential for advancing midwives' professional autonomy and recognition within health-care systems [71].

Regulation and Levels of Authority

Midwifery in Europe is a regulated profession, but the level of authority and scope of practice for midwives varies significantly between countries. While there are EU-wide directives setting minimum standards for education and professional recognition, national laws and health-care systems determine the actual authority and autonomy of midwives in practice.

The midwifery regulation framework is determined by the (1) EU Directives: The European Union has established minimum standards for midwifery education and practice through European Union Directives (notably EEC/80/154 and

EEC/80/155, updated in 2013). These set requirements for education duration, content, and professional activities, supporting mutual recognition of qualifications and freedom of movement for midwives across member states [42, 59, 74] and (2) National implementation: Each country implements these directives differently. While most have moved midwifery education into higher education institutes, the degree of professional autonomy, regulatory oversight, and leadership roles for midwives still vary widely [42, 74, 76].

In many Western and Northern European countries, midwives have a high degree of autonomy, particularly in managing normal pregnancies and births. In some countries, midwife-led care is the standard for low-risk pregnancies, with midwives serving as the primary caregivers [20, 74, 75]. In contrast, in some Eastern and Southern European countries, midwives have less authority, with doctors required to be present during births or to oversee care. The scope of practice may be poorly defined or restricted by national law, limiting midwives' visibility and influence [20, 42]. While most countries have codes of ethics and professional associations, midwives' leadership roles and influence in health-care policy remain limited in many regions [20, 75].

Perspectives on Midwifery Care

Research into European midwifery highlights the importance of personalized, continuous care and effective communication among midwives, patients, and other health-care providers. Women across several European countries value the trust and empowerment fostered by midwives, especially when care is individualized and consistent throughout pregnancy, childbirth, and early parenthood [31, 40]. However, women often encounter fragmented care, inconsistent information, and a lack of emotional support, which can undermine their experiences and outcomes [15, 31]. Both patients and health-care team members emphasize the need for better interprofessional collaboration, standardized information, and involvement of family members, particularly partners, in the care process [15, 31, 40]. Barriers to implementing midwifery-led models include hierarchical health-care structures, a dominant medical model, and insufficient awareness of the safety and benefits of midwifery care, though national guidelines and collaborative engagement can facilitate progress [7]. In special settings, such as prisons or refugee camps, women face additional challenges like limited choice and disempowerment, but continuity of midwifery care remains crucial for their well-being [68]. Overall, improving midwifery care in Europe requires addressing systemic issues, enhancing communication, and supporting midwives to deliver comprehensive, individualized care that meets the diverse needs of women and their families [31, 40, 78].

Conclusion

While midwifery is firmly established as a profession across Europe, significant challenges persist. Despite strong regulatory frameworks in many countries, Europe continues to face regional disparities and workforce shortages. These challenges are further compounded by concerns about fair remuneration and the recognition of midwives' independent roles. While midwifery autonomy is improving, particularly in the realm of education, substantial barriers may still exist in practice, regulation, and professional recognition. Effective workforce planning, better data collection, and targeted policy leadership are critical to ensuring equitable access to midwifery care across all regions. Professional development remains a key focus, with many midwives required to participate in continuing education programs to maintain and enhance their skills. Overcoming these challenges will require concerted policy changes, robust education, and stronger interprofessional collaboration. The disparities in midwifery numbers and the ongoing need for effective planning underscore the challenges in workforce distribution and health-care delivery across Europe.

Perspectives for a Future of Midwifery

The International Confederation of Midwives (ICM) defines the global scope of midwifery practice as the "autonomous care of women and newborns," emphasizing midwives as primary providers of reproductive, maternal, and newborn health services. This framework is intentionally rights-based, client-centered, and grounded in professional independence. However, realizing this scope of practice in clinical settings—particularly in postcolonial, hierarchical health systems—remains a challenge.

Many midwives, from the diploma to the graduate school educated, continue to face restricted clinical autonomy due to regulatory, institutional, or sociocultural barriers. In some countries, midwifery remains embedded within the nursing profession, limiting midwives' ability to practice independently. Similarly, in other countries, midwifery is impeded under medicine, which also limits practice potential.

In some locales, outdated legislation or physician-led protocols prevent midwives from fully exercising skills such as initiating life-saving interventions or making referrals. These constraints are in direct contradiction to the vision of midwives as autonomous, accountable practitioners.

Leaders from around the globe are asked to ponder the following questions related to realizing the expansion of full scope midwifery practice.

1. How do you define clinical autonomy in nurse-midwifery practice, and why is it essential for delivering high-quality, respectful maternal and newborn care?
   Purpose: To explore the philosophical and practical meaning of autonomy from a midwifery leadership perspective, grounded in care quality, safety, and rights-based approaches.

2. In your experience, what systemic or cultural barriers most commonly limit midwives' clinical autonomy—and how have you or your organization addressed them?
   Purpose: To surface real-world constraints (e.g., regulatory, institutional, gender-based) and solutions, offering practical and inspirational insights from leadership and advocacy work.
3. Looking ahead, what bold shifts or commitments are needed globally and locally to strengthen midwives' clinical decision-making authority within health systems?
   Purpose: To provoke visionary, future-forward responses that inform global discourse on midwifery-led models of care, professional respect, and health system reform.

Snapshot from a Regional Professional Association Leader

Clinical autonomy is not a privilege bestowed upon midwives—it is the ethical recognition of their preparation, expertise, and the trust placed in them by the women and communities they serve. It is the ability to act, lead, and decide independently within one's full scope of practice, grounded in professional standards and core competencies. An advanced practice midwife is not merely a provider, but a mentor, a clinical strategist, a policy interpreter, and a driver of innovation across leadership, management, education, and research.

And yet, this autonomy remains systemically and culturally constrained. Outdated regulations, resistant medical hierarchies, and unsupportive policies often undercut the very midwives trained to deliver evidence-based, life-saving care. Even within our profession, those who ascend to advanced levels of practice may find themselves met with skepticism rather than solidarity. Culturally, biases persist—whether toward male midwives or toward younger professionals seeking to serve their communities with integrity.

Dr. Glory S. Msibi

East Central and South Africa colleges of Nursing and Midwifery (ECSACONM) PRESIDENT

The tension between the aspirational scope of midwifery and its practical limitations speaks to deeper issues of professional recognition, gender dynamics, and health system design. Midwives are often caught in systems that undervalue their training and expertise, resulting in fragmented care, delayed interventions, and burnout. Without structural support, such as updated legislation, midwife-led units, and independent regulatory bodies, global competencies may remain more aspirational than actionable.

In essence, clinical autonomy is not simply a professional privilege; it is a cornerstone of safe, evidence-based care that requires both political will and system-level reform to dismantle the barriers that constrain midwives and, ultimately, the communities they serve. Clinical autonomy is not a technical privilege; it is the operationalization of trust in midwives' expertise, education, and evidence-based practice. Yet in many health systems, autonomy remains conditional—granted through layers of approval, constrained by hierarchies and institutional protocol.

We must boldly reimagine health systems where clinical midwives write the protocols, shape the legislation, and mentor the next generation into a model of care that centers humanity and evidence in equal measure. Autonomy must not be the exception; it must be the expectation.

Future-Forward and Provocative Questions on Clinical Autonomy in Midwifery

1. What if midwives—not physicians—were the default primary providers of all low-risk maternity care globally? Would outcomes improve? Would systems collapse or transform?
2. In what ways does the current legal definition of "autonomy" limit midwives' true independence—and who benefits from that limitation?
3. Should the ICM Scope of Practice become a legally binding standard within national regulatory frameworks—rather than aspirational guidance?
4. How can midwifery be reimagined as a full-spectrum, life-course profession beyond maternity—without being subsumed by general nursing or medicine?
5. What systemic shifts are needed for midwife-led care models to become the global norm rather than the exception?
6. What would it take for midwives to be recognized as prescribers and independent health practitioners in every country—without physician oversight?
7. What are the ethical implications of regulating midwives within male-dominated medical boards or under ministries that do not represent them?
8. How can midwives build collective power and political capital to influence national scopes of practice and clinical guidelines directly?
9. To what extent is the lack of clinical autonomy a reflection of broader gender inequities?
10. What might the future of autonomous midwifery look like in a world without borders—where digital care, migration, and global licensing are possible?

References

1. Accreditation Commission for Midwifery Education. ACME-accredited programs; 2023. Available from: https://theacme.org/accredited-midwifery-education-programs/
2. Accreditation Commission for Midwifery Education. Criteria for programmatic accreditation of midwifery education programs (Final criteria); 2019. Available from: https://theacme.org/wp-content/uploads/2024/02/Preaccreditation.pdf
3. Altınayak SÖ, Apay SE, Vermeulen J. The role of midwifery associations in the professional development of midwifery. Eur J Midwifery. 2020;4(July) https://doi.org/10.18332/ejm/122388.
4. American Association of Colleges of Nursing. The Doctor of Nursing Practice (DNP) fact sheet; n.d. https://www.aacnnursing.org/news-data/fact-sheets/dnp-fact-sheet
5. American College of Nurse-Midwives. About midwives: CNMs and CMs; 2023. Available from: https://www.midwife.org/About-Midwives

6. Auerbach S. The origins of modern public health in Caribbean slavery, 1764–1790. Soc Hist Med. 2018;31(3):505–28.
7. Batinelli L, McCourt C, Bonciani M, Rocca-Ihenacho L. Implementing midwifery units in a European country: situational analysis of an Italian case study. Midwifery. 2023;116:103534. https://doi.org/10.1016/j.midw.2022.103534.
8. Breckinridge M. Wide neighborhoods: a story of the frontier nursing service. Lexington: University Press of Kentucky; 1981.
9. Brumley J, Kessler JL, Boys A. Professional Foundation of Midwifery. In: Varney's midwifery. 7th ed. Jones & Bartlett Learning; 2024.
10. Bryant A, Reynolds NR, Hart L, Johnson PG, Kalula A, Gokul B, et al. A qualitative study of fourteen African countries' nursing workforce and labour market. Int Nurs Rev. 2022;69(1):20–9. https://doi.org/10.1111/inr.12670.
11. Calvert B, Homer CSE, Bar-Zeev S, Ferguson A, Scarf V. A scoping review mapping economic evaluations of midwifery service provision and the midwifery workforce. Appl Health Econ Health Policy. 2025; https://doi.org/10.1007/s40258-025-00962-z.
12. Canadian Association of Midwives. Midwifery in Canada: Fact sheet; 2023. Available from: https://canadianmidwives.org/about-midwifery/
13. CARICOM. Human Resource Development 2030 Strategy: Unlocking Human Potential. Caribbean Community (CARICOM). 2017. Available from: https://caricom.org/documents/16065-caricom-hrd-2030-strategy-viewing.pdf
14. CARICOM. Calls for more investment in nurses as shortage hurts region. Caribbean Community (CARICOM); 2025, April 30. Available from: https://caricom.org/calls-for-more-investment-in-nurses-as-shortage-hurts-region
15. Chauvet C. Editorial. Nordic J Nurs Res. 2021;41:1–2.
16. Chirwa MD, Nyasulu J, Modiba L, et al. Challenges faced by midwives in the implementation of facility-based maternal death reviews in Malawi. BMC Pregnancy Childbirth. 2023;23:282. https://doi.org/10.1186/s12884-023-05536-2.
17. Cohen R, Patterson O. The sociology of slavery: black Society in Jamaica, 1655–1838. Cambridge: Polity Press; 2022. p. 314. (First published in 1967). Soc [Internet]. 2022 Oct [cited 2025 Nov 15];59(5):617–9. Available from: https://link.springer.com/10.1007/s12115-022-00775-z
18. Davis-Floyd R, Cheyney M. Birth in eight cultures: a crosscultural investigation of childbirth practices. Long Grove: Waveland Press; 2019.
19. da Gama SGN, Viellas EF, Torres JA, Bastos MH, Brüggemann OM, Theme Filha MM, Leal MC. Labor and birth care by nurse with midwifery skills in Brazil. Reprod Health. 2016;13(Suppl 3):123.
20. El-Ardat M, Galijašević N, Lačević-Mulahasanović L, Šaldo D, Imamović F. The role and importance of the midwife before, during and after birth and their status in the health system. J Comm Med Pub Health Rep. 2025;6(01)
21. Elmer D, Endrei D, Németh N, Csákvári T, Kajos LF, Molics B, Boncz I. Changes in the number of healthcare professionals in European healthcare systems between 2000 and 2018. Orv Hetil. 2022;163(41):1639–48.
22. Emons J, Luiten M. Midwifery in Europe: an inventory in fifteen EU-member states. Deloitte & Touche; 2001.
23. Endalamaw A. Health workforce development and systems strengthening: global perspectives on nursing and midwifery. Springer; 2024.
24. European Commission Directorate-General for Employment, Social Affairs Inclusion. Spark Legal Policy Consulting Mapping and assessment of developments of one of the sectoral professions under Directive 2005/36/EC – The profession of midwife. Publications Office of the European Union. 2025. Available from: https://op.europa.eu/en/publication-detail/-/publication/9585c119-5e0a-11f0-a9d0-01aa75ed71a1/language-en
25. European Parliament Council of the European Union, 2005. EU Directive 2005/36/EC of the European Parliament and of the Council of 7 September 2005 on the recognition of professional qualifications; 2005

26. Goemaes R, Embo M, Hernandez-Garcia AB, De Koster K, Castiaux G, Hammoucha N, Sulejmani F, Beeckman K, Bogaerts A. The future of midwifery care and education in Belgium: a discussion paper. Midwifery. 2025;141:104237. https://doi.org/10.1016/j.midw.2024.104237.
27. Goode CJ, Williams CA. History of nurse-midwifery in the United States. J Nurse Midwifery. 1993;38(5):325–30.
28. Green-Stewart SL. Disease and empire: women & caregiving in colonial Jamaica. Doctoral thesis. Hamilton: McMaster University; 2022. Available from: https://macsphere.mcmaster.ca/bitstream/11375/27443/2/Green-Stewart_Sandria_L_finalsubmission202203_PhD.pdf
29. Hamilton, A. Midwifery still relevant, important career, says assn head. Daily Observer (Jamaica); 2025. pressreader.com/jamaica/daily-observer-jamaica/20200524/28716246458756
30. International Council of Nurses. Guidelines on advanced practice nursing. Geneva: International Council of Nurses; 2020.
31. Janke TM, Makarova N, Schmittinger J, Agricola CJ, Ebinghaus M, Blome C, Zyriax BC. Women's needs and expectations in midwifery care – results from the qualitative MiCa (midwifery care) study. Part 1: preconception and pregnancy. Heliyon. 2024;10(4):e25862. https://doi.org/10.1016/j.heliyon.2024.e25862.
32. Jordan B. Birth in four cultures: a crosscultural investigation of childbirth in Yucatan, Holland, Sweden, and the United States. 4th ed. Long Grove: Waveland Press; 1993.
33. Kemp J, Maclean GD, Moyo N. Global midwifery: principles, policy and practice. Cham: Springer International Publishing; 2021.
34. Kieft RA, De Brouwer BB, Francke AL, Delnoij DM. How nurses and their work environment affect patient experiences of the quality of care: a qualitative study. BMC Health Serv Res. 2014;14(1):249.
35. Kimani RW, Gatimu SM. Nursing and midwifery education, regulation and workforce in Kenya: a scoping review. Int Nurs Rev. 2023;70(3):444–55.
36. Lillo E. Midwifery in Chile – a successful experience to improve women's sexual and reproductive health: facilitators & challenges. JAMA. 2016;3(1):4–20.
37. Loudon I. Maternal mortality in the past and its relevance to developing countries today. Am J Clin Nutr. 2000;72(1 Suppl):241S–6S. https://doi.org/10.1093/ajcn/72.1.241S.
38. International Confederation of Midwives. International definition and scope of practice of the midwife. The Hague: International Confederation of Midwives; 2025.
39. MacKay RE, et al. Nurse- and midwife-led HIV services in Eastern and Southern Africa: challenges and opportunities for health facilities. J Assoc Nurses AIDS Care. 2020;31(4):392–404.
40. Makarova N, Janke TM, Schmittinger J, Agricola CJ, Ebinghaus M, Blome C, Zyriax BC. Women's expectations, preferences and needs in midwifery care – results from the qualitative midwifery care (MiCa) study: childbirth and early parenthood. Midwifery. 2024;132:103990. https://doi.org/10.1016/j.midw.2024.103990.
41. Marzalik PR, Feltham KJ, Jefferson K, Pekin K. Midwifery education in the U.S. – certified nurse-midwife, certified midwife and certified professional midwife. Midwifery. 2018;60:9–12. https://doi.org/10.1016/j.midw.2018.01.020.
42. Moravcová M. Midwifery–how are we doing in The Czech Republic with the regulation of the profession? Cent Eur J Nurs Midwifery. 2022;13(4):728–9.
43. Muhayimana A, Kearns I. Healthcare providers' perspectives on sustaining respectful maternity care appreciated by mothers in five hospitals of Rwanda. BMC Nurs. 2024;23(1):442.
44. Muraraneza C, Mukamana D, Katende G, Bazirete O, Wolvaardt L. Academic partnerships in transforming nursing and midwifery education in Africa: a systematic scoping review protocol. Syst Rev. 2024;13(1):262.
45. Murdock M, Durant S. Settler midwifery: a colonial tool in Canada's reproductive healthcare system. Birth. 2025;52(3):370–5. https://doi.org/10.1111/birt.12888.
46. Nagórska M. Medical Professions in International Perspective. Midwife. Rzeszów: Rzeszow University Publishing House; 2024.
47. National Council of Indigenous Midwives (NCIM). Available at https://indigenousmidwifery.ca/mission-vision-values/; n.d.

48. Nawagi F, Kneafsey R, Modber M, Mukeshimana M, Ndungu C, Bayliss-Pratt L. An overview of nursing and midwifery leadership, governance structures, and instruments in Africa. BMC Nurs. 2023;22:168. https://doi.org/10.1186/s12912-023-01336-3.
49. Niyigena A, Girukubonye I, Barnhart DA, Cubaka VK, Niyigena PC, Nshunguyabahizi M, et al. Rwanda's community health workers at the front line: a mixed-method study on perceived needs and challenges for community-based healthcare delivery during COVID-19 pandemic. BMJ Open. 2022;12(4):e055119.
50. Nove A, Ten Hoope-Bender P, Boyce M, Bar-Zeev S, de Bernis L, Lal G, Matthews Z, Mekuria M, Homer CSE. The state of the world's midwifery 2021 report: findings to drive global policy and practice. Hum Resour Health. 2021;19(1):146. https://doi.org/10.1186/s12960-021-00694-w.
51. Nove A, Friberg IK, de Bernis L, Cameron M, et al. Potential impact of midwives in preventing and reducing maternal and neonatal mortality and stillbirths: a lives saved tool modelling study. Lancet Glob Health. 2020;8(1):e24–33.
52. Ngunyulu S, Mulaudzi F. African indigenous beliefs and practices during pregnancy, birth and postnatal care. In: Indigenous knowledge systems and cultural dimensions of school nursing care; 2022. Available from: https://www.ncbi.nlm.nih.gov/books/NBK601353/
53. Nyawira L, Tsofa B, Musiega A, Munywoki J, Njuguna RG, Hanson K, et al. Management of human resources for health: implications for health systems efficiency in Kenya. BMC Health Serv Res. 2022;22:1046. https://doi.org/10.1186/s12913-022-08432-1.
54. Pan American Health Organization (PAHO). New PAHO report reveals 14 countries in the Americas face health worker shortages; 2025, April 30. Available from: https://www.paho.org/en/news/30-4-2025-new-paho-report-reveals-14-countries-americas-face-health-worker-shortages
55. Parizad N, Almasi L, Cheraghi R, Piran M. Job stress and its relationship with nurses' autonomy and nurse-physician collaboration in intensive care unit. J Nurs Manag. 2021;29(7):2084–91. https://doi.org/10.1111/jonm.13343.
56. Pezaro DS, Zarbiv G, Jones J, Feika ML, Fitzgerald L, Lukhele S, et al. Characteristics of strong midwifery leaders and enablers of strong midwifery leadership: an international appreciative inquiry. Midwifery. 2024;132:103982.
57. Pitter CP, Hewitt H, McWhinney-Dehaney L, Williams D, Vassell-Murray I. Blooms and mushrooms: midwifery experience in Jamaica. In: Gray M, Kitson-Reynolds E, Cummins A, editors. Starting life as a midwife. Cham: Springer International Publishing; 2019. p. 141–53.
58. Pop-Tudose ME, Radu MC. Similarities in midwifery education, regulation, and practice across Europe – a literature review. Eur J Midwifery. 2023;7(Supplement 1) https://doi.org/10.18332/ejm/172978.
59. Power A. Beyond Brexit: cross-border collaborations in pre-registration midwifery education. Brit J Midwifery. 2018;26(1):57–9.
60. Raddatz M, Hellmers C, zu Sayn-Wittgenstein F, Stelzig S. Midwifery in Germany – the necessity of developing a workforce and service planning approach. Eur J Pub Health. 2019;29(Supplement_4) https://doi.org/10.1093/eurpub/ckz186.419.
61. Relyea MJ. The rebirth of midwifery in Canada: an historical perspective. Midwifery. 1992;8(4):159–69. https://doi.org/10.1016/S0266-6138(05)80002-6.
62. Ricchi A, Covezzi IP, Di Biase L, Saccani G, Galli C, Molinazzi MT, Putignano A, Neri I. Midwives autonomy in discharge women after physiological childbirth. Gazzetta Medica Italiana Archivio Per Le Sci Med. 2019;178(7–8):534–7.
63. Sandall J, Fernandez Turienzo C, Devane D, et al. Midwife continuity of care models versus other models of care for childbearing women. Cochrane Database Syst Rev. 2024;4(4):CD004667.
64. Saralegui-Gainza A, Soto-Ruiz N, Escalada-Hernández P, Arregui-Azagra A, García-Vivar C, San Martín-Rodríguez L. Density of nurses and midwives in sub-Saharan Africa: trends analysis over the period 2004–2016. J Nursing Management. 2022;30(8):3922–32.
65. Sarmiento I, Atkin L, Keith-Brown K, Rees M, Sesia P. Maternal health and indigenous traditional midwives in Mexico: a scoping review. Glob Health Res Policy. 2021;6:24.

66. Sauvegrain P, Schantz C, Rousseau A, Gaucher L, Dupont C, Chantry EAA. Midwifery research in France: current dynamics and perspectives. Midwifery. 2024;131:103935. https://doi.org/10.1016/j.midw.2024.103935.
67. Schiebinger L. Secret cures of slaves: people, plants, and medicine in the eighteenth-century Atlantic world. Stanford: Stanford University Press; 2017.
68. Triantafyllou E, Vivilaki V. What are the challenges midwives face working with refugee women and how can they be addressed? Eur J Midwifery. 2023;7:18. https://doi.org/10.18332/ejm/168942.
69. Vedam S, et al. Mapping integration of midwives across the United States: impact on access, equity, and outcomes. PLoS One. 2018;13(2) https://doi.org/10.1371/journal.pone.0192523.
70. Verderese MdL, Turnbull LM. World Health Organization, Geneva (Switzerland). The Traditional Birth Attendant in Maternal and Child Health and Family Planning [microform]: A Guide to Her Training and Utilization / Maria de Lourdes Verderese and Lily M. Turnbull Distributed by ERIC Clearinghouse [Washington, D.C.] 1975. https://eric.ed.gov/?id=ED118873
71. Vermeulen J, Buyl R, Luyben A, Fleming V, Tency I, Fobelets M. How to promote midwives' recognition and professional autonomy? A document analysis study. Midwifery. 2024;138:104138. https://doi.org/10.1016/j.midw.2024.104138.
72. Vermeulen J, Fobelets M, Fleming V, Luyben A, Stas L, Buyl R. How do midwives view their professional autonomy, now and in future? Healthcare. 2023;11(12) https://doi.org/10.3390/healthcare11121800.
73. Vermeulen J, Luyben A, Buyl R, Debonnet S, Castiaux G, Niset A, Muyldermans J, Fleming V, Fobelets M. The state of professionalisation of midwifery in Belgium: a discussion paper. Women Birth. 2021;34(1):7–13. https://doi.org/10.1016/j.wombi.2020.09.012.
74. Vermeulen J, Luyben A, Jokinen M, Matintupa E, O'Connell R, Bick D. Establishing a Europe-wide foundation for high quality midwifery education: the role of the European midwives Association (EMA). Midwifery. 2018;64:128–31. https://doi.org/10.1016/j.midw.2018.06.009.
75. Vermeulen J, Luyben A, O'Connell R, Gillen P, Escuriet R, Fleming V. Failure or progress? The current state of the professionalisation of midwifery in Europe. Eur J Midwifery. 2019;3:22. https://doi.org/10.18332/ejm/115038.
76. Vermeulen J, Vivilaki VG. A value-based philosophy debate on academic midwifery education in Europe. Eur J Midwifery. 2021;5(November):1–3. https://doi.org/10.18332/ejm/143528.
77. Winkelmann J, Muench U, Maier CB. Time trends in the regional distribution of physicians, nurses and midwives in Europe. BMC Health Serv Res. 2020;20(1):937.
78. WHO European Region. Strengthening the skills of future midwives. 2024. Available from: https://www.who.int/europe/news/item/03-05-2024-strengthening-the-skills-of-future-midwives
79. World Health Organization. Global strategic directions for nursing and midwifery 2021–2025. Geneva: World Health Organization; 2021.
80. World Health Organization. Midwives' Voices, Midwives' Realities; 2016
81. United Nations Population Fund [UNFPA], World Health Organization [WHO], International Confederation of Midwives [ICM]. The State of the World's Midwifery; 2021. Available from: https://www.unfpa.org/sites/default/files/pub-pdf/21-038-UNFPA-SoWMy2021-Report-ENv4302_0.pdf
82. WBRC News. Midwifery and maternal outcomes in Alabama; 2025, June 23. Available from: https://www.wbrc.com/2025/06/23/study-shows-states-that-utilize-midwives-have-better-maternal-outcome
83. WSNA. The state of midwifery in Washington; 2024. Available from: https://www.wsna.org/news/2024/the-state-of-midwifery
84. Zug KE, Cassiani SHB, Pulcini J, Bassalobre Garcia A, Aguirre-Boza F, Park J. Advanced practice nursing in Latin America and the Caribbean: regulation, education and practice. Rev Lat Am Enfermagem. 2016;24:e2807. https://doi.org/10.1590/1518-8345.1615.2807.

Clinical Autonomy for Nurse Anesthetists Globally

Sandra Maree Ouellette, Nico Decock, Assumpta Yamuragiye, and Hui-Ju Yang

Introduction

Autonomy in anesthesia care refers to the degree of independent decision-making power given to health-care professions like nurse anesthetists. It encompasses both clinical autonomy and professional autonomy. Clinical autonomy allows health-care professionals such as nurse anesthetists to make independent decisions based on education, licensure, and expertise. It empowers nurse anesthetists to tailor anesthesia plans, manage unexpected surgical developments, and adjust anesthesia in real time to optimize outcome and patient safety [1]. Professional autonomy allows the nurse anesthetist to work within their defined scope of practice to provide high-quality individualized timely patient care with or without extensive physician supervision. It can lead to greater access to surgical care, excellent patient outcomes, and patient satisfaction.

S. M. Ouellette (✉)
Adjunct Faculty, School of Medicine, Department of Academic Nursing, Wake Forest University, Winston-Salem, NC, USA

N. Decock
Centre Hospitalier Regional Universitaire de Nancy, Regional University Hospital of Nancy, Nancy, France
e-mail: n.decock@chru-nancy.fr

A. Yamuragiye
College of Medicine and Health Sciences, School of Health Sciences, Department of Anestheisa, University of Rwanda, Kigali, Rwanda
e-mail: a.yamuragiye@ur.ac.rw

H.-J. Yang
Department of Anesthesiology, Taipei Veteran General Hospital, Taipei, Taiwan

Nursing Department, National Yang Ming Chiao Tung University, Hsinchu, Taiwan

A. Kapu et al. (eds.), *A Global View on Clinical Autonomy for Advanced Practice Nurses*, Advanced Practice in Nursing,
https://doi.org/10.1007/978-3-032-21458-4_3

The journey to clinical autonomy in any country can be a long one. At its core is organizational strength through establishing a national organization dedicated to high educational standards, credentialing, political advocacy with support of laws, statutes, or regulations aimed at the ability of the nurse anesthetist to be recognized in their country and be allowed to work at the top of their licensure and expertise without unnecessary dependence on other providers. It supports a collaborative model where all team members work according to their licensure, skill, and expertise for enhanced patient outcomes and safety.

This chapter begins with the journey to anesthesia practice autonomy in four countries associated with the International Federation of Nurse Anesthetists: United States of America; France; Rwanda; and Taiwan. The discussion includes historical evolution of nurse anesthetist in WHO regions, workforce considerations in the region, education and training considerations, impact of optimal autonomy in practice, and regulation and levels of authority in the country allowing practice autonomy. The American story is the oldest and perhaps best recorded. For that reason, it outlines steps necessary to reach the goal of practice autonomy for the nurse anesthetist.

The Road to National Autonomy for Nurse Anesthetists

The American Story: Long Journey, Nearing the Destination

The wonderous story of anesthesia began on October 16, 1846, when a dentist, William Morton, provided ether anesthesia for Dr John Collins Warren who proceeded to excise a tumor from a patient's neck at the Massachusetts General Hospital. While news spread quickly in the USA and abroad regarding success of Morton's demonstration, surgical morbidity and mortality remained high, largely because of infections and mishaps associated with the occasional anesthetist who was untrained. There was no anesthesia specialist [2].

By 1867, Joseph Lister had developed a method for antiseptic surgery and surgical outcomes improved [3, 4]. However, there still was the question regarding who should administer the anesthesia? There was no financial incentive to a physician to become the anesthesia specialist and the job often fell on poorly trained interns or house officers who were more interested in watching the surgery than watching the patient. At times dropping ether or chloroform fell on whoever was available and might include orderlies, hospital porters, medical students, and other surgeons and nurses. The occasional anesthetist did not know the science of anesthesia and was unpracticed in the art of its administration. It came as no surprise then that there was a high rate of morbidity and mortality associated with anesthesia.

The administration of anesthesia by nurses in the United States dates back to the Civil War between 1861 and 1865. In her autobiography, Catherine Lawrence, the first recorded nurse to administer anesthesia, reported she administered chloroform to wounded soldiers during that war [5]. During the period 1875–1899, increased awareness of the need for an anesthesia specialist to decrease morbidity and mortality associated with anesthesia led to the recruitment of Catholic Sisters and graduate nurses for these services. Sister Mary Bernard, in 1877, may have been the first nurse to specialize in anesthesia making her the first advanced practice nurse in the USA [6].

Based on an excellent record of nurse specialist in anesthesia, surgeons at reputable institutions began to recruit nurses and selected a nurse to administer anesthesia for their patients. Early notable nurses who devoted their practice principally to anesthesia included the Graham sisters, Alice McGaw and Agatha Hodgins.

Edith and Dinah Graham worked with the Mayo brothers at St Mary's Hospital, Rochester, MN, during the period 1887–1893 [7]. Edith Graham later married Dr. William Mayo and recruited Alice McGaw who worked with the Mayo brothers for a number of years. Alice McGaw utilized ether and chloroform for her patients and in the St Paul Medical Journal in 1900, she reported on 1092 cases requiring anesthesia without an accident, need for artificial respiration, or pneumonia. In 1904, she reported on over 11,000 cases and, in 1906, over 16,000 cases without a death directly related to anesthesia [8]. This was an exceptional feat for the time and Dr. William Mayo named her the Mother of Anesthesia [9]. At the time, St Mary's Hospital, now Mayo Clinic, was a leader in surgical discovery and care and surgeons from all over the country and other parts of the world came there to observe the work of the Mayo brothers. An unexpected surprise was the anesthesia delivered by Alice McGaw. It was said that McGaw was the most observed individual at the institution with the exception of the Mayo Brothers.

Dr. George Crile at Lakeside Hospital, Cleveland, OH, recruited Agatha Hodgins as his anesthetist [10]. He was interested in thyroid surgery and very progressive in management of the patient in shock. Miss Hodgins pioneered an anesthetic technique consisting of oxygen, nitrous oxide, and ether. McGaw and Hodgins taught other nurses and some physicians to administer anesthesia. Increased utilization of nurses as the anesthesia specialist led to the inclusion of anesthesia content in nursing curricula and the development of four formalized postgraduate nurse anesthesia courses: St Vincent's Portland, OR 1909; St John's, Springfield, IL in 1912; New York Postgraduate Hospital, New York, 1912; and Long Island College Hospital, Brooklyn, NY 1914 [11].

Dr. Crile and Agatha Hodgins started an educational program at Lakeside Hospital in 1915 after she returned from service in World War I. In 1916, physicians working with the Medical Board of Ohio challenged Dr. Crile's use of nurses in administering anesthesia and the school closed. After a hearing, nurse anesthesia practice was found to be legal. An amendment to the Medical Practice Act stated nothing in the act could be construed to prevent nurses from administering anesthesia under the direction and supervision of a physician. This was the first recognition of nurse anesthetists in any health practice act in the USA. The school, which had closed due to legal action, reopened in 1917 [12].

Nurse anesthetists assisted surgeons care for the wounded in every war and conflict since the Civil War. Although World War I or the Great War occurred during the period 1914–1918, the USA did not enter the war until 1917.Serving in both the Army and the Navy, they were assigned to ambulance companies, field surgical

Table 1 Early landmark cases challenging the nurse anesthesia specialty in the USA

1917	Frank vs. south in Kentucky. In this case, the Kentucky court of appeals ruled that nurse anesthetist Margaret Hatfield was not engaged in the practice of medicine when she administered anesthesia for surgeon Louis frank's cases
1934	Charmers-Francis vs. Nelson in California. The California supreme court affirmed the superior court finding for nurse anesthetist Dagmar Nelson by confirming the legality of nurse anesthesia practice

units, and base hospitals. They taught nurses and physicians to administer anesthesia. Noted nurse anesthetists who were deployed to the front-line administering anesthesia included Anne Penland, Agatha Hodgins, and Sophie Winton. Rapid growth of nurse anesthetists and the strong alliance between them and many surgeons stimulated challenge from a few physicians who planned to make anesthesia solely a medical specialty. The first such physician challenges occurred in Ohio and Kentucky. See Table 1 for a brief discussion of Frank versus South and Dagmar Nelson, two early landmark cases [13]. The Dagmar Nelson trial, the only legal case to test the legality of nurses administering anesthesia, was won in 1934.

Challenges to Nurse Anesthesia Practice Continue—So Let's Organize

With continued antinurse anesthetist activity, much of it led by a physician anesthesia specialist Dr. Francis McMechan and his wife Laurette, it was time for nurse anesthetists to organize [14, 15]. On June 17, 1931, 40 anesthetists representing 17 states met in a classroom in the Anesthesia Department of Lakeside Hospital in Cleveland, Ohio. Led by Agatha Hodgins, they founded the International Association of Nurse Anesthetists. In a few months, the name was changed to the National Association of Nurse Anesthetists (NANAs) and in 1939, it became the American Association of Nurse Anesthetists (AANAs) [16]. In 2020, a membership-driven resolution to rebrand the association passed and it is now known as the American Association of Nurse Anesthesiology [17].

Advancement of the profession through AANA spanned decades. Table 2 lists landmark achievements, which served as steppingstones for advancement in education, practice, and autonomy. These achievements paved the way for recognition of the nurse anesthetist at the national and state levels and resulted in the freedom to practice autonomously. These achievements are briefly summarized as follows:

1. Standardization of education was the primary objective following founding of the National Association of Nurse Anesthetists. At the time, all programs were hospital based with no standards of education or practice instruction for entry into the profession. Visionary leaders at the time such as Agatha Hodgins, Gertrude Fife, and Helen Lamb knew that survival was dependent on excellence in education and practice as well as standardization of education in all programs. They worked with Helen Lamb, a student of Agatha Hodgins and Chief Nurse

Table 2 Landmark achievements of AANA in building the bridge to clinical autonomy

1.	Early development and support of standardization of the specialty through development of education and practice standards
2.	National Certification by examination in 1945
3.	Quality assurance in education through program accreditation in 1952. The AANA accreditation program was recognized by the U.S. Office of Education in 1955
4.	In 1975, the Council on Accreditation of Nurse Anesthesia Educational Programs and the Council on Certification of Nurse Anesthetists were created. The credentialing functions of AANA were transferred to these autonomous councils
5.	Membership approved continuous professional development and in 1978, the Council on Recertification was established. In 2007, the Council on Certification and the Council on Recertification became the National Board of Certification Recertification Nurse Anesthetists or NBCRNAs
6.	In 1989, AANA became one of the 11 countries to sign the founding charter of the International Federation of Nurse Anesthetists (IFNAs)
7.	Movement of educational programs from hospital-based certificate programs to universities. All programs transitioned to university-based master's degree entry by 1998 and doctoral entry by 2025
8.	In 1986, the U.S. Congress passed legislation providing CRNAs direct reimbursement under Medicare Part B, making nurse anesthetists the first nursing specialty/nonphysician group to be accorded direct reimbursement rights under the Part B Medicare federal program. Direct reimbursement under Medicare was implemented by regulation in 1989. This achievement was a seven-year process with 4 years devoted to legislation and three years to acceptable regulation with parity in payment
9.	In 2020, the U.S. Congress passed legislation, the Affordable Care Act, that included nondiscrimination provisions to prohibit health plans from discriminating against licensed health-care professionals such as CRNAs and other nonphysician providers solely based on their licensure
10.	In 1997, the Health Care Financing Administration (HCFA) administration proposed a ruling that would remove physician supervision requirements for CRNAs under Medicare regulations. Debated heavily by physicians, in 2001, HCFA again made a final ruling that removed physician supervision from CRNAs. In the end, however, the Bush administration introduced "opt-out" requiring state governors to request a removal in their state. To date, 25 states and Guam and DC have opted out

Anesthetist at Barnes Hospital, St Louis, MO. Today, Helen Lamb is known as the Mother of Nurse Anesthesia Education [18].

2. The AANA administered the first qualifying (certification) examination on June 4, 1945. The 38-page examination was taken by 90 women in 39 hospitals in 28 states, plus one in the territory of Hawaii. It was called the qualifying examination then, because it qualified successful candidates for membership in the AANA [19].
3. The AANA began its quality assurance or accreditation program for schools of nurse anesthesia in 1952. In 1955, the U.S. Department of Health, Education, and Welfare recognized the AANA as the accrediting agency for schools of nurse anesthesia. This milestone effectively standardized education for all programs throughout the USA [19, 20].
4. In 1975, restructuring of education and recognition of credentialing entities by the U.S. Office of Education led to creation of autonomous councils for the nurse anesthesia programs and individuals. The Council on Certification of Nurse

Anesthetists and the Council on Accreditation of Nurse Anesthetists Educational Programs were created, and the credentialing functions of the AANA were transferred to these autonomous councils [21].

5. In 1970s, AANA membership approved mandatory continuing education and in 1978, the Council on Recertification was formed to administer the mandatory continuing education program of AANA. In 2007, the Council on Certification and the Council on Recertification incorporated to become the National Board of Certification and Recertification of Nurse Anesthetists (NBCRNA). This entity now is responsible for initial certification and continuing recertification [22]. Its credentialing program is called MAC or Maintaining Anesthesia Certification. Initial certification and continued recertification must be maintained to work as a Certified Registered Nurse Anesthetist in the USA.
6. In 1989, representatives of AANA joined ten other country representatives in establishing and signing the founding charter for the formation of the International Federation of Nurse Anesthetists (IFNAs). Globalization of the specialty of nurse anesthesia practice through educational, practice, and monitoring standards was a goal, and remarkable progress has been made toward improved education and practice authority in all member countries [23].
7. The initiation to move all nurse anesthesia educational programs from hospitals to institutions of higher learning at the baccalaureate and graduate levels began in 1969. By 1998, all U.S. programs were affiliated with a university and offered a Master's degree at graduation. By 2025, all programs had transitioned to doctoral entry at graduation. Today, there are approximately 150 programs in the USA with over 2500 clinical sites for education of the next generation of CRNAs [24].
8. In an attempt to control spiraling health-care costs in the USA, the Federal Government introduced reimbursement regulations in 1983 that negatively impacted CRNAs. In short, there was not a pathway for reimbursement for CRNA services given to Medicare and Medicaid patients. AANA leadership then began a seven-year journey lobbying the Federal Government for direct reimbursement in Part B Medicare and appropriate regulation for parity in payment. The first 4 years was devoted to legislation, and the last 3 years was devoted to regulation. In 1986, President Ronald Regan and the U.S. Congress passed legislation providing CRNAs direct reimbursement under Part B Medicare. Nurse anesthetists became the first nursing specialty in the USA to be accorded direct reimbursement rights under the federal program and the first nonphysicians recognized in the Part B payment pool. Following intense efforts with suitable federal regulators, Medicare Direct Reimbursement was implemented in 1989 [25].
9. In 1997, the U.S. Health Care Financing Administration (HCFA) proposed a ruling that would remove physician supervision requirements for CRNAs under Medicare Part A regulations. As expected, this was debated heavily by physician anesthesiologist, but in 2001, HCFA again made a final ruling that removed physician supervision from CRNAs at the federal level. Although U.S. President Bill Clinton had signed the regulation, it was forwarded to the President George

Bush administration in the closing days of the Bill Clinton Presidency. The Bush White House delayed blanket removal of supervision for CRNAs. What was later supported by the Bush administration was not across-the-board removal of supervision for CRNAs but substituted by "opt-out" by governors in states that wished to remove this supervision requirement, effectively moving legislation from the national level to the state level. To date, 25 states as well as Guam and Washington DC have opted out of supervision for CRNAs. Many other states do not have federal supervision requirements in state law but are eligible for opt-out should a governor wish to do so. Below are several recent examples of regulatory changes at the state or regional levels addressing regulatory authority and promoting practice autonomy for CRNAs [26].

1. Idaho Bill 289:

   This bill was unanimously passed by the House and Senate and was signed by Governor Little on March 28, 2025. It states "CRNAs provide the full spectrum of anesthesia care and related services……and are responsible for the care they provide. The law further states physicians are not liable for the action or omission relating to these anesthesia services provided solely and independently by a CRNA acting within the scope of CRNA licensure, education, training and experience and in accordance with state and federal laws" [27].
2. Kansas Bill 67:

   On April 1, 2025, Kansas Governor signed Senate Bill 67 granting CRNAs prescriptive authority. The law allows CRNAs to prescribe durable equipment and prescribe and administer any drug consistent with Registered Nurse Anesthetist education and qualifications in accordance with state nursing and controlled substance laws [28].
3. New Mexico Bill 78:

   This Bill was signed April 10, 2025. The bill was introduced at the request of the New Mexico Association of Nurse Anesthetists (NMANAs). It states that CRNAs shall function in an independent role or in collaboration with other health-care providers in accordance with others in a health-care facility. The law defines independent role as performing any action including determining, preparing, administrating, or monitoring anesthesia care or anesthesia-related services without the supervision of another health-care provider [29].

   Legislative gains are made annually promoting CRNA autonomy in the USA.

The Certified Register Nurse Anesthetist as an APRN

In the APRN model of regulation in the USA, there are four roles: certified registered nurse anesthetist (CRNA), certified nurse mid-wife (CNM), clinical nurse specialist (CNS), and certified nurse practitioner (CNP). The definition of an APRN was defined in 2008 and can be found on Table 3 [30].

The Certified Registered Nurse Anesthetist is prepared to provide the full spectrum of patients' anesthesia care and anesthesia-related care for individuals across

Table 3 Definition of advanced practice nurse in the united states

An APN is a nurse:
1. Who has completed an accredited graduate-level education program preparing him/her for one of the four recognized APN roles;
2. Who has passed a national certification examination that measures APN role and population-based competencies and who maintains continued competencies as evidenced by recertification in the role and population through the national certification program;
3. Who has acquired clinical knowledge and skills preparing him/her to provide direct care to patients as well as component of indirect care; however, the defining factor for all APNs is that a significant component of the education and practice focuses on direct care of individuals;
4. Whose practice builds on the competencies of registered nurses by demonstrating a greater depth and breadth of knowledge, a greater synthesis of data, increased complexity of skills and interventions, and greater role autonomy;
5. Who is educationally prepared to assume responsibility and accountability for health promotion and/or maintenance as well as the assessment, diagnosis, and management of patient problems, which include the use and prescription of pharmacologic and nonpharmacologic interventions;
6. Who has clinical experience of sufficient depth and breadth to reflect the intended license; and
7. Who has obtained a license to practice in one of the four APN roles: Certified registered nurse anesthetist (CRNA), certified nurse-midwife (CNM), clinical nurse specialist (CNS), or certified nurse practitioner (CNP)

the life span. This includes patients that are healthy through all levels of acuity. This care is provided in diverse settings, including hospital surgical suites, obstetrical delivery rooms, critical access hospitals, acute care, pain management centers, ambulatory surgical centers, and offices of dentist, ophthalmologists, podiatrist, and plastic surgeons. Licensed APNs are independent practitioners with no regulatory requirements for collaboration, direction, or supervision [30].

Workforce, Manpower Issues, and Solutions

There are three providers credentialed to administer anesthesia in the United States: physicians who commonly are referred to as physician anesthesiologists; certified registered nurse anesthetists or CRNAs/nurse anesthesiologists; and anesthesiology assistants (AAs). Anesthesiologist Assistants were introduced in the 1960s with two major programs based at Emory University, Atlanta, Georgia, and Case Western Reserve University, Cleveland Ohio. Anesthesiologist Assistants work only with anesthesiologists, are not independent, autonomous providers, are not a solution to anesthesia services in rural states that are often CRNA practice only, and are not recognized/licensed to work in all states. While these anesthesia providers have been educated for many decades, their numbers remain approximately 2000 to 4000 total. While the American Society of Anesthesiologist (ASA) remained neutral on this provider for many decades, that view has changed. In August 2000, the ASA House of Delegates endorsed efforts to obtain licensure and reimbursement for AAs practicing under the onsite direction of an anesthesiologist and the following year, they endorsed efforts to educate, train, and allow practice of AAs in as many states as anesthesiologists request the service. Now there are 18 programs that train AAs and they can practice in 19 states, the District of Columbia, Guam, and the Veterans Administration [31].

The practice of anesthesia in the USA has been recognized as a nursing specialty for more than 100 years. There are 150 plus Council on Accreditation of Nurse Anesthesia Programs accredited in the USA utilizing more than 2500 clinical sites. To be accepted into one of these programs, the applicant must be a Registered Nurse with a Bachelor of Science in Nursing (BSN) or an RN with another appropriate bachelor's degree. The programs are very competitive and a GPA of 3.5 or higher is desired. Programs require at least 1 year of full-time critical care nursing experience and many applicants have 2- or 3-years' experience in high acuity areas prior to admission. Nurse anesthetists are the only anesthesia professional requiring critical care experience prior to beginning formal anesthesia education [32].

All CRNA educational programs today award a doctoral degree at graduation. The programs are 36–51 months in length depending on university requirements and from the Bachelor Science in Nursing (BSN) to graduation, it is 8-to-10-year educational process. Graduates must pass the National Certification Examination to enter practice and comply with maintenance of certification requirements. Both credentialing programs are administered by the National Board of Certification and Recertification (NBCRNA) and must be complied with continuously to work in the USA.

The job market for CRNAs is robust. Jobs are plentiful in both large and small hospitals, outpatient facilities, surgical and dental offices, and in urban and rural communities. CRNAs may work in the ACT or Anesthesia Care Team Model where one anesthesiologist may direct up to four rooms for reimbursement. This was established in 1983 under TEFRA and speaks only to reimbursement and not quality of care [33]. CRNAs may work without an anesthesiologist, which is a common model in office-based practice, dental offices, and rural America.

CRNAs are unusual in that their practice of anesthesia is recognized as both a nursing and medical specialty unified by the same standards of care. There are over 60,000 employed CRNAs, and the market is expected to grow 38% between 2022 and 2032. There are approximately 52,400 active anesthesiologists with an average age in 2020 of 52.6 years. The average age of CRNAs is 47.5 and 12% plan to retire by 2027 [34].

The market for all anesthesia professionals looks good as we move into the future. As an advanced practice nurse anesthetist, the CRNA/nurse anesthesiologist practice with a high degree of autonomy and respect. Qualified to make independent judgements regarding all aspects of anesthesia care based on education, licensure and certification, and nearly 100 years of history, CRNAs can be the solution to the nations concerns in providing high-quality anesthesia care for all. In 2001, the Center for Medicare and Medicaid (CMS) allowed states to opt out of the requirement for reimbursement that a surgeon or anesthesiologist oversee the provision of anesthesia by CRNAs for Medicare Part A, facility payment. An analysis of

Medicare data for 1999–2005 found no evidence that opting out of physician oversight resulted in increased inpatient deaths or complications [35]. In addition, a publication in 2010 stated that both anesthesiologists and certified nurse anesthetists provide high-quality, efficient anesthesia care in the USA. CRNAs, however, are less costly to train, can perform the same set of anesthesia services, and their compensation lags behind the physician anesthesia specialist [36]. A closer look at efficiency, access, and cost indicates that CRNAs are clearly the solution to the nation's anesthesia coverage problem.

In summary, the road to practice autonomy is a long process with many building blocks conquered before it becomes a reality. It is not given. It is earned and is based on organizational structure for nurse anesthetists, education, strong practice standards, licensure and certification, mandatory continuous professional development, political advocacy, title protection, recognition, and, above all, unquestioned competency in the specialty. Practice models vary from solo to anesthesia care team. There are no quality-of-care outcome studies in anesthesia in the USA that demonstrate different outcomes based upon the anesthesia provider. The CRNA enjoys clinical practice autonomy within both practice models while working together with the perioperative team in keeping the patient as the focus of all care.

The Journey in Africa Toward Clinical Autonomy

Rwanda is small landlocked country with a surface area of a 26,338 km^2 located in East African region. The total population is around 13 million. The country faces a critical shortage of health-care professionals including anesthesia providers.

Safe anesthesia care is a cornerstone of effective surgical and obstetric services, yet many low- and middle-income countries, including Rwanda, continue to face a critical shortage of trained anesthesia providers. In response to this challenge, Rwanda has relied heavily on non-physician anesthetists, particularly nurse anesthetists to deliver essential care across its health facilities. These professionals, trained through formal academic and clinical pathways, are the primary providers of anesthesia services in most district and provincial hospitals, especially where physician anesthesiologists are scarce or absent [37].

The current anesthesia profession in Rwanda dates back to colonial times, when anesthesiologists from foreign countries provided anesthesia in Rwandan hospitals which were very few at that time. Before the 1994 Genocide, only one Rwandan anesthesiologist, who was trained in Belgium, was practicing in one University teaching hospital. Few Rwandans were sent to be trained outside the country. As surgical volume increased, on-the-job training for nurse anesthetists began [38].

The formal training of anesthesia started in 1996 with the former Kigali Health Institute (now University of Rwanda). Graduates of the program at that time were an advanced diploma holder in anesthesia and the program's entry profile was an enrolled nurse (A2) with a certain clinical experience. However, as the country reviewed the structure of nursing education in Rwanda, the A2 nursing program was phased out, and the recruitment profile shifted to high school graduates with background in sciences that must include biology in their combination. The program was upgraded to a bachelor's degree level in anesthesia with different reviews to ensure graduates are equipped with necessary skills and competency to provide anesthesia in the country, especially those graduates who worked alone in different hospitals across the country. It was later in 2006 that a residency in anesthesiology started in partnership with Canadian Society of Anesthesiologist.

Currently as of June 2025, there are only 45 anesthesiologists and around 557 nurse anesthetists for over 13 million of the Rwandan population. Those nurse anesthetists are working in public and private health-care settings including referral and district hospitals.

Over 95% of anesthesia care services in Rwanda are covered by nurse anesthetists. Considering the Rwandan context where anesthesia practice, especially in district hospitals, are performed by nurse anesthetists without supervision of anesthesiologists, the existing training programs of nurse anesthetists in Rwanda train them to become solo care providers. Nurse anesthetists can work *alone* or under supervision of a physician anesthetists depending on the level of care. In referral hospitals, there could be one physician anesthesiologist supervising 10 operating theatres. However, in every operating theatre, there must be a nonphysician anesthetist per every patient [39].

The shortage of health-care providers including anesthesia providers in the country is huge and the Rwanda ministry of health started a strategy known as four by four (4 × 4) aiming at quadrupling the number of health-care professionals in 4 years. In line with that, two universities started training nurse anesthetists at a bachelor's degree level. The University of Rwanda has long been the primary institution training anesthesia providers at the bachelor's level, and its graduates have become integral to the country's surgical and emergency care system [40]. It is expected that the new programs along with graduates from the University of Rwanda will contribute to increasing the number of nurse anesthetists who will provide safe anesthesia care to contribute to quality care and achievement of health-related sustainable development goals [41].

Recognizing the persistent gap in anesthesia personnel and the increasing complexity of surgical care, the Ministry of Health has recently intensified efforts to scale up training and strengthen the professional autonomy of nurse anesthetists. In a major milestone, Rwanda's first Master of Science in Nursing Anesthesia program was recently accredited in May 2025 and is enrolled its first cohort in September 2025. This advanced program aims to elevate clinical expertise and enhance decision-making autonomy, empowering nurse anesthetists to independently manage complex anesthesia cases and contribute to leadership within surgical teams [42]. It is expected that the graduates of the master's in nurse anesthesia at master's level will function as advanced nurse practitioners who will contribute to advanced nurse anesthesia practice. Expanding the training pipeline not only increases workforce numbers but also supports enhanced autonomy by equipping nurse anesthetists with rigorous clinical knowledge and decision-making skills essential for independent practice.

As nurse anesthetists gain greater autonomy, they are poised to play a pivotal role in achieving national health goals and advancing universal health coverage. The current scope of nurse anesthetist in Rwanda covers the anesthesia in different types of surgeries and is not discussing the role of nurse anesthetists in intensive care units. However, during Covid 19 and the recent Marburg outbreak, nurse anesthetists played an important role indicating their usefulness in patient management in acute settings. The scope needs review to expand on nurse anesthetists' scope and contribute to achieving access to health-care services to the Rwandan population [43].

Overview of Health-Care System in Rwanda

Health-care system in Rwanda is a pyramidal structure composed of tertiary hospitals and provincial and district hospitals. Health centers and health posts are the levels for basic care. There are in total 57 hospitals in Rwanda. Recent structure has upgraded some district hospitals to make them level two teaching hospitals to enable them to train a big number of students in health-related domains. Some health centers have also been medicalized to allow them to provide surgery and obstetric care. Overall, there are 5 national referral hospitals, which provide tertiary care, 27 hospitals that achieve Level II recognition, indicating they meet a higher standard of quality and service. Furthermore, there are 33 district hospitals, which are the primary level of care within the health-care system [44].

Nurse anesthetists are involved at all levels of care, especially levels that provide surgical interventions. Additionally, some nurse anesthetists in Rwanda work in prehospital care such as what is commonly known in Rwanda SAMU or Service d'Aide Medical Urgence.

Importance of Nurse Anesthetist's Autonomy in Improving Surgical and Obstetric Care

Rwanda has improved many health-care indicators. For instance, maternal death rates have been reduced from 210 to 201 per 100,00. One of the factors that contributed to that achievement was accessibility to service in terms of time and quality. For example, Cesarean sections are the most common surgical intervention performed at district hospitals and medicalized health centers and at those levels of care, nurse anesthetists cover anesthesia services as solo providers.

Nurse anesthetists have contributed to increasing surgical volume and addressing surgical workforce shortages, especially in rural and district hospitals. In 2015, around 58% of the Rwandan population did not have access to surgical care and one of the factors contributing to that gap was a shortage of anesthesia providers including nurse anesthetists. Currently, the surgical volume has increased to 786/100,000 even though the access is still low compared to 5000 procedures per 100,000 population recommended by the lancet commission of Global surgery [44].

Also, nurse anesthetists have contributed to improving access to safe anesthesia and reducing surgical wait times. They have also contributed to enhanced perioperative and patient safety outcome as well as cost-effective anesthesia care [45].

Challenges

Although Rwanda is advancing toward nurse anesthetist clinical autonomy, the current practice, which is a physician-led model, is still challenging the full autonomy in many ways. For instance, the current public health insurance scheme pays certain services when they have been provided by a physician. Another potential challenge related to achieving full autonomy is the fact that as the number of physician anesthetists increases, especially in referral and urban hospitals, the nurse anesthetists working in this tertiary level of care do not function at their full scope of practice. Physicians appear not to trust the knowledge that nurse anesthetists exhibit and tend to feel like increasing the competencies and allowing nurse anesthetists to function at their full scope is a threat to physician practice. However, the collaboration is not bad when considering that the current practice, a nurse anesthetist is taking care of a patient with a ratio of one by one while it is technically impossible for anesthesiologist to have that ratio considering their critical shortage.

Another potential challenge is the shortage of nurse anesthetists to the extent that some work in more than two health-care facilities. The critical shortage leads to increased workload, which can lead to poor job satisfaction. The surgical volume increases progressively with the availability of surgeons, and this should go together with the increase in the number of anesthesia providers. However, the gaps are still existing and will progressively be addressed as the MOH is committed to continue increasing the number of nurse anesthetists. One of the steps is to open training programs in addition to the UoR.

Lastly, nurse anesthetists complain about not finding career pathway advancement which sometimes encourages them to leave the profession and register in other professions which offer career growth opportunities. Lack of continuous professional development such as training opportunities and mentorship are also some of the key challenges faced by nurse anesthetists in Rwanda.

Clinical Autonomy of Nurse Anesthetists in France

The clinical autonomy of nurse anesthetists in France (Infirmiers Anesthésistes Diplômés d'État, IADE) has evolved significantly since the profession's inception in 1947. This evolution is deeply rooted in a dynamic interplay among national regulation, educational reform, and international standards for advanced practice nursing. Over time, IADEs have shifted from a role of technical assistance under strict medical supervision to one of recognized advanced clinical expertise and leadership in multidisciplinary teams. Autonomy of nurse anesthetists in France explores the historic and regulatory pathway to recognition, the central importance of rigorous education, the growing political awareness of nurse anesthesia care, and the realization of clinical autonomy within the anesthesia care team [46].

The Pathway to Recognition

Early Development and Regulation

Globally, nurse anesthesia traces its roots to the nineteenth century, when nurses began administering anesthesia after the discovery of ether. In France, the formal journey began in 1947 with the introduction of the first official anesthesia courses for nurses, initially positioning them as technical assistants to anesthesiologists [45]. By 1949, dedicated training programs led to the creation of the assistant anesthetist qualification, marking the profession's first regulatory milestone [47].

The 1960s and 1970s saw further structuring: the Certificate of Aptitude for Assistant Anesthetist (CAF AA) was established in 1960, extending training to 18 months, and then to 24 months in 1972, with a prerequisite of 3 years of prior nursing experience. These changes reflected a growing recognition of the need for specialized knowledge and skills in anesthesia nursing, though autonomy remained limited and always under medical supervision.

Professionalization and Legal Protection

A decisive shift occurred in the 1980s and 1990s. The 1988 decree introduced the Certificate of Aptitude for Specialized Nurse in Anesthesia and Resuscitation (CAFISAR), granting exclusive rights to practice anesthesia to those with this specialization. In 1991, the State Diploma of Nurse Anesthetist (DE IADE) formalized the profession and integrated it into the French public hospital system, signaling a transition from technical assistance to advanced clinical responsibility [46]. Legal protection of the IADE title became a priority, ensuring that only those with the appropriate education and credentials could practice, thus safeguarding public safety and professional standards.

International Influence and Modern Regulation

The founding of the International Federation of Nurse Anesthetists (IFNA) in 1989 and the adoption of international standards for education and practice further shaped the French regulatory landscape. The IFNA and International Council of Nurses (ICN) advocated for master's-level education, formal program recognition, and lifelong professional development, all of which were gradually integrated into French policy [48].

The 1994 decree established the doctor-IADE partnership, requiring the presence of an anesthesiologist for every procedure—a model balancing increased autonomy with patient safety [47]. Subsequent reforms, including the 2002 and 2012 decrees, aligned the IADE curriculum with the European higher education system and the master's degree framework [48]. The 2017 decree further clarified IADE competencies, emphasizing their role in clinical analysis, anesthetic planning, and patient management in high-risk settings, while maintaining the requirement for medical supervision [49].

By 2025, the adoption of a new nursing law marked a significant step forward [49]. This law recognized the advanced practice of nurse anesthetists, explicitly referencing their clinical expertise, decision-making capacity, and the ability to perform certain acts independently within a regulated framework [50]. While the profession now enjoys greater autonomy, particularly in patient assessment, anesthetic planning, and emergency response, the legal framework still ensures patient safety by requiring collaboration with physicians for the most complex procedures [48].

The Importance of Education in Nurse Anesthesia

Education is the cornerstone of IADE clinical autonomy. According to ICN and IFNA guidelines, nurse anesthetists must complete a basic generalist nursing education, followed by a recognized postgraduate anesthesia program at the master's level or higher [48]. In France, the IADE curriculum reflects these international standards: access to the program is reserved for experienced nurses, and the 24-month program (3640 hours) combines advanced theoretical coursework with extensive clinical placements.

The curriculum is structured around seven teaching units, covering advanced anatomy, physiology, pharmacology, monitoring, airway management, and the full range of anesthesia techniques for diverse patient populations. Clinical practicum requirements ensure that students acquire hands-on experience in real-world settings, preparing them to independently assess, plan, and deliver anesthesia care.

Competency assessment is rigorous and ongoing, involving exams, professional simulations, and the completion of a professional project. This pedagogical rigor, aligned with the master's level, equips IADEs with the expert knowledge base, complex decision-making skills, and clinical competencies necessary for advanced practice. Continuous professional development is mandated, reflecting the need for IADEs to stay abreast of advances in science, technology, and clinical practice.

Formal recognition and accreditation of educational programs are essential for ensuring quality and consistency. The IFNA's Anesthesia Program Approval Process (APAP) provides international accreditation, and the first school to receive this status was the Ecole des Infirmiers Anesthésistes Hôpital Salpêtrière in Paris, France. Through this robust educational framework, IADEs are empowered to deliver safe, high-quality anesthesia care and to assume leadership roles within the health-care system.

Political Awareness of Nurse Anesthesia Care

The political dimension of nurse anesthesia care has gained prominence as governments and health organizations recognize the essential role of nurse anesthetists in achieving universal health coverage and addressing workforce shortages. The integration of IADEs into prehospital emergency teams (SAMU) exemplifies their critical contribution to public health [49]. Their advanced training in pharmacology, airway management, and resuscitation enables them to provide high-level care in both hospital and prehospital settings.

Professional associations, such as the IFNA and national nurse anesthesia organizations, have been instrumental in advocating for the recognition, regulation, and protection of the nurse anesthetist role. These organizations engage with policymakers to develop standards, influence legislation, and promote public and professional awareness of the value of nurse anesthetists. In France, the legal protection of the IADE title and scope of practice reflects the success of these advocacy efforts [49].

Political awareness also extends to the need for appropriate credentialing, licensure, and title protection, which safeguard the public from unqualified practitioners and ensure that only those with the requisite education and competencies can practice as nurse anesthetists. The ongoing evolution of the IADE role in France is closely linked to these political and regulatory developments, which support the profession's growth and its alignment with international best practices.

Clinical Autonomy Within the Anesthesia Care Team

Clinical autonomy for nurse anesthetists in France is characterized by a high degree of responsibility and accountability within the anesthesia care team. IADEs are advanced practice nurses who plan and deliver anesthesia, pain management, and related services across the perioperative continuum—preoperative, intraoperative, and postoperative care. Their scope of practice includes patient assessment, development of anesthesia plans, administration of anesthesia, monitoring, management of complications, and postoperative evaluation.

IADEs collaborate closely with physician anesthesiologists, surgeons, and other health-care professionals, ensuring a patient-centered, holistic, and evidence-based approach to care. Their advanced assessment, critical thinking, and decision-making skills enable them to respond effectively to complex clinical situations and emergencies. In settings such as prehospital emergency care, IADEs often function with significant autonomy, making critical decisions in the absence of immediate physician oversight.

The IFNA and ICN emphasize that nurse anesthetists should be authorized to practice to the full extent of their education and competencies, including prescriptive authority, diagnosis, and referral, as permitted by national regulations [50, 51]. In France, while IADEs operate within a collaborative model, their clinical autonomy is supported by legal frameworks, educational standards, and professional guidelines that recognize their expertise and leadership [52].

Research evidence demonstrates that anesthesia care provided by nurse anesthetists is as safe and effective as that provided by physician anesthesiologists, particularly when supported by rigorous education and professional standards. This evidence underpins the continued expansion of clinical autonomy for IADEs in France and internationally.

Perspectives and Future Directions: The PEPPA Model in France

As the demand for advanced practice roles in nursing grows, ensuring successful and sustainable implementation requires more than regulatory reform and education alone. The Participatory, Evidence-based, Patient-focused Process for Advanced Practice Nursing (PEPPA) model offers a structured, sequenced, and participatory methodology to guide the evolution of advanced practice nursing roles, particularly for IADEs in France [53].

The PEPPA model is built on several foundational principles [54]:

Foundation on Real-world Clinical Needs: The deployment of advanced practice roles is steered by actual clinical data, ensuring organizational changes meet both patient and service requirements.

Participatory and Interdisciplinary Engagement: The model mandates the involvement of all key stakeholders—including IADEs, anesthesiologists, hospital management, policymakers, and patients—throughout the process. This inclusive approach ensures that new or expanded roles are accepted, sustainable, and correctly tailored to context.

Structured and Sequenced Planning: Clearly defined transitional phases guide role definition, implementation, and evaluation, avoiding hazards such as fragmented responsibilities or poor stakeholder engagement.

Sustainable Role Development

By integrating continuous evaluation and iterative improvement, the PEPPA model ensures that IADEs' expanded roles align with evolving health-care needs and regulatory standards. Ongoing assessment of effectiveness, patient outcomes, and institutional impact is seen as critical for long-term success and adaptation.

Toward Greater Autonomy and Recognition

The use of frameworks like PEPPA facilitates professional recognition, interprofessional collaboration, and the institutionalization of clinical leadership among French nurse anesthetists. Through the blending of advanced training, regulatory clarity, and participatory planning, the pathway is set for IADEs to expand their scope further, aligning more closely with global best practices.

Conclusion

The clinical autonomy of nurse anesthetists in France has been forged through a combination of historical evolution, rigorous education, political advocacy, and alignment with international standards. IADEs are recognized as advanced practice nurses, equipped with the knowledge, skills, and competencies to deliver safe, high-quality anesthesia care in diverse settings. Their clinical autonomy is both a reflection of their professional expertise and a response to the evolving needs of the health-care system. As the profession continues to advance, supported by robust education, credentialing, and political engagement, nurse anesthetists in France are poised to play an increasingly central role in ensuring access to safe anesthesia care for all [47].

Professional Autonomy of Nurse Anesthetists in Taiwan: Perspectives on Policy, Culture, and Practice

As global health-care systems face the challenges of population aging, workforce shortages, and the need for higher-quality care, Advanced Practice Registered Nurses (APRNs) have emerged as essential providers to bridge the care gap. Among them, Nurse Anesthetists (NAs) play a critical role, especially in regions with limited anesthesiologist availability. However, unlike the independent practice models seen in the U.S. and Nordic countries, Nurse Anesthetists in Taiwan face legal and institutional restrictions that constrain their professional autonomy. This discussion explores the current status and challenges of professional autonomy for nurse anesthetists in Taiwan through the lens of legal frameworks, educational pathways, clinical roles, institutional support, health-care culture, and international comparisons, and suggests pathways for reform.

Legal and Institutional Frameworks

Taiwan began training Nurse Anesthetists in 1958, but their status has long lacked formal legal recognition, creating risks of unauthorized practice. In instances of adverse events, NAs have often been accused of practicing medicine without a license. The Taiwan Association of Nurse Anesthetists (TANAs), the only national organization representing NAs, has consistently advocated for legal practice rights. However, anesthetic procedures are still legally restricted to physicians.

The Nurse Practitioner (NP) system in Taiwan was the first APRN framework developed. While 16 specialties were initially proposed, anesthesia lacked standardized national regulations. As a result, each hospital defined NA responsibilities differently, causing role ambiguity and inconsistencies in accountability [55].

It was not until 2020 that the Ministry of Health and Welfare (MOHW), under Article 7-1-3 of the Nurses Act and the "Regulations for Nurse Practitioner Subspecialty and Qualification Examinations," formally included anesthesia as a certified NP specialty [56]. The "Regulations Governing the Practice of NPs under Physician Supervision" stipulate that NAs must operate under physician oversight [57]. Notably, "supervision" does not require physical presence, allowing anesthesiologists to concurrently manage multiple patients with Certified Registered Nurse Anesthetists Nurse Practitioner (CRNANP) support.

Education and Certification

According to current regulations, CRNANP may receive training through hospital-based programs or master's degree tracks; however, Taiwan is yet to establish a dedicated graduate program for NA education [56]. Current curricula of hospital-based programs are largely skill-oriented, with insufficient emphasis on clinical judgment, risk assessment, and leadership [58]. Consequently, while many NAs are clinically competent, they lack the foundational training to collaborate with physicians on an equal footing or practice independently.

Clinical Practice and Scope of Responsibility

In clinical settings, CRNANP perform key functions such as preoperative reassessments, anesthesia induction and maintenance, intraoperative monitoring, and postoperative recovery [59]. However, their actions are generally limited to following explicit physician instructions, restricting independent decision-making.

Chang et al. describe this as a "high execution, low decision-making" model, where CRNANPs bear clinical responsibility without corresponding authority or protection [60]. The ambiguity of responsibilities also increases legal risks and professional stress, leading many to adopt overly conservative practices.

Current regulations allow CRNANPs to perform certain tasks traditionally reserved for physicians, including extubation, LMA removal, arterial line management, and maintenance of anesthesia. However, they are explicitly prohibited from initiating anesthesia, including intubation and insertion of spinal needle or epidural needle.

Interprofessional Collaboration and Cultural Barriers

The NA role remains shaped by hierarchical medical culture, where physician-led models dominate and nurses are primarily seen as implementers. Even experienced CRNANPs with strong clinical skills often find their input undervalued [55] Additionally, many patients mistakenly believe all anesthesia is administered by physicians, weakening public recognition and professional confidence among CRNANPs.

Organizational Support and Institutional Mechanisms

While some hospitals have established clear scheduling and role delineation systems, most lack formal mechanisms for delegation, limiting CRNANPs participation in clinical decisions and policymaking. Moreover, opportunities for continuing education, career advancement, and institutional engagement remain scarce, hindering professional development [61].

International Comparison and Reform Opportunities

In contrast, U.S. Certified Registered Nurse Anesthetists (CRNAs) enjoy full practice authority in many states, and Nordic countries similarly allow NAs to independently administer anesthesia. Taiwan could benefit from adopting international best practices to revise legislation, improve education, and redefine CRNANP roles. Especially in rural or underserved areas, expanding CRNANPs' clinical autonomy could enhance patient safety and optimize resource use [58].

CRNANPs in Taiwan have demonstrated high levels of professional competence in clinical practice. However, their autonomy remains constrained by systemic limitations. A comprehensive reform across legal, educational, organizational, and cultural dimensions is essential to legitimize their role and empower their practice, ultimately contributing to a more efficient and equitable health-care system.

Summary

The road to practice autonomy for the nurse anesthetists globally is long and often filled with barriers that appear insurmountable. There are many steps to achieve this goal for global nurse anesthetists and often begins with the founding of a national organization to represent and guide nurse anesthetists. Once this is established, attention is turned toward adoption of educational, practice, monitoring standards and clinical experience that builds minimum entry level competence in the graduate of anesthesia programs. Throughout the career of an advanced practice nurse anesthetist, knowledge and skills will grow, especially if the country or professional organization mandates continuous professional development. In addition to education, the anesthesia national organization can lobby for legislative and regulatory policy that will increase recognition and title protection of the nurse anesthetist in the country. Through membership in the International Federation of Nurse Anesthetists and the 2024 updated global anesthesia manpower study [62, 63], there is documented evidence of nurse anesthetists practicing in 90 countries which span all six WHO regions (Table 4). Nurse anesthetist practice is critical to increasing access to safe anesthesia care and surgery. Global nurse anesthetists must never give up or take their eye off the goals in this journey. The rewards for the patients, country, and region as well as the individual far outweigh the time, energy, and, at times, frustration that come with gaining practice autonomy.

Table 4 WHO regions and countries

Africa	Americas	Eastern Mediterranean	Europe	Southeast Asia	Western Pacific
Algeria	Belize	Iran	**Austria***	Bhutan	**Australia***
Benin*	El Salvador	Libya	**Bosnia***	**Indonesia***	**Cambodia***
Burkina	Guyana	Morocco	**Croatia***	Thailand	China
Burundi*	Honduras	Palestine	**Cyprus***	Timor-Leste	**Japan***
Cameroon*	**Jamaica***	Saudi Arabia	**Denmark***		Lao
Chad	Nicaragua	**Tunisia***	**Finland***		Marshall Islands
Democratic Republic of Congo	Paraguay		Marshall		Malaysia
Eritrea	**United States of America***		**France***		Micronesia
Ethiopia*			**Germany***		Palau
Faso			**Greece***		Papua New Guinea
Gabon			**Hungary***		Philippines
Gambia			**Iceland***		Solomon Islands
Ghana*			**Luxembourg***		**South Korea***
Ivory Coast*			**Macedonia***		Sudan
Kenya*			**Montenegro***		**Taiwan***
Lesotho			**The Netherlands***		Tonga

(continued)

Table 4 (continued)

Liberia*	**Norway***	Vanuatu
Madagascar	**Poland***	Vietnam
Malawi	Romania	
Morocco*	**Serbia***	
Mozambique	**Slovenia***	
Niger	**Spain***	
Nigeria*	**Sweden***	
Rwanda*	**Switzerland***	
Senegal	**Turkey***	
Sierra	**United**	
Leone*	**Kingdom***	
Somaliland		
Tanzania*		
Togo		
Uganda*		
Zambia*		

Bold* Identifies Member Countries in IFNA

References

1. Mrayyan MT, Khait AA, Rabab AM, et al. Professional autonomy in nursing: a concept analysis. SAGE Open. 2024:1–17.
2. Eger EI, Westhorpe RN, Seidman LJ. The half century before ether day. In: The Wonderous story of anesthesia. New York: Springer; 2014. p. 22.
3. Seidman LJ, Westhorpe RN, Eger EI. History reflected in the evolving approaches for a patient undergoing cholecystectomy. In: The Wonderous story of anesthesia. New York: Springer; 2014. p. 71.
4. Bankert M. The mother of anesthesia. In: Watchful care: a history of America's nurse anesthetists. New York: The Continuum Publishing Company; 1989. p. 18.
5. Lawrence C. Autobiography. James B Lyon Printer; 1896. p. 114.
6. Bankert M. The mother of anesthesia. In: Watchful care: the history of America's nurse anesthetists. New York: The Continuum Publishing Company; 1989. p. 25.
7. Bankert M. The mother of anesthesia. In: Watchful care the history of America's nurse anesthetists. New York: The Continuum Publishing Company; 1989. p. 30.
8. Bankert M. The mother of anesthesia. In: Watchful care: a history of America's nurse anesthetists. New York: The Continuum Publishing Company; 1989. p. 31.
9. Bankert M. The mother of anesthesia. In: Watchful care: a history of America's nurse anesthetists. New York: The Continuum Publishing Company; 1989. p. 38.
10. Bankert M. Up against that sort of thing. In: Watchful care: a history of America's nurse anesthetists. New York: The Continuum Publishing Company; 1989. p. 39–41.
11. Bankert M. Up against that sort of thing. In: Watchful care: a history of America's nurse anesthetists. New York: The Continuum Publishing Company; 1989. p. 42–3.
12. Bankert M. A very personal property right. In: Watchful care: a history of America's nurse anesthetists. New York: The Continuum Publishing Company; 1989. p. 61–2.
13. Bankert M. A very personal property right. In: Watchful care: a history of America's nurse anesthetists. New York: The Continuum Publishing Company; 1989. p. 62–3.
14. Bacon DR. Francis Hoeffer McMechan, MD: creator of modern anesthesiology. Anesthesia Analgesia. 2012;115(5):1393–400.

15. Calmes SH. Laurette McMechan (1878-1970): mother of anesthetists. Anesthesia Analgesia. 2012;115(6):1401–9.
16. Bankert M. A matter of felicitation. In: Watchful care: a history of America's nurse anesthetists. New York: The Continuum Publishing Company; 1989. p. 67–8.
17. Warden P. Looking forward (1910-1922). In: Watchful care: a history of America's nurse anesthetists Vol II. The Sheridan Group Inc.; 2023. p. 219–21.
18. Koch E. Helen Lamb: the mother of anesthesia education. AANA NewsBulletin. 2002:24.
19. Bankert M. Worlds at war. In: Watchful care: the history of America's nurse anesthetists. New York: The Continuum Publishing Company; 2025. p. 128.
20. Horton B, Kramer M. Commitment to quality: The history of nurse anesthesia accreditation Part One: 1930–1982. AANA journal online; 2020. Available www.aana.com/aanajournalonline, p. 8–12
21. Horton B, Kramer M. Commitment to quality: the history of nurse anesthesia accreditation part Two. 1983–2019. AANA Journal online; 2021. Available www.aana.com/aanajournalonline, p. 4–19
22. Warden PA. A new millennium of watchful care. (2001-2010). In: Watchful care: a history of America's nurse anesthetists, vol. II. The Sheridan Group Inc; 2023. p. 161–71.
23. Bjorkman K, Horton BJ, Riesen M, Yang J, Anang S. History of the IFNA education committee. In: The global voice for nurse anesthetists: International Federation of Nurse Anesthetists (1989–2021). Park Ridge: AANA; 2021. p. 201–31.
24. Warden P. A new millennium of watchful care (2001-2010). In: Watchful care: a history of America's nurse anesthetists, vol. II. The Sheridan Group Inc; 2023. p. 158–60.
25. Warden P. The history of anesthesia and nurse anesthetists to 1989. In: Watchful care: a history of America's nurse anesthetists, vol. II. The Sheridan Group Inc; 2023. p. 38–42.
26. Warden P. A new millennium of watchful care (2001-2010). In: Watchful care: a history of America's nurse anesthetists, vol. II. The Sheridan Group Inc; 2023. p. 114–25.
27. AANA Anesthesia Essentials, (Online), April 25, 2025.
28. AANA Anesthesia Essentials, (Online), April 17, 2015.
29. AANA Advocacy Hotline, (Online), April 18, 2025.
30. APRN Consensus Work Group& National Council State Boards of Nursing APN Advisory Committee. Consensus Model for APN Regulation: Licensure, Accreditation, Certification & Education; 2008, pp. 1–41
31. Warden P. A new millennium of watchful care: (2001-2010). In: Watchful care: a history of America's nurse anesthetist, vol. II. The Sheridan Group Inc; 2023. p. 130–3.
32. Gaines K. Nurse anesthetists (CRNA) schools by state/programs online; 2025
33. Bruton-Maree N. Federal healthcare policy: how the AANA advocates for its members. In: A Preprofessional study and resource guide for CRNA's. 2nd ed. Park Ridge: AANA; 2011. p. 308–9.
34. AANA. What is the CRNA/nurse anesthesiology job outlook. Online; 2025
35. Dulisse B, Cromwell J. No harm found when nurse anesthetists without supervision by physicians. Health Aff. 2010;29(8):1469–75.
36. Hogan PF, Seifert R, Moore C, Simonson B. Cost effectiveness analysis of anesthesia providers. Nurs Econ. 2010;28(3):159–69.
37. Rwanda Ministry of Health. 19220. Republic of Rwanda Standards for Safe Practice of Anesthesia. Vol 10. Rwanda.
38. Enright A. Anesthesia training in Rwanda. Canadian J Anaesthesia. 2007;54(11):935–9.
39. Ministry of Health. Rwanda national surgical, obstetric, and anesthesia plan, Strategic Plan www.Moh.Gov.Rw17 of 82; 2018
40. Rwanda Allied Health Professionals Councils. Non Physician Anaesthetists in Rwanda Scope of Practice [Internet]; 2017. Available from: https://rahpc.org.rw/storage/documents/January2018/Cr6UXIIDnHz5jkdApoRH.pdf
41. Ministry of Health. Rwanda healthcare future RSSB 4x4Scholarship Scheme; 2024

42. Ministry of Health. The 4x4 Reform: A Path to Quality Health Care in Rwanda [Internet]; 2023. Available from: https://www.moh.gov.rw/news-detail/the-4x4-reform-a-path-to-quality-health-care-in-rwanda
43. Rwanda Allied Professionals Councils. Nonphysician Anesthetists in Rwanda Scope of Practice; 2017
44. Rwanda Ministry of Health. Rwanda National Surgical, Obstetrics, and Anesthesia plan. Strategies Plan www.Moh.Gov17 of 82; 2018
45. Rwanda ministry of Health. Republic of Rwanda standards for the practice of anesthesia Vol 10. Rwanda; 2022
46. SNIA Historique profession IADE
47. https://www.elsevier-masson.fr/media/wysiwyg/France/PDF/9782294780158.pdf
48. Décret n° 94–1050 du 5 décembre 1994 relatif à la sécurité en anesthésie.
49. Arrêté du 23 juillet 2012 relatif à la formation conduisant au diplôme d'État d'infirmier anesthésiste, modifié par l'arrêté du 17 janvier 2017.
50. Décret n° 2017–1248 du 7 août 2017 relatif à l'exercice de la profession d'infirmier anesthésiste diplômé d'État.
51. ICN_Nurse-Anaesthetist-Report_EN_WEB.pdf
52. Assemblée nationale, Sénat: Rapports sur la place des IADE dans la loi de modernisation du système de santé (2025).
53. Code de la santé publique: Statut, compétences, autonomie et collaboration des IADE.
54. International Federation of Nurse Anesthetists (IFNA). Guidelines and Standards for Education and Practice.
55. Webinaire CNPIA de la vision à l'action
56. Lu MC. A policy review of the nurse practitioner system in Taiwan: challenges and perspectives. J Prev Med. 2018;6:41–71.
57. Ministry of Health and Welfare. Regulation for Nurse Practitioner Subspecialty and Qualification Examinations; 2023a. https://law.moj.gov.tw/LawClass/LawAll.aspx?pcode-L0020199
58. Ministry of Health and Welfare. Regulations Governing the Practice of Nurse Practitioners Under Physician Supervision; 2023b. https://dep.mohw.gov.tw/DONAHC/cp-1043-5254-104.html
59. Liu HL, Wang SY, Chen Y. Professional role perception and practice barriers among nurse anesthetists in Taiwan. Asian Nurs Res. 2020;14(2):101.
60. Huang HT, Chen CH. Exploring the clinical role and legal responsibility of nurse anesthetists. Taiwan Clin Nurs J. 2019;21(3):35–42.
61. Chang YW, Lee JH, Tsai MH. Teamwork and autonomy in nurse anesthesia practice: a qualitative study in Taiwan. J Clin Nurs. 2021;30(5–6):e1132. https://doi.org/10.1111/jocn.15567.
62. IFNA. Country Members 2025. https://ifna.org/practice/countrymembers/.
63. Law TJ, Lipnick MS, Morriss W, Gelb AW, Mellin-Olsen J, Filipescu D, Rowles J, Rod P, Khan F, Yazbeck P, Zoumenou E, Ibarra P, Ranatunga K, Bulamba F; Collaborators. The global anesthesia workforce survey: updates and trends in the anesthesia workforce. Anesth Analg. 2024;139(1):15–24. Epub 2024 Mar 12. PMID: 38470828. https://doi.org/10.1213/ANE.0000000000006836.

Clinical Autonomy for Clinical Nurse Specialists (CNSs)

Jennifer Manning

Introduction

The Clinical Nurse Specialist (CNS) role, a form of Advanced Practice Nursing (APN), is recognized globally for its potential to improve patient outcomes, enhance care quality, and drive health-care innovation [6]. Central to realizing this potential is clinical autonomy—the authority to act, make independent decisions, and be accountable for practice within a defined scope of practice. However, the extent and nature of CNS autonomy vary dramatically across the globe, shaped by its autonomy, context, regulatory frameworks, and professional power dynamics [5].

Defining CNS Autonomy in a Global Context

Autonomy in nursing is a multi-faceted concept, encompassing professional competence, independent decision-making, and professional interactions. Globally, the CNS role is often defined by graduate-level education (minimum master's degree) and expertise across three spheres of impact: patient, nurse (nursing practice), and organization/system (Fig. 1) [6].

The Clinical Nurse Specialist (CNS) role is defined by its strategic impact across three interconnected domains, commonly referred to as the spheres of impact: the Patient/Client, the Nursing Practice, and the Organization/System. The Patient/Client sphere represents the core function of the CNS as an advanced clinical practitioner. Here, the focus is on providing expert, direct care to individuals and

J. Manning (✉)
School of Nursing, Louisiana State University Health Sciences Center, New Orleans, LA, USA
e-mail: jmanni@lsuhsc.edu

A. Kapu et al. (eds.), *A Global View on Clinical Autonomy for Advanced Practice Nurses*, Advanced Practice in Nursing,
https://doi.org/10.1007/978-3-032-21458-4_4

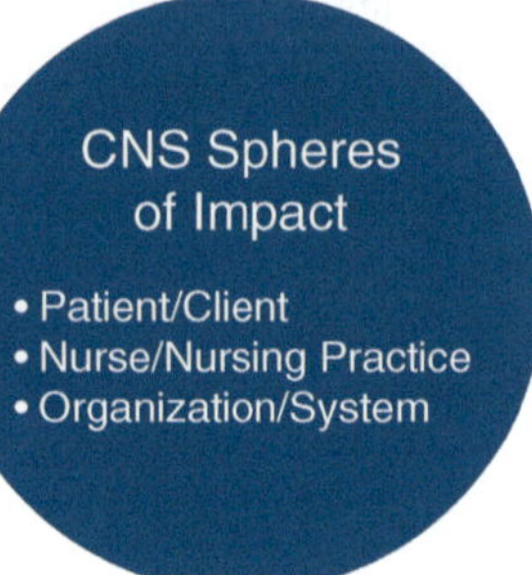

Fig. 1 CNS Three Spheres of Impact

families, particularly those with complex or chronic conditions. The CNS utilizes advanced assessment, diagnosis, and intervention skills, often acting as a consultant to the direct care team to manage challenging cases and ensure high-quality patient outcomes, while also providing essential education and coaching to empower patients in their self-management [8].

The second sphere of impact centers on the Nurse/Nursing Practice. In this capacity, the CNS functions as a change agent, educator, and mentor, elevating the competency and professional standards of the nursing staff. This involves translating complex research into actionable, evidence-based practices (EBP) and integrating these into daily nursing care. By providing mentorship, formal education, and coaching, the CNS helps staff nurses develop critical thinking skills and clinical expertise. This systematic approach to practice improvement ensures that the entire unit or department provides consistent, high-quality care, ultimately raising the standard of nursing delivery across the organization [6].

Finally, the CNS impacts the Organization/System sphere by addressing structural barriers to quality care and promoting continuous improvement. This sphere involves macrolevel interventions, such as leading quality improvement (QI) initiatives, developing new policies and procedures, and evaluating the efficient use of health-care resources. By analyzing system-level data (e.g., readmission rates, infection rates) and advocating for changes in organizational policy, the CNS ensures the environment is optimized for both patient safety and effective nursing practice. The successful operation within these three complementary spheres enables the Clinical Nurse Specialist to drive holistic, sustainable improvements in health-care delivery and ultimately enhance patient outcomes across the entire system [5].

Differentiating CNS from Other APN Roles

Internationally, CNS roles often overlap with or are confused with Nurse Practitioner (NP) roles, leading to significant challenges with autonomy. Key distinctions exist between the two roles, first in the scope of practice. Legally and functionally, NPs are authorized to operate independently in diagnosing and prescribing for patients.

CNS roles emphasize expert consultation and the ability to shape the environment in which care is delivered. The CNS role is crucial for elevating the standard of care for all patients on a unit or across an organization by improving processes and staff competency [2]. The NP is vital for providing direct access to advanced medical management for individual patients. The CNS role evolved to focus on clinical expertise applied broadly to nursing practice and systems. In contrast, the NP role was developed to increase access to primary and specialty medical care [5].

As an Advanced Practice Nurse (APN), the CNS operates with a level of specialized clinical expertise that significantly exceeds the depth and breadth of a standard Registered Nurse scope. Their advanced status is demonstrated through high-level autonomy, specifically in the development of evidence-based standards of care and the provision of expert clinical consultation and mentorship to nursing staff. Unlike generalist roles, the CNS serves as a strategic leader in quality improvement and system-level change initiatives, utilizing expert diagnostic and treatment skills within their specialty to optimize patient outcomes. While they are highly skilled in complex clinical decision-making, their advanced practice is often distinguished and sometimes constrained by the regional variations in their legal authority to prescribe or independently initiate medical orders [6].

Global Variations in CNS Autonomy and Scope

The level of autonomy a Clinical Nurse Specialist (CNS) can exercise is highly contextual and fundamentally depends on the macrolevel health-care system structure of the country or region in which they practice. This structural influence dictates whether the CNS operates under an Autonomous Model, characterized by independent practice and prescriptive authority (common in parts of North America), a Collaborative/Supervised Model, where autonomy is limited by physician oversight and hierarchical structures (common in many European and Asian systems), or a model constrained by systemic deficits, such as a lack of formal regulation and necessary resources (common in developing economies) [9]. Therefore, the actual scope and impact of the CNS role are less about the individual's education and more about the legal and organizational environment that either grants or withholds practice independence [11].

High Autonomy/Full Practice Models

The Autonomous Model represents the highest level of practice authority achieved by Clinical Nurse Specialists (CNSs) in certain health-care systems, particularly within evolving models found in North America. This model signifies the successful institutionalization of the role, in which the CNS's practice authority is legally recognized and closely aligned with their advanced education and specialized competencies. The defining characteristic of this model is Independent Practice, meaning the CNS operates without the mandatory requirement of a written collaborative agreement or direct supervision from a physician (MD/DO). This independence empowers the CNS to function as a self-directed advanced practitioner, making complex clinical decisions autonomously within their defined scope [6].

A key marker of true clinical autonomy within this model is the granting of Prescriptive Authority. In certain jurisdictions, the CNS is authorized to prescribe medications, including drugs and durable medical equipment, independently. This prescriptive ability is crucial because it fully integrates the diagnostic and assessment phase of care with the implementation of a comprehensive treatment plan. When a CNS can diagnose a condition and immediately initiate the necessary pharmaceutical or equipment-based intervention without requiring a physician's sign-off, they streamline care delivery, enhance patient access, and solidify their role as a primary decision-maker in the patient's care trajectory [13].

In Scotland, the Clinical Nurse Specialist (CNS) role is characterized by a high degree of functional autonomy, often operating at an advanced level within the NHS career framework. A prominent example of this independence is found in the Rapid Cancer Diagnostic Service (RCDS), where CNS practitioners act as clinical leads, performing independent histories and physical assessments to formulate differential diagnoses for patients with suspicious symptoms. Unlike many European models that require physician sign-off, Scottish CNSs who qualify as Independent Prescribers have the authority to prescribe medications from the British National Formulary and can independently order diagnostic investigations, such as CT scans. This model allows the CNS to function as a primary decision-maker and "change agent," directly managing the diagnostic pathway and leading nurse-led triage clinics to improve system-level efficiency and patient outcomes.

Ultimately, the successful advocacy for and achievement of the Autonomous Model reflects a significant evolution in nursing's professional recognition and a strategic response to modern health-care demands. By operating independently and exercising prescriptive authority, CNSs maximize their impact across the Patient, Nurse, and System spheres. This level of autonomy is essential for the CNS to lead clinical quality improvement efficiently, swiftly implement evidence-based practices, and provide expert management for complex patient populations, thereby optimizing overall system performance and ensuring timely, holistic patient care [14].

Collaborative/Supervised Models

The Collaborative/Supervised Model describes the CNS role in regions, such as many parts of Europe and Asia, where health-care systems adhere to a more traditionally hierarchical medical model. This structure places the physician at the apex of decision-making, which fundamentally influences the scope and autonomy of CNS. Although these advanced practice nurses possess high levels of clinical competence and can diagnose and initiate complex nursing interventions, their practice is often constrained by the need for formal physician oversight. This may manifest as mandatory collaboration agreements, required medical sign-off for actions such as advanced diagnostics or prescribing medications, or a hierarchical structure that subordinates the CNS to the medical team [7].

A significant challenge within this model is the resulting limited autonomy and potential for inefficiency in practice. Unlike fully autonomous CNS models, the requirement for physician involvement can slow down care delivery and reduce the CNS's ability to act on their advanced assessment skills independently. Despite their specialized education and expert role within the CNS spheres of impact (Patient, Nurse, and System), their functional independence is often capped. This structural limitation prevents the CNS from maximizing their potential to drive clinical change and deliver seamless, rapid care, thereby mitigating the full value they could bring to the patient care team [8].

In China, the Clinical Nurse Specialist (CNS) role is currently transitioning from a purely collaborative, hospital-based model toward one with more formal legislative support, particularly in regional pilot programs. While national regulations such as the Prescription Management Measures still strictly limit prescribing rights to registered physicians, the Shenzhen Special Economic Zone Medical Regulations (effective January 2023) marked a significant breakthrough by authorizing qualified specialist nurses to prescribe certain medications and order examinations within their specific areas of expertise. These eligible nurses must typically hold a bachelor's degree in nursing, have at least five years of experience (including two in a specialty field), and complete a three-month certification program. Despite these advancements, the role still faces challenges with conceptual ambiguity and a lack of unified national standards, which can lead to a "helper" perception among other medical professionals. Looking forward, the 15th Five-Year Plan (2026–2030) and the proposed Nurse Act are expected to further define nursing rights and practice conditions to address the high demand for specialized care in an aging population [10].

Furthermore, CNSs operating under this collaborative structure frequently encounter pervasive role ambiguity. Research indicates that even highly skilled CNSs struggle with how their role is perceived by other professionals, especially physicians and hospital managers [3]. Instead of being recognized as an independent advanced practitioner responsible for specific outcomes, the CNS role is often mistakenly viewed as merely "helping" or augmenting the physician's workload. This lack of clarity and defined boundaries undermines the CNS's authority, complicates team dynamics, and hinders the full integration of the advanced nursing role into the health-care organization's core operational and clinical processes [14].

Emerging/Developing Economies

The implementation of the Clinical Nurse Specialist (CNS) role in Emerging/Developing Economies is fundamentally shaped by the need to shift tasks to address significant health-care workforce shortages. In these lower-income settings, CNSs or nurses in equivalent advanced roles become crucial for filling critical service gaps. However, the potential for these advanced practitioners to function autonomously is often constrained by two major systemic factors. The primary constraint is a lack of formal regulation; the absence of clear, national legislation defining the CNS scope of practice, protecting their title, or setting standardized educational requirements prevents these roles from being fully institutionalized and recognized. Without formal legal backing, their advanced practice is vulnerable to restriction by other health-care cadres or the organizational hierarchy.

In Germany, the Clinical Nurse Specialist (CNS) role is currently undergoing a significant legislative transformation through the Nursing Competence Act (*Pflegekompetenzgesetz*), which officially enters into force on January 1, 2026. This landmark legislation marks a shift from a strictly collaborative model toward one that legally empowers specialist nursing staff to exercise their own responsibility in medical practice. Under the new law, CNSs and other advanced practice nurses will be authorized to independently manage specific clinical areas—such as wound management, diabetes, and dementia—and even issue follow-up prescriptions, tasks previously reserved exclusively for doctors. To support this expanded autonomy, the German government is establishing a "model scope of practice" in coordination with nursing professional organizations to clearly define these new powers and ensure the role is systematically integrated into the national health-care infrastructure. This reform aims not only to alleviate the workload of physicians but also to formalize the status of academically trained nurses, providing them with the legal authority and professional recognition necessary to drive high-quality, patient-centered care [16].

The second significant challenge is the pervasive lack of infrastructure and resources, which directly impedes autonomous practice and the ability to enact system-wide changes. This includes limited organizational support, such as a lack of protected time for complex, non-direct care activities, inadequate equipment, or insufficient access to necessary diagnostic and prescribing tools. While a CNS may be educated to perform at an advanced level, the system's inability to provide the required resources and supportive structures means their practice is often limited to basic gap-filling tasks. Consequently, despite the dire need for their expertise, the full impact of the CNS across all three spheres (Patient, Nurse, and System) is severely hampered by these resource and regulatory deficits [8].

Factors Enabling and Constraining Global CNS Autonomy

The extent of Clinical Nurse Specialist (CNS) autonomy worldwide is determined by a complex interplay of three key factors operating at the system (macro), organizational, and individual levels. The journey toward achieving greater independence in practice is fundamentally enabled or hindered by the regulatory frameworks and cultural norms present in each country. Understanding these diverse influences is key to successfully integrating the CNS role and maximizing its impact on patient care and efficiency globally [6].

1. **System-Level Enablers and Constraints**

At the macrolevel, the most significant factor enabling Clinical Nurse Specialist (CNS) autonomy is the Regulatory Environment. Strong, supportive national legislation that clearly defines the CNS's scope of practice, establishes rigorous credentialing standards, and provides title protection serves as the single greatest enabler of independence. Conversely, autonomy is severely constrained by regulatory ambiguity or national laws that explicitly favor the practice of competing advanced roles, such as Nurse Practitioners (NPs). Furthermore, National Health Workforce Policy can either create crucial opportunities for role expansion, for instance, when addressing severe physician shortages—or restrict it in areas with saturated labor markets or where traditional medical roles are highly protected [14, 15].

A powerful and often overlooked systemic barrier is the Cultural Context. In cultures where nursing has historically been devalued or strongly associated with traditional femininity and subordination, health-care structures tend to be paternalistic. This environment actively works to devalue autonomous advanced nursing practice, leading to perceptions that the CNS's specialized expertise threatens the existing professional balance of power. These deep-seated cultural and historical biases create systemic resistance that often undermines formal policy attempts to grant CNSs greater independence, making it difficult for the role to gain genuine acceptance at both the patient bedside and within executive boardrooms [7, 11].

2. **Organizational-Level Factors**

Within the specific health-care setting, Organizational-Level Factors determine whether a facility is prepared to fully utilize the Clinical Nurse Specialist (CNS). Key enablers include strong Leadership and Champions—particularly active support from executive nurses, such as the Chief Nursing Officer (CNO)—who understand and advocate for the CNS role. Equally vital is achieving crystal-clear Role Clarity within the institution. A lack of an agreed-upon job description can lead to confusion and duplication of effort with other advanced roles (like NPs) or specialty nurses, thereby limiting the CNS's perceived and actual authority to lead and implement necessary system changes effectively [15].

Crucial to the successful integration and functional autonomy of the CNS are positive Interprofessional Relationships. Establishing positive working relationships and fostering early, continuous engagement with physician colleagues is essential for functional autonomy. When the medical team respects the CNS's expertise and competence, collaboration flourishes, and the CNS is empowered to act on their advanced skills. Conversely, significant barriers arise when there is active resistance from medical professional associations or a perception that the CNS is "eroding" the physician's domain. Overcoming this resistance requires consistent, demonstrated competence and the cultivation of mutual respect built at the local clinical level [2, 13].

Individual-Level Factors

Finally, the Clinical Nurse Specialist's (CNS) personal success in claiming and exercising autonomy rests on Individual-Level Factors. Autonomy is fundamentally earned through demonstrated professional competence, complex clinical decision-making skills, and continuous, specialty-specific education. The CNS's individual capacity for effective Professional Interaction—meaning the ability to engage in advocacy, act as a role model, and collaborates key to gaining peer respect and expanding impact. However, constraints such as heavy clinical workloads and associated Burnout can functionally reduce autonomy by consuming time needed for crucial non-direct care activities, such as research integration, systems leadership, and the development of evidence-based protocols [4, 14].

3. **Impact and Future Trajectories**

The extent of Clinical Nurse Specialist (CNS) autonomy worldwide is determined by a complex interplay of factors operating at the system, organizational, and individual levels. The CNS's ability to achieve and maintain greater independence in practice is fundamentally enabled or hindered by the regulatory frameworks and cultural norms specific to each country. Understanding these diverse influences—which range from national laws to individual professional skills—is key to successfully integrating the CNS role into global health-care systems and maximizing its powerful impact on patient care and overall system efficiency [11].

In Saudi Arabia, the Clinical Nurse Specialist (CNS) role is a vital component of the Vision 2030 health-care transformation, where it is increasingly recognized for managing complex conditions such as diabetes and cardiovascular disease through comprehensive assessments and diagnostic management. Although the Saudi Commission for Health Specialties (SCFHS) defines the role as one capable of working autonomously, true functional independence remains a dynamic negotiation against traditional medical hierarchies. Practitioners in the region frequently encounter "top-down" management styles and a lack of national laws protecting their specific professional duties, which can lead to physician domination over clinical decision-making. While there is a push for expanded authority, full prescriptive rights are not yet a national standard, often leaving the CNS to operate under strict institutional protocols or in a collaborative capacity. Consequently, the success of the CNS in the Arab context is heavily dependent on overcoming cultural biases regarding nursing subordination and establishing the legal frameworks necessary to protect their advanced scope of practice [1].

The extent of Clinical Nurse Specialist (CNS) autonomy globally is shaped by a complex interplay of factors across system, organizational, and individual levels. At the system level, strong national legislation and title protection act as primary enablers, while paternalistic cultural norms and regulatory ambiguity often serve as significant barriers. Organizationally, success depends on clear role definitions, executive leadership support, and the cultivation of positive interprofessional relationships with physicians to prevent role erosion. Individually, autonomy is earned through demonstrated clinical competence and professional advocacy, though it is frequently constrained by heavy workloads and burnout. Ultimately, successfully integrating the CNS role and maximizing its impact on global health-care efficiency requires navigating these diverse influences to align educational foundations with supportive legal frameworks.

Conclusion

In conclusion, clinical autonomy for the CNS is not a static endpoint but a dynamic achievement contingent on strong educational foundations, supportive legislation, and successful navigation of interprofessional relationships on a global stage marked by significant structural variance.

References

1. Almukhaini S, Weeks L, Macdonald M, Martin-Misener R, Ismaili Z, Macdonald D, Al-Fahdi N, Rasbi S, Nasaif H, Rothfus M. Advanced practice nursing roles in Arab countries in the Eastern Mediterranean region: a scoping review. JBI Evid Synth. 2022;20(5):1209–42. https://doi.org/10.11124/JBIES-21-00101.
2. Ares TL. Role transition after clinical nurse specialist education. Clin Nurse Spec. 2018;32(2):71–80. https://doi.org/10.1097/NUR.0000000000000357.
3. Bachiller-Barquín A, Martín-Martín J, Vázquez-Calatayud M. Implementing the clinical nurse specialist role in hospital settings: a scoping review. Clin Nurse Spec. 2025;39(2):65–81. https://doi.org/10.1097/NUR.0000000000000884. PMID: 39969808
4. Bryant-Lukosius D, Carter N, Kilpatrick K, Martin-Misener R, Donald F, Kaasalainen S, Harbman P, Bourgeault I, DiCenso A. The clinical nurse specialist role in Canada. Nurs Leadersh (Tor Ont). 2010;2010:140–66. https://doi.org/10.12927/cjnl.2010.22273. PMID: 21478691
5. DiLibero J, Mohr LD, Burton-Williams KM, Calvert PL, Dresser S, Mason TM, Schaefer KA, Tidwell J. The clinical nurse specialist: maximizing return on investment. Nurs Adm Q. 2024;48(4):286–96. https://doi.org/10.1097/NAQ.0000000000000652. Epub 2024 Aug 30. PMID: 39213402
6. Fulton JS. Standards, competencies, and clinical nurse specialist role. Clin Nurse Spec. 2024;38(4):157–8. https://doi.org/10.1097/NUR.0000000000000834. PMID: 38889054
7. Gabbard ER, Klein D, Vollman K, Chamblee TB, Soltis LM, Zellinger M. Clinical nurse specialist: a critical member of the ICU Team. Crit Care Med. 2021;49(6):e634–41. https://doi.org/10.1097/CCM.0000000000005004. PMID: 34011837
8. Jokiniemi K, Kärkkäinen A, Korhonen K, Pekkarinen T, Pietilä AM. Outcomes and challenges of successful implementation of the clinical nurse specialist role: participatory action research. Nurs Open. 2023;10(2):704–13. https://doi.org/10.1002/nop2.1336. Epub 2022 Sep 5. PMID: 36065161; PMCID: PMC9834530
9. Klein TA. Implementing autonomous clinical nurse specialist prescriptive authority. Clin Nurse Spec. 2012;26(5):254–62. https://doi.org/10.1097/NUR.0b013e318263d753.
10. Lian X, Qian W, Zhang Y. The development of nurse-led clinics in China: current status and future perspectives. Medicine (Baltimore). 2024;103(46):e40527. https://doi.org/10.1097/MD.0000000000040527. PMID: 39560592; PMCID: PMC11576046
11. Manning JM. Implications of the future of nursing report on clinical nurse specialists. Clin Nurse Spec. 2022;36(4):179–80. https://doi.org/10.1097/NUR.0000000000000684.

12. Miller J, Cornell M, Foley A. The history of clinical nurse specialists in emergency care. Adv Emerg Nurs J. 2024;46(4):363–8. https://doi.org/10.1097/TME.0000000000000535.
13. Osborne J, Kerr H. Role of the clinical nurse specialist as a non-medical prescriber in managing the palliative care needs of individuals with advanced lung cancer. Int J Palliat Nurs. 2021;27(4):205–12. https://doi.org/10.12968/ijpn.2021.27.4.205. PMID: 34169745
14. Ray MM, Mittelstadt P. Prescriptive authority and independent practice progress for the clinical nurse specialist: changes since 2010. Clin Nurse Spec. 2016;30(5):302–3. https://doi.org/10.1097/NUR.0000000000000242.
15. Ulit MJ, Eriksen M, Warrier S, Cardenas-Lopez K, Cenzon D, Leon E, Miller JA. Role of the clinical nurse specialist in supporting a healthy work environment. AACN Adv Crit Care. 2020;31(1):80–5. https://doi.org/10.4037/aacnacc2020968.
16. Wheeler KJ, Miller M, Pulcini J, Gray D, Ladd E, Rayens MK. Advanced practice nursing roles, regulation, education, and practice: a global study. Ann Glob Health. 2022;88(1):42. https://doi.org/10.5334/aogh.3698. PMID: 35755314; PMCID: PMC9205376

Definitions and Models of Collaboration in Healthcare Worldwide

Ashley Love, Rene Love, Steven Pryjmachuk, and Beatriz Rosana Gonçalves de Oliveira Toso

Collaboration in advanced practice nursing occurs at the intersection of regulation, workplace policy, and day-to-day team relationships. In this chapter, "collaboration" refers to coordinated, respectful interprofessional practice that supports safe, timely care; it is distinct from legal requirements such as supervisory or collaborative agreements. Importantly, effective collaboration is person centered: it enables shared decision-making and reduces delays or fragmentation that can arise when roles, authority, or communication pathways are unclear.

Advanced Practice Nursing in the United States

Advanced Nursing Practice in the United States

Currently, advanced practice in the United States (USA) exhibits substantial variability. Unlike many other nations, regulatory agencies in the USA are decentralized and primarily operate at the state level, resulting in significant differences across the

A. Love
Private Practice, Boulder, CO, USA

Ellmer School of Nursing at Old Dominion University, Virginia Beach, VA, USA

R. Love (✉)
Ellmer School of Nursing at Old Dominion University, Virginia Beach, VA, USA
e-mail: rlove@odu.edu

S. Pryjmachuk
The University of Manchester, Manchester, UK
e-mail: steven.pryjmachuk@manchester.ac.uk

B. R. G. de Oliveira Toso
Wester Paraná State University-UNIOESTE, Cascavel, Brazil

A. Kapu et al. (eds.), *A Global View on Clinical Autonomy for Advanced Practice Nurses*, Advanced Practice in Nursing,
https://doi.org/10.1007/978-3-032-21458-4_5

country. Regulation can even vary among APN specialties within a state. Numerous governmental and nongovernmental organizations guide each state's specific regulatory framework for advanced practice.

When referencing the term collaboration, the APN often interprets it as working together with a physician for practice, as required by state regulations. This section extends beyond regulation to discuss the various models that nurses employ to collaborate both intra- and interprofessionally to improve health outcomes. To fully understand this and the interplay between multiple models of collaboration in healthcare, the reader must first be familiar with the role that state regulatory bodies play in health-care delivery and the variations in state laws that influence the scope of advanced practice nursing.

Regulation of US Health-Care Professions

State governments largely govern the regulation of advanced practice nursing in the USA. This regulation leads to considerable variation in prescribing practices, collaborative requirements, interstate mobility, and licensure. In recent years, an increasing number of states have granted nurse practitioners (NPs) full practice authority. While the regulation may vary, the national scope of APNs includes assessment, diagnosis, treatment, and management of patients.

As of 2025, 35 states and the District of Columbia have granted NPs full autonomy to evaluate, diagnose, prescribe, and order medical tests for patients; however, the other 16 states have either reduced or restricted practice conditions [1]. Here, "full practice authority" indicates that state law does not require a formal supervisory or collaborative agreement for core NP functions; however, NPs remain accountable to professional standards, institutional policies, and interprofessional teamwork. Under reduced practice, state law limits at least one element of NP practice and may require regulated collaboration with another discipline for specific functions, which can affect workflow and timeliness of care. Still, the state law places limits on the APN's ability to engage in all elements of NP practice, such as the need for regulation requiring the NP to have a collaborative agreement with another provider for certain aspects of their care throughout their entire career or limiting how the NP can practice in varying settings. Restricted practice restricts the ability of APNs even further, as state law requires supervision by another provider, most often a physician, throughout their practice career [1]. Barriers to practice persist in states with reduced or restricted practice, despite data indicating that full autonomy improves access and health outcomes [2].

Definitions and Collaborative Model Development

The World Health Organization defines interprofessional collaboration as health-care providers from different professions working together on behalf of patients, families, and communities to deliver the highest quality of care [3]. The history of collaboration in United States healthcare emerged from a need to ensure ongoing quality care in the context of shifting disease models, growing medical knowledge, technological advancements, and rising health-care costs, as well as expanding populations [4]. There are a variety of collaborative care models utilized, but all work toward enhancing the health outcomes while minimizing costs.

The Institute of Medicine's (IOM) report, Crossing the Quality Chasm: A New Health System for the twenty-first century, believed that interprofessional collaboration was imperative for patient safety, quality care, and cost containment [5]. The IOM's The Future of Nursing report supports advanced practice nurses in practicing to their full capabilities and training, being full partners with physicians and other health-care providers [6]. APNs will often be the lead on the collaborating team, especially as the primary care provider, collaborating and coordinating care on behalf of their patients.

The work toward collaborative care has provided a foundation for interprofessional education among a wide variety of health-care providers. Nurse practitioners' knowledge and areas of expertise can play unique roles in the collaboration process [7]. The American Association of Colleges of Nursing (2021) embedded interprofessional partnerships as one of the domains in competency-based education for nurses. Nurse practitioners' knowledge and areas of expertise can play unique roles in the collaboration process [7]. Domain 6: Interprofessional Partnerships involves "intentional collaboration across professions and with care team members, patients, families, communities, and other stakeholders to optimize care, enhance the healthcare experience, and strengthen outcomes" [7]. This educational domain supports certification exam questions on interprofessional practice, regardless of the certifying body.

Interprofessional practice is enhanced even further in areas where nurse practitioners can practice to the full extent of their licensure. Within these geographical areas, health-care providers increase patient access to high-quality care, lower health-care costs, boost patient satisfaction, and improve health-care collaboration and efficiency [8–10]. As the most trusted profession, advanced practice nurses hold a unique role in healthcare and the community to facilitate the coordination of care. While many faculty are excited about interprofessional education, there is some hesitation about how to implement this across professions [11]. Educational institutions often accomplish interprofessional education by having various health students participate together in simulation activities and case studies.

Interprofessional Collaboration

Working interprofessionally has become even more critical over the last few years. With the increase in complexity of the aging population, in addition to limited financial resources, it is essential to work together to provide efficient and effective evidence-based care. The APN who provides holistic, evidence-based care is well suited to connect a team from a variety of professions to serve a patient best. As primary care providers who often lead these teams, a significant part of the challenge lies in acting as a liaison rather than being the team leader, ensuring patients and their families remain connected to all providers and team members.

Qualitative research synthesized over 10 years identified the following vital concepts in interprofessional collaboration: communication, trust, respect, mutual acquaintanceship, power, patient-centeredness, task characteristics, and environment [12]. Researchers determined that essential concepts include the need for professional role clarity, a formal structure for interorganizational collaboration, and the need for team identity and differentiation of individual roles for interprofessional collaboration [12]. Taken together, these findings suggest that collaboration is most effective when roles and decision pathways are explicit and when communication is structured rather than ad hoc. Patient-centeredness is not only an outcome of good teamwork but also a driver of it, because shared goals and shared decisions can reduce duplication, conflicting advice, and avoidable delays for patients and families.

There are varying models of intra- and interprofessional collaboration in practice. These include the interorganizational collaboration, collaborative care model, integrated care model, coordinated care model, colocated model, and cross-sector collaboration. These will be described below, along with opportunities for APNs to be involved in research and academia as part of collaboration.

Interorganizational Collaboration

There are many ways to implement interorganizational collaboration. Most frequently, this occurs when a patient transitions between settings and organizations. Interorganizational collaboration allows for opportunities for providers to work together for the benefit of the patient, such as admission from a primary care setting to acute care or vice versa. Other possibilities exist when patients are.

Transitioning services between organizations, for instance, pediatric care to adult care for patients with intellectual disabilities. These all require providers to work together among organizations to provide the most efficient and effective care.

Sometimes interorganizational collaboration occurs when like providers, APNs, come together for a common cause. When APNs come together to address a common issue for the population, positive outcomes can occur. For example, several years ago, during the COVID pandemic, a national collaboration was formed by APNs to target high-value care and implement initiatives that optimize clinical practices. Promote evidence-based practice at varying clinical patient care sites. Ultimately, this initiative was successfully implemented in a variety of sites across 14 different states, utilizing evidence-based care in a cost-effective, efficient, and effective manner, which resulted in improved health outcomes while reducing patient care costs [13].

Other exciting ways that advanced practice nurses are engaging in interorganizational collaboration are by being the conduit for research between academic institutions and community partners. As advanced practice nurses (APNs) and community providers, the APN can facilitate research between the two organizations to improve patient outcomes. They can conceptualize research ideas based on gaps in care, bring the multidisciplinary team together, assist in study design, help design the study, and recruit the patient participants. They have in-depth knowledge of disparate populations and how to engage these individuals, leading to improvements in care for the vulnerable and medically underserved populations [14]. APNs and researchers collaborate to generate new knowledge and then disseminate it back to the practice site.

Additionally, there are opportunities for varying organizations and practice settings to collaborate and share their expertise with others. Such opportunities often occur when organizations are deficient in providing care to specialty patients. The two organizations may agree to provide specialty services as needed through telehealth or phone consultations.

There has been a particular push over the last several years for nursing academia to work with academic partners and not remain siloed. This type of interorganizational collaboration includes partnerships between health-care organizations and nursing schools that define the goal of nursing graduates to meet the demands in healthcare, especially as schools move toward competency-based education. Academic institutions can invite an APN specialist to deliver guest lectures to nursing or health-care students. This type of collaboration often occurs with the development of a relationship between two organizations based on the students' needs. This collaboration enables interprofessional education on the diverse roles and their interplay across settings and organizations.

These types of interorganizational collaborations allow for opportunities to emerge that are bigger than individual people. They address education, research, and practice at the organizational level. This work improves cost while making healthcare more efficient and effective.

Collaborative Care Model

The collaborative care model provides mental health and primary health-care services concurrently through basic collaboration on-site or close collaboration with some system integration [15]. Typically, the primary care provider first sees a patient to address any physical health complaints. If the primary care provider identifies any behavioral health concerns, they then refer the patient to a behavioral health-care manager (BHCM). The BHCM conducts an initial evaluation to assess the severity of symptoms and creates a provisional diagnosis and treatment plan, which the consulting psychiatric provider then reviews. Based on recommendations, resources may be provided for counseling and/or medications [16]. Throughout this process, the BCHM updates an interorganizational registry to prioritize which patient cases to review more frequently with the consulting psychiatric provider. They also continue to work as a liaison between the health-care providers. When behavioral health providers are available for care and consultation, such as is the case in this collaborative care model, the overall competence and confidence of primary care providers can be improved when addressing and managing their patients' mental health needs [17–19].

As the number of physicians continues to decline and physician shortages increase, APNs will be essential in implementing this type of care model. When APNs work to the full extent of their licensure, they best utilize the necessary resources. When this occurs, the APN can assist in increasing access to health-care services, decreasing overall health-care costs, and improving patient outcomes [20].

Coordinated Care Model

A coordinated care model requires professionals to work together to develop relationships between themselves and their clinical sites to serve the community's needs. This model functions like a generalist-to-specialist model [22]. The primary care provider would assess and screen for illness and then deliver care up to their scope of practice. If the type of illness or treatment were beyond the advanced practice nurse's scope of practice, the primary care APN provider would then refer out to a specialist. An example of this would be when a health-care provider refers a mental health diagnosis to a psychiatric mental health advanced practice nurse for specialist care. The specialist may either treat the patient, act as a consultant and refer to the primary care provider, or they may stabilize the treatment before referring to the primary care provider.

The coordinated care model is most effective when providers can continue practicing in their sites while providing the necessary care for patients. While they coordinate the care, it often lacks proper integration. The providers work in separate locations, and communication about the patient may occur either formally or informally between the two providers. This model requires a concentrated effort on the part of both providers to ensure that care is not fragmented when using this model. Interprofessional communication and transfer of information between the two providers/sites is critical for improved patient outcomes [21].

Colocated Care Model

Colocated care models place primary and behavioral health-care services in the same facility. This care model moves beyond just coordination and increases opportunities for communication to occur among specialty teams through the sharing of resources. The care providers each assume roles within their prospective specialties while eliminating the traditional silo of specialty practice [22]. The integration and colocation of a shared space and resources, such as medical records and scheduling operations, promote both formal and informal collaboration and educational opportunities within the respective care services. When mental health patients receive referrals to behavioral health providers in a colocated space, no-show rates decrease significantly [23]. This type of colocation can occur in a primary care setting. It can also occur in a chronic disease specialty clinic, such as a diabetes or sickle cell clinic, where patients may require the additional services of a separate specialty provider, such as a psychiatric mental health nurse practitioner advanced provider.

The colocated model presents unique and advantageous opportunities for nurse practitioners due to their specialty expertise and growing number in the United States [24, 25]. Federally Qualified Health Centers most often implement colocated care models [26]. The majority of APNs working at these centers are in health professional shortage areas (HPSAs) [27]. From 2011 to 2023, the number of nurse practitioners working at these sites increased significantly, demonstrating how APNs can successfully implement and carry out these models [28].

Integrated Care Model

In an integrated care model, both primary care and behavioral health-care providers are colocated, working in tandem to create and implement a shared treatment plan for their patients [22]. This approach can reduce the time required to attend appointments and improve access to care.

Appointments improve health-care access, decrease emergency room admissions, lower the burden placed on primary and mental health providers, and lead to successful patient outcomes [29]. The culture of this care model focuses on simultaneously addressing the holistic care needs of each patient. It functions best when care providers deliver in a population-based setting where they can track treatment interventions and outcomes [22]. This model allows providers to look at mental health and medical diagnoses together for the benefit of the patient, instead of addressing them separately.

The American Psychiatric Nurses Association (APNA) has encouraged primary care settings to adopt this type of integrated care model, which very often requires a system-level approach to change [29]. However, the health-care setting must first understand the barriers and challenges patients face that influence their health behaviors [29]. Additionally, interprofessional teams must understand the roles of each member of the team. To help address these implementation barriers, APN education requirements now include the development of interprofessional collaboration skills. One such example of this is the creation of collaborative clinical practice experiences for family nurse practitioners and psychiatric-mental health nurse practitioner students in the primary care setting [29].

Cross-Sector Collaboration

Cross-sector collaboration involves active participation and harmonization of diverse stakeholders, including patients and their families, municipal agencies, health-care professionals, and other paraprofessionals working in tandem to inform and direct decision-making as it pertains to patient treatment and care [30]. This collaborative approach enables comprehensive patient treatment plans and patient care by combining diverse perspectives and bridging current gaps in care.

Additionally, it can assist in facilitating a more therapeutic alliance by increasing communication and a holistic understanding of what the patient's needs are from a biopsychosocial perspective [31]. The overarching benefit of cross-sector collaboration is the ability to work together to address complex societal issues.

In 2016, the US Department of Health and Human Services released the Public Health 3.0 initiative, which emphasized the need for the development of new cross-sectional partnerships among community stakeholders and public health agencies [32]. Through the combination of money and expertise, the opportunity to address larger issues in the community that impact healthcare is possible. This model included community partners and sectors that could improve and address social determinants of health [32]. Nurse practitioners play a crucial role in the development, facilitation, and leadership of cross-sectoral collaborations given their knowledge, clinical expertise, and advocacy [33].

Nursing education builds its foundations upon holistic care. Holistic care involves addressing all aspects of care for a patient beyond treating their medical diagnosis. This training supports the nurses as being the crux of the work that can be done through cross-sector collaboration.

By bringing together partners in healthcare, patients, and the community, we address larger health issues, including social determinants of health and environmental factors.

Summary

Advanced practice nurses play a critical role in collaborative care at multiple levels, including interprofessional and interorganizational collaboration and the use of collaborative, coordinated, colocated, integrated, and cross-sector care models. Across these approaches, APNs help strengthen communication, continuity, and role clarity to improve quality, access, and outcomes. The foundation is started in education and continues throughout an APN's career as they deliver holistic care and contribute to system improvement. Central to these efforts is person-centered care, in which patients and families are active partners in goal setting, care planning, and shared decision-making.

Advanced Practice Nursing in the United Kingdom

At the time of writing, advanced practice in the United Kingdom (UK) is somewhat messy. It lacks a clear regulatory steer, with many governmental and nongovernmental organizations across the UK's four constituent nations—England, Wales, Scotland, and Northern Ireland—seeking to influence its direction. To understand the current position regarding advanced *nursing* practice in the UK, the reader will need to know a little about the health-care professions in the UK and their various regulators, how healthcare is delivered in the UK, nongovernmental organizations with vested interests in advanced practice, and the unique position of UK preregistration nursing.

Regulation of UK Health-Care Professions

The regulation of health-care professions in the UK largely occurs at a national (i.e., UK-wide) level. There are several regulators (see Fig. 1), each regulating the training and practice of their respective professions. All are "statutory bodies" in that they are established by UK law, and each maintains a register of licensed (i.e., registered) practitioners for their respective professions. The regulators in turn are overseen by a "super-regulator," the Professional Standards Authority (PSA).

Two of the regulators—the Nursing and Midwifery Council (NMC) and the Health and Care Professions Council (HCPC)—are particularly relevant to a discussion of advanced nursing practice in the UK. The NMC's relevance is obvious given

Regulator	Regulates
General Medical Council (GMC) www.gmc-uk.org	Physicians (usually called 'doctors' in the UK); more recently, physician associates and anaesthesia associates
General Dental Council (GDC) www.gdc-uk.org	Dental professionals, including dentists, dental nurses, dental technicians, and dental hygienists
Nursing & Midwifery Council (NMC) www.nmc.org.uk	Nurses, midwives and nursing associates
Health and Care Professions Council (HCPC) www.hcpc-uk.org	Allied health professionals (AHPs) such as physiotherapists (physical therapists), dieticians, paramedics, and radiographers
General Pharmaceutical Council (GPhC) www.pharmacyregulation.org	Pharmacists and pharmacy premises in England, Wales and Scotland
Pharmaceutical Society NI www.psni.org.uk	Pharmacists and pharmacy premises) in Northern Ireland
General Optical Council (GOC) www.optical.org	Optometrists, dispensing opticians, and optical businesses
General Chiropractic Council (GCC) www.gcc-uk.org	Chiropractors
General Osteopathic Council (GOsC) www.osteopathy.org.uk	Osteopaths
Professional Standards Authority for Health and Social Care (PSA) www.professionalstandards.org.uk	Regulates and oversees the work of the healthcare regulators

Fig. 1 UK health-care regulators

its role as the nursing regulator. The HCPC is relevant, because, together with the NMC, it regulates the largest proportion of "nonmedical" health professionals in the UK.

For historical and political reasons, health-care professionals in the UK are categorized as either "medical" or "nonmedical," with the medical professions being those regulated by the General Medical Council (GMC) and the General Dental Council (GDC), and the nonmedical professions being all others. The medical professions (i.e., physicians and dentists) have somewhat ambivalent views about advanced practice. On one hand, they may argue that the debate about advanced practice is irrelevant to them. They might claim they already operate at an advanced level, because, compared to the nonmedical professions, their initial training requires many more years of study, including postgraduate study. On the other hand, since much of the advanced practice debate in the UK has been, rightly or wrongly, about the use of medical associates and non-medical professionals with advanced practice qualifications as (low-cost) substitutes for physicians, they are not entirely detached from the debate. Indeed, the debate has intensified recently given the GMC was tasked with regulating physician and anesthesia associates at the end of 2024. The medical professions' contributions to the debate are not always positive: physician associates and advanced practitioners have been pejoratively called "noctors" (i.e., not a doctor) by their medical colleagues [34], and the doctors' trade union, the British Medical Association, mounted an unsuccessful legal challenge to the GMC's regulation of medical associates [35].

UK Health-Care Provision

Although insurance-based private and not-for-profit health-care provision exists in the UK, most healthcare is provided by the UK's National Health Service (NHS). The NHS is a state health-care system, funded by general taxation and largely free at the point of delivery. Healthcare is a "devolved" function, so each of the UK's four nations operates its own version of the NHS, which leads to some anomalies, for example, prescriptions are free for residents of Scotland, Wales, and Northern Ireland; yet, in England, most working-age adults have to pay a set fee per item.

Each of the four nations has an NHS department that deals with workforce education and training. These departments mostly focus on *continuing* (postregistration) education and training, because the education standards for initial registration are set by the regulatory bodies. Healthcare being devolved means workforce education and training can be different in each of the four nations. This also produces anomalies, for example, while preregistration nursing students in England generally take out student loans to cover the tuition fees and living costs associated with their courses, the Welsh NHS will pay the tuition fees of nursing students studying in Wales if they agree to work in Wales for 2 years following graduation.

Since the NHS dominates health-care provision across the four nations, it heavily influences health-care education and training, often in collaboration with the regulatory bodies. Sometimes, however, the NHS can be at odds with the regulatory bodies. The remits of the regulatory bodies cover the *whole* of the UK and *all* healthcare professionals whether they work for the NHS or for the private or not-for-profit sectors. Again, this can lead to anomalies: in the mid-2010s, NHS Health Education England pressured the NMC to introduce and regulate a new nursing role below that of the registered nurse (RN), the "nursing associate." At the time, the NHS in Wales, Scotland, and Northern Ireland choose not to support this role [36]; so, the NMC created and regulated the role in England only, though the NMC approved the role in Wales in 2024 and, at the time of writing, Scotland is exploring its introduction.

Preregistration Nursing in the UK

One factor that influences UK *specialist*—if not advanced—nursing practice is that, unlike most of the rest of the world, nursing at initial registration is already specialist. To gain initial registration as an RN in the UK, students study for an NMC-approved, 3-year bachelor's (baccalaureate) degree at a university of their choice selecting, *at the point of starting their courses*, one of four specialist areas or "fields" of nursing: adult, mental health, children, and learning (developmental) disability. Thus, newly qualified UK RNs will already be specialist in one of these four areas. There are arguments for and against this specialist position [37, 38], and over the years, the NMC has moved increasingly toward the genericism of the rest of the world [39] but, at the time of writing, the four specialist fields still exist.

Note that midwifery is a separate profession in the UK. It is available as a direct-entry specialty, that is, a prior RN qualification is not required to become a midwife. As with nursing, students study for an NMC-approved, 3-year bachelor's degree, the completion of which leads to qualification as a registered midwife, RM.

There is a further complication in UK pre-registration nurse education that has implications for advanced practice. The NMC insists that the *minimum* academic entry point for an RN is a bachelor's degree; however, in a bid to increase interest in nursing, some universities offer NMC-approved pre-registration *master's* courses. This means a newly qualified RN completing a pre-registration master's will enter the NMC Register already holding a master's degree. While a master's may signify the RN has advanced-level *intellectual* abilities, it does not, however, signify advanced level *practice*: the communication and relationship management skills and nursing procedures the NMC requires for initial registration [40] are the same regardless of whether initial registration was gained via a bachelor's or a master's degree.

Other Bodies with Vested Interests

A few other bodies have some influence over the education and training of nurses in the UK. The most well-known is the professional association (and trade union), the Royal College of Nursing (RCN; www.rcn.org.uk). The Royal College of Midwives (RCM; www.rcm.org.uk) is lesser known internationally but has some influence over the education and training of midwives. The Council of Deans of Health (www.councilofdeans.org.uk) represents universities delivering nonmedical health-care education (mostly nursing schools) and is an influential lobbying body with close contacts in both government and the regulatory bodies.

In addition, each of the four nations has a government-employed Chief Nursing Officer who offers clinical and workforce advice to their respective government, advice that often has implications for education and training.

Finally, the Royal Pharmaceutical Society (RPharmS; www.rpharms.com) shapes UK advanced practice as it is the body that sets the standards for prescribing in advanced practice [41]. Interestingly, the RPharmS is a *professional* body, not a regulatory body, though it was the regulatory body for pharmacists prior to the establishment of the GPhC in 2010.

The Current Regulatory Position

Advanced practice in the UK is currently not regulated by any of the regulatory bodies, which is unusual by international standards [42]. There are a few reasons why the regulatory progress of advanced practice in the UK has been slow. Firstly, up until recently, there appears to have been little appetite for the regulation of advanced practice from the regulatory bodies themselves: indeed, in 2009, the Council for Health-care Regulatory Excellence (the forerunner of the PSA), argued against the introduction of national regulation, because it felt advanced practice was merely an extension of skills assessed at initial registration [43]. Secondly, from an advanced *nursing* practice perspective, allegations of organizational inefficiency and dysfunction within the NMC, dating as far back as 2008 [44], may have meant the NMC had no capacity to consider further regulatory roles, because it could not cope with the roles it already had.

However, in the last few years, the question of regulation has returned to the advanced practice agenda with many stakeholders now seeing a need for regulation. Several factors are behind this renewed interest: the increasing number of advanced practice roles; 'competitors' encroaching on the business of the regulators; inconsistencies in the education standards for advanced practice; and some worrying trends in the use of "advanced" in health worker job titles.

The demand for advanced practitioners in the UK has grown over the last decade and is likely to grow further in the future. Both "top-down" and "bottom-up" factors have driven this demand [42]. Top-down drivers stem from national and local policy initiatives, for example, NHS England's 2023 *Long-Term Workforce Plan* [45] sees more advanced practitioners as a solution to a shortage of doctors and changes in population morbidity, such as the growth in the number of people living with long-term conditions and an increasingly ageing population. Bottom-up drivers stem from employers concerned about the increasing costs of healthcare and from professions seeking to motivate their members through more fulfilling roles and clearer career pathways.

Regarding competition, in the absence of regulation, several organizations have attempted to accredit advanced practice as a way of demonstrating that the practitioner has met certain standards. NHS England's "Centre for Advancing Practice" provides a "digital badge" [46] that individual practitioners (from any discipline) who have completed an accredited advanced practice master's courses can use. UK-wide, the RCN also provides accreditation of advanced nursing practice [47]. However, unlike regulation, accreditation has no legal standing: while a poorly performing advanced practitioner might lose accreditation or even their job, they would not necessarily lose their statutory license to practice. Regarding inconsistencies in education standards, confusion over a "master's level" requirement for advanced practice courses means that some advanced practice courses had significant content at bachelor's level, while others were full master's degree [48]. Regarding worrying trends in job titles, unlike "registered nurse," titles associated with advanced practice (such as "advanced clinical practitioner" or "advanced nurse practitioner") are not protected titles in the UK, meaning that they can be used legally (if unethically) by individuals without any relevant qualifications. Indeed, a 2017 study [49] reported that around four percent of UK "nursing" jobs involved titles alluding to specialist and advanced levels of practice despite the individuals holding those jobs having no nursing registration!

Consensus and Frameworks

Not only is there renewed interest in regulating advanced practice, but there is also an emerging consensus around what such regulation should encompass. Firstly, there is agreement that advanced practice should build on the initial registration qualification (normally a bachelor's degree) and be at minimum a *master's* degree. For advanced nursing practice, this is in line with International Council of Nurses (ICN) guidance [50]. Secondly, each of the four UK nations has published a framework for advanced practice. Within each framework, there is a reasonable consensus of there being four "pillars" of advanced practice, despite the naming and ordering of these pillars varying and the terminology for any standards being different (see Fig. 2).

Thirdly, there is a consensus that advanced practitioners need to be a "nonmedical" prescriber (NMP). In the UK, there are three classes of NMP—supplementary, community practitioner nurse, and independent. Supplementary prescribers can prescribe only under protocol, usually in partnership with a medical practitioner; community practitioner nurse prescribers can only prescribe from the nursing formulary section of the *British National Formulary* [52]; independent prescribers are, like physicians, allowed to prescribe from the entirety of the *British National Formulary*. Advanced practitioners are expected to be *independent* prescribers. In the UK context, "independent prescriber" is a legal prescribing qualification and does not imply practicing outside governance structures, multidisciplinary pathways, or clinical accountability. Despite not currently regulating advanced practice, both the NMC and HCPC regulate prescribers within their professions, using the standards within the RPharmS's competency framework [41].

	England	Wales	Scotland	Northern Ireland
Framework	Multi-professional framework for advanced practice in England (18)	Professional framework for enhanced, advanced and consultant clinical practice (19)	Nursing, midwifery and allied health professionals' development framework (20)	Advanced nursing practice framework (21)
Year	2025	2023	No date	2016 (under review)
Standards terminology	capabilities	competencies	competence	core competencies
Pillar names (numbers reflect order presented in framework)	1. Clinical practice	1. Clinical practice	1. Clinical practice	1. Direct clinical practice
	2. Leadership and management	3. Leadership and management	3. Leadership and management	2. Leadership and collaborative practice
	3. Education	2. Education	2. Facilitating learning	3. Education and learning
	4. Research	4. Research and audit	4. Evidence, research and development	4. Research and evidence-based practice

Fig. 2 Advanced practice frameworks in the UK nations

Despite the consensus, there are still a few obstacles to the regulation of advanced practice. For example, there is no agreement over whether job titles should be protected or, indeed, what title should be used. In the early days of establishing advanced practice, there seems to have been a preference for "advanced clinical practitioner (ACP)," but more recently, there have been calls to simply use "advanced practitioner," because the term "clinical" may not be relevant in some settings and professional contexts where advanced practice may take place [51]. Moreover, there is the question of whether the definitions of, and standards for, advanced practice should be profession-specific or multiprofessional. Currently, the frameworks for England, Wales, and Scotland are multiprofessional though Northern Ireland's is not. While many stakeholders support a multiprofessional approach to the regulation of advanced practice [42], the various regulators have different priorities and, thus, the likelihood is that the regulators will go at their own pace, collaborating with each other where they can. This approach appears to be the one adopted by the NMC.

The NMC Review and Principles for Advanced Practice

The demand for advanced practitioners coupled with potential risks to the public from unstandardized training, confusion over job titles, and lack of public awareness of what advanced practice is led the NMC to instigate an advanced practice review in 2023 [53]. As part of this review, the NMC commissioned a report from The Nuffield Trust [42], an independent health-care research agency. The Nuffield Trust report outlined the risks and benefits of regulation and the various options available. Following this report, and after consultation with those working in advanced practice roles, the NMC outlined a roadmap for the regulation of advanced practice in nursing and midwifery. However, while the NMC has set out to regulate advanced practice, the HCPC remains skeptical: it currently does not support regulation, though it continues to engage with the NMC [54].

The NMC's roadmap starts with a set of principle for advanced practice [55], which were published as this chapter was being written (mid-2025). Future elements of the roadmap include a consideration of how advanced practice will fit into a scheduled 2026 revision of the NMC Code (the professional standards of practice and behavior for UK nurses and midwives) and, in 2027, starting the process of setting the standards for advanced practice and any associated advanced practice courses. This means that full regulation of advanced nursing practice might not happen until at least 2028.

Some key elements from the NMC's principles for advanced practice are listed below and give an indication of what the regulation of advanced nursing practice in the UK might look like:

- Currently, they are merely *principles*, not regulatory standards.
- Advanced practice is seen as *level of practice* rather than a job title or role.
- The four pillars outlined earlier are intrinsic to advanced practice.
- They explicitly define advanced practice through professional and public definitions of *nurses and midwives working at an advanced level* (see Fig. 3). Note how they use "nurses and midwives working at an advanced level" rather than advanced (nursing/midwifery) practitioner.
- Principles for employing organizations sit alongside principles for individual professionals, presumably to try and get some consistency across employers in supporting the delivery of advanced practice.

Professional version:
A registered nurse or midwife working at an advanced level is an expert professional with additional post-graduate education and experience. They use their evidence-informed knowledge, skills and capability to influence, shape, deliver and lead safe and effective care, while managing risk, uncertainty and complexity

Public version:
A registered nurse or midwife working at an advanced level of practice is a professional who has completed extra post-qualification education to increase their knowledge and skills, allowing them to deliver and lead expert, higher-level care.

Fig. 3 The NMC's definition of advanced practice [55]

Collaboration and Advanced Practice

Collaboration permeates two aspects of advanced practice in the UK: (a) collaboration between those with a vested interest in advanced practice to expedite its regulation; and (b) expectations that collaboration is an inherent aspect of the work of advanced practitioners.

Dealing with the latter first, the NMC principles acknowledge that advanced level practice is underpinned by interconnected systems and interprofessional working and learning. There are also explicit and implicit requirements for collaboration within each of the four pillars across the four nations' frameworks.

Considering Each Pillar in Turn

Clinical Practice While expressed differently in each of the four nations' frameworks, all four see collaboration between professionals as a critical element of advanced practice. There is an expectation that much of the work of advanced practitioners will be unpredictable and complex, so both intra- and interprofessional collaboration will be important, as will collaboration with individuals and agencies outside of the professions. The frameworks see the sharing of accurate, concise and timely information as essential for patient safety and good clinical outcomes. As an example, an advanced-level psychiatric/mental health nurse dealing with a young person who has taken an overdose may need to liaise and collaborate with physical health colleagues, pathology departments, and poisons centers to ensure the young person's physical well-being. They may also need to liaise with parents and other family members, with peers, the young person's school or college, and any other organization important to the young person (e.g., a religious community) to ensure their psychological and social well-being. The practitioner will need skills to balance opposing demands on information, such as when anxious parents want updates on the young person's progress, but the young person does not want the parents to know, or where there is suspicion of dating abuse.

Leadership and Management Collaboration here largely revolves around team building and teamwork. There is an expectation that advanced practitioners will lead and/or manage teams and that they will contribute to—if not lead—the collaborative development of practices, processes, and systems that improve health-care outcomes and health-care delivery. Consider what collaboration might be needed in the design and establishment of a nurse-led hypertension clinic. The advanced nurse practitioner here would need to identify premises and any appropriate physical resources, they will need to secure a team to work within the clinic and ensure that colleagues are appropriately trained and supported, and they would need to liaise with physician and pharmacy colleagues to ensure continuity of care for patients. They may even need to write standard operating procedures for the service and ensure that the service meets any necessary quality and regulatory standards.

Education Collaboration in the education pillar focuses on the advanced practitioner's role in creating and supporting an organizational culture that encourages both colleagues and patients to learn and develop. For patients, this will mean ensuring that patients are given enough information about their conditions and any available options for treatment so that they can make fully informed decisions. As an example of truly "coproduced" care, an advanced nurse practitioner working with elderly patients might outline the pros and cons of surgery against medication for heart failure in a 70-year old man, ensuring that he understands what heart failure is and the range of options available, that any questions he or family members might have are answered honestly and in nontechnical language, and, where practicable, he is given ample time to make a decision. For colleagues, collaboration might mean informal or formal teaching and learning opportunities in the clinical setting (either delivered or organized by the advanced practitioner), peer support and mentoring, or offering clinical supervision to others. Alternatively, it might mean a formal relationship with an education institution, for example, delivering lectures and conducting theoretical and practical assessments at a local university nursing school or even a joint appointment between a health-care provider and educational institution.

Research The focus on this pillar is using collaboration to enhance the links between clinical practice and research. At its simplest level, this might mean collaborating—if not taking the lead—on local audit and quality improvement initiatives; at a more complex level, it might mean collaborating on externally funded research projects. As with education, the advanced practitioner would benefit here from close links with local universities and research institutes. Dissemination of research is also relevant in that the frameworks encourage advanced practitioners to publish from the research they are involved in, ideally in collaboration with colleagues and through the peer review process. In the UK, the National Institute for Health and Care Research (modelled on the US National Institutes of Health) offers opportunities for clinicians to both lead and be collaborators on funded research projects, as well as offering competitive fellowship opportunities for clinicians. Some of the fellowship opportunities—the Doctoral Award, for example—are suitable for advanced practitioners who want research to be a greater part of their responsibilities. These awards allow the clinician to conduct a PhD project while remaining in clinical practice, providing their salary costs, the costs of the research project, and tuition fees. Successful awards require collaboration with a university or research institute and with academic and clinical colleagues conducting similar research elsewhere.

Collaboration Among Stakeholders

If the regulation of advanced practice in the UK is not to be stymied further, it is essential that all those with a vested interest in advance practice work together. This may not necessarily be easy given that some organizations who have invested heavily in driving the advanced practice agenda (e.g., NHS England and RCN) may have to concede control to the regulatory bodies. Indeed, the RCN has already indicated that it will stop credentialling as a result of the NMC's move to regulation [47].

It is also important that the various regulatory bodies continue to work together on advanced practice even if their timelines vary. If the NMC becomes the first body to regulate advanced practice, the other regulatory bodies should be encouraged to borrow from the NMC and learn from its experiences when customizing regulation for their professions. There is every indication from the NMC's roadmap that it intends to do this, particularly with the HCPC and, in addition, the RPharmS will be a necessary agent in the regulation of independent prescribing in advanced practice.

The provision of advanced practitioner education also requires collaboration with those bodies that have the authority to award master's degrees, that is, the universities. However, as in many countries, the UK university sector is struggling financially [56]; so, universities are unlikely to support the provision of advanced practice education without financial incentives. Unlike the USA, obtaining an advanced practice qualification does not necessarily come with a significant salary increase in the UK; so, individuals may not be willing to fund themselves. A major funding initiative for education and training, the apprenticeship levy, was seen as a potential source of funds for advanced practice qualifications. This levy, introduced in April 2017, is a tax on large employers to fund work-based apprenticeship qualifications, with the hope it might encourage employers to develop the skills of their workers. Employers with an annual pay bill of £3 ($4) million or more (this includes the NHS in all four nations) are levied 0.5% of their payroll, which is held as digital credits, which can be spent on apprenticeships including degree apprenticeships, that is, those that also lead to a bachelor's, master's or doctoral degree. Most of the existing advanced practice courses at UK universities have been designed to attract levy funding, which required collaboration between employers (usually the NHS) and the university. However, accusations of a "middle-class grab" of apprenticeships—older, already qualified workers taking up master's apprenticeships at the expense of lower-level apprenticeships for younger, unqualified workers [57]—means the UK Government will withdraw levy support for master's and doctoral apprenticeships early in 2026, and so, advanced practice courses will become ineligible for levy funding.

That the NMC has set advanced practice principles for employers alongside those for professionals reinforces the importance of engaging and including employers. Many employers rightly recognize the value of advanced practice in enhancing patient outcomes and employer engagement is necessary to set up an advance practice apprenticeship. However, employers need to recognize the value of advanced practice to their organizations by remunerating practitioners appropriately. The NMC has no authority over the pay or grading of staff. Individual NHS providers (known as "trusts") locally set the pay and grading of their staff, using a UK-wide agreed banding framework known as "Agenda for Change." Under this framework, the minimum an RN can be graded at is Band 5 (which is what newly qualified RNs start at), and it is generally accepted that the minimum grade for an advanced practitioner should be Band 7. However, there is significant variation across the UK in advanced practice banding. The Nuffield Trust report for the NMC [42] found most advanced practitioners in Scotland were paid at Band 7; in England and Wales, pay varied between Bands 7, 8a, and 8b; and in Northern Ireland, pay was mostly at B and 8a. This variance is not explained by differences in the job and is probably down to the value placed on the role by individual trusts. Indeed, there is a history of UK nursing roles being devalued and downgraded, particularly when money is tight [58].

Finally, it is important that the medical professions are on board with any plans for the regulation of advanced practice. Since advanced practice in the nonmedical professions is designed to *complement* the work of physicians, it will be somewhat difficult to work collaboratively with, and be accepted by, physicians if they perceive advanced practitioners as a threat or they do not understand what advanced practice is and how it can help with their workloads [59].

Conclusion

It looks like the regulation of advanced practice in the UK is finally on its way though it may only be for nursing and midwifery in the immediate future. Earlier hopes of multiprofessional approach to regulation were perhaps optimistic, though there remains the opportunity for collaboration between the various regulators, assuming they continue to engage with one other. Collaboration with other bodies with vested interests in advanced practice in the UK will hopefully continue even though regulation may irritate those like NHS England and the RCN that have invested time and effort on accrediting advanced practice. Funding may be an obstacle given the upcoming changes to levy support for master's apprenticeships. However, if employers were to standardize Band 8a as the appropriate band for a qualified advanced practitioner, RNs may see the uplift in salary this would offer as an incentive to pay their own fees.

Advanced practice deals with uncertain and complex situations within interconnected and multiprofessional systems of health and social care. To deliver safe and effective care, the advanced practitioner requires collaborative clinical, interpersonal and intellectual skills that cut across all four pillars of advanced practice: they will need to collaborate with colleagues in their own and other professions, both within and outside of their immediate teams, with educational, research, and other scholarly institutions, and, lastly but perhaps most importantly, with patients and those close to them. Advanced practice clearly has a positive future in UK healthcare provision; whether the same can be said for the *regulation* of advanced practice remains to be seen.

Advanced Practice Nursing in Brazil

In Brazil, advanced practice nursing is not yet officially acknowledged, but nurses with advanced degrees practice in advanced roles. Despite the absence of legal recognition and a standardized regulatory framework, Brazilian nurses are increasingly engaging in activities characteristic of Advanced Practice Nursing (APN). These practices occur in diverse settings, particularly within Primary Health Care (PHC), where nurses perform expanded roles that align closely with the competencies and responsibilities of APN as defined by the International Council of Nurses [60]. To better understand the pathway to build APN in Brazil, we present a brief description about Brazilian unified health system (SUS—Sistema Único de Saúde), followed by nursing education characteristics and the current status about APN implementation in Brazil.

Health System in Brazil: Structure, Principles, and Challenges

The Brazilian Unified Health System (Sistema Único de Saúde—SUS) is one of the largest publicly funded health-care systems in the world. Created by the Brazilian Federal Constitution of 1988, SUS was established with the objective of providing universal, comprehensive, and equitable healthcare to all citizens, grounded in the principles of universality, integrality, and equity [61].

SUS is structured across three levels of care: primary, secondary, and tertiary. Primary Health Care (PHC) serves as the foundation and entry point of the system. It is delivered through the Family Health Strategy (FHS), which involves multidisciplinary teams responsible for promoting health, preventing disease, and managing chronic conditions in defined geographical areas [62].

Secondary care encompasses more specialized outpatient services and diagnostic support, while tertiary care includes high-complexity procedures offered in specialized hospitals. The organization of SUS is decentralized, with responsibilities shared among federal, state, and municipal governments. The federal government provides policy direction and funding, while municipalities are largely responsible for service delivery [63].

In parallel to SUS, a private health sector coexists, accessed mainly through private insurance plans or out-of-pocket payments. Although approximately 25% of the population has private coverage, the majority rely solely on public services [64]. The dual nature of Brazil's health system has raised concerns about equity and the potential for segmentation, as those with higher socioeconomic status are often able to access more timely and comprehensive care through private providers [65].

Despite its challenges, SUS has been instrumental in improving health indicators in Brazil. Programs such as the National Immunization Program and the expansion of PHC have contributed to reductions in infant mortality and increased life expectancy [66]. During the COVID-19 pandemic, SUS played a central role in testing, vaccination, and hospitalization, demonstrating its critical value in public health emergencies [67].

Nevertheless, persistent issues such as workforce shortages, long waiting times, and inadequate infrastructure continue to hinder the system's efficiency and quality. Strengthening governance, increasing public investment, and integrating innovative practices—such as telehealth and advanced nursing roles—are considered essential to ensuring sustainability and improved health outcomes [68].

Nursing Education in Brazil: Structure and Challenges at the Undergraduate and Graduate Levels

Nursing education in Brazil is structured into two main academic levels: undergraduate (bachelor's degree) and graduate (stricto sensu and lato sensu programs). Its development has been guided by national educational policies, health-care demands, and the professionalization of nursing within the broader context of the SUS.

Undergraduate Nursing Education

The undergraduate nursing program in Brazil leads to the title of *Enfermeiro* (Registered Nurse) and requires a minimum of 5 years (4000 h) of academic and practical training, as established by the National Curriculum Guidelines (DCNs) defined by the Ministry of Education (MEC) [69]. These guidelines emphasize the formation of generalist nurses, capable of acting at all levels of care—promotion, prevention, treatment, and rehabilitation—based on ethical principles, scientific evidence, and humanized care.

Undergraduate education includes theoretical instruction and practical training in hospital settings, primary health-care units, and community-based services. The SUS serves as a central axis for professional training, ensuring that nursing students experience real-world health contexts [70]. In recent decades, the expansion of private higher education institutions has significantly increased the number of nursing programs. While this democratized access, it also introduced concerns about the quality and uneven geographic distribution of educational institutions [71].

Graduate Nursing Education

Graduate education for nurses in Brazil comprises two modalities: *lato sensu* (specialization and residency programs) and *stricto sensu* (master's and doctoral degrees). *Lato sensu* programs are typically 1–2 years in duration and aim to deepen professional skills in specific areas, such as family health, obstetric nursing, or intensive care. These programs are regulated by the MEC but are not equivalent to academic degrees [72].

Stricto sensu graduate programs include academic and professional master's and doctoral degrees. These programs are evaluated and accredited by the Coordination for the Improvement of Higher Education Personnel (CAPES). Academic master's and doctoral degrees focus on research, theory, and the development of new scientific knowledge, while professional master's degrees emphasize the application of knowledge to improve health-care services, focusing recently in APN [73].

Brazil has made substantial progress in developing graduate nursing programs. According to CAPES data, the country hosts over 40 graduate programs in nursing, many of which are internationally recognized for their scientific productivity and contribution to evidence-based practice [74]. Graduate education is also essential for the development of faculty, researchers, and advanced practitioners who can contribute to health-care innovation and leadership within the SUS.

Despite these advances, graduate nursing education faces challenges such as regional concentration in the Southeast and South regions, funding limitations, and the need for greater integration between academic research and service needs [75]. Furthermore, some proposals for APN education were submitted to appreciation of CAPES in recent years, nonetheless being approved. By this reason, we don't have until now educational programs for APN [76].

Regulation of the Nursing Career in Brazil

Nursing in Brazil is regulated primarily by the Federal Nursing Council (Conselho Federal de Enfermagem—Cofen) and the Regional Nursing Councils (Conselhos Regionais de Enfermagem—Coren), which operate under Law No. 5.905/1973, establishing their structure, responsibilities, and authority [77].

The core legal document that governs nursing practice is the Nursing Professional Practice Law (Law No. 7.498/1986), which defines the scope of practice for nursing professionals, including nurses (enfermeiros), nursing technicians (técnicos de enfermagem), and nursing assistants (auxiliares de enfermagem). This legislation delineates professional activities, such as administration, care planning, health education, and coordination of the nursing team, which are exclusive to registered nurses [78]. Furthermore, Decree No. 94.406/1987 regulates the execution of this law, further specifying professional attributions and the legal responsibilities of each category [79].

To legally practice nursing in Brazil, professionals must hold a diploma from a recognized educational institution and obtain registration with the appropriate Regional Nursing Council. This registration process ensures the professional's adherence to ethical codes and continuous professional development, as defined by Resolution Cofen No. 564/2017, which updates the Code of Ethics for Nursing Professionals in Brazil [80].

Cofen and the Corens are responsible for overseeing professional conduct, issuing licenses, promoting continuing education, and handling disciplinary processes. The councils are also proactive in regulating emerging fields within nursing, issuing resolutions that define advanced roles and specialties. For example, Cofen Resolution No. 640/2020 recognizes the performance of advanced nursing practices, particularly in primary healthcare, although Brazil does not yet have national legislation formally recognizing the Nurse Practitioner (NP) role [81].

Despite advancements, the regulatory environment faces challenges such as disparities in professional autonomy across regions, inconsistencies in implementing scope-of-practice policies, and limited legal recognition of advanced practice nursing. Therefore, there is a growing debate about the need to reform regulatory frameworks to accommodate the evolving responsibilities of nurses, especially in response to health system demands and the expansion of primary care [82].

Nursing regulation in Brazil is well established but requires ongoing updates to reflect the professional evolution and health system needs. To perform as APN, a specific regulatory mark needs to be created by Cofen. Strength of regulatory bodies and alignment with international standards are essential for enhancing nursing practice and improving health-care delivery.

Interprofessional Collaboration in Brazil

Interprofessional collaboration between nurses and physicians is a key component of effective PHC, particularly in Brazil, where the SUS is based on principles of universality, comprehensiveness, and equity. The Family Health Strategy (ESF), Brazil's main model for PHC, encourages teamwork among health professionals, with nurses and physicians as central members of multidisciplinary teams [83].

The collaboration between nurses and physicians within PHC is grounded in a shared goal of improving patient outcomes through coordinated care, task sharing, and mutual respect. Nurses in the ESF are responsible for clinical care, health education, nursing consultations, chronic disease management, and home visits, often acting as the first point of contact for patients [84]. Physicians focus on diagnosis, treatment, and technical supervision, but increasingly rely on nurses to manage routine and preventive care. The institutionalization of collaborative practices is facilitated by Ministerial Ordinance No. 2.488/2011, which defines responsibilities for team members within the ESF and encourages interdisciplinary actions [85].

However, interprofessional collaboration in Brazil still faces challenges related to professional hierarchies, unclear role boundaries, and power asymmetries between physicians and nurses [86]. Despite policies promoting teamwork, the traditional biomedical model continues to influence practice, sometimes limiting nurses' autonomy and contribution to decision-making processes. Studies have shown that effective collaboration depends not only on structural and normative frameworks but also on interpersonal dynamics, leadership, communication, and mutual recognition of competencies [87].

Efforts to strengthen interprofessional collaboration include continuing education programs, interprofessional training in undergraduate curricula, and team meetings for case discussions and care planning. Expanding collaborative competencies and strengthening the legitimacy of nursing roles are necessary steps toward a more equitable and effective PHC model, including APN.

Advanced Practice Nursing Competencies Currently Performed by Nurses in Brazil

Although the role of the nurse practitioner (NP) or APN has not yet been formally regulated in Brazil, nurses in various regions already perform activities that align with internationally recognized APN competencies. These include clinical decision-making, patient assessment, diagnosis, prescription of medications, chronic disease management, and leadership in care coordination, particularly within the framework of the ESF in the Brazilian PHC [82, 88].

The ICN defines an APN as a registered nurse who has acquired expert knowledge base, complex decision-making skills, and clinical competencies for expanded practice, the characteristics of which are shaped by the context and country where they are credentialed [60]. In Brazil, despite the absence of a formal title, many nurses already exercise competencies such as conducting autonomous nursing consultations, requesting and interpreting diagnostic tests, and managing chronic conditions like hypertension, diabetes, and prenatal care, particularly in underserved and rural areas where access to physicians is limited [89].

These expanded competencies are supported by Law No. 7.498/1986, which regulates nursing practice in Brazil and grants nurses' autonomy to perform health education, prescribe medications from institutional protocols, and provide comprehensive nursing care [78]. Additionally, the *Protocolos de Enfermagem na Atenção Primária à Saúde* issued by the Ministry of Health in partnership with Cofen provide clinical guidelines that authorize nurses to act in areas such as women's health, child care, and management of communicable diseases [90].

Several studies indicate that nurses in PHC demonstrate advanced competencies in clinical judgment, leadership, and interprofessional collaboration. For example, they often lead case discussions, coordinate multidisciplinary care, and implement health surveillance and risk stratification strategies [91, 92]. Despite their crucial role, the lack of formal recognition of APN as a specific career path in Brazil has limited the development of specialized postgraduate programs and regulatory frameworks, which are essential for consolidating advanced practice [82].

Freire et al. [93] found that 83.5% of nurses surveyed in southern Minas Gerais reported performing advanced practice activities, such as wound evaluation, prescription of dressings, and participation in the development of care protocols. However, despite these practices, a significant portion of the respondents had little to no formal knowledge of the APN concept, highlighting a gap between practice and conceptual understanding.

Similarly, Carrer et al. [94] conducted a multicenter observational study that analyzed nursing consultations in PHC settings across four Brazilian states. The study revealed that nurses partially applied APN competencies—particularly in domains related to care focus, provision, and assessment and diagnosis—yet faced limitations in areas such as clinical reasoning, cultural sensitivity, and advanced communication skills. The average identification rate of APN competencies across all domains was 47.6%, suggesting that while APN-aligned practices are present, their application remains inconsistent and often unsystematic.

The literature also reveals that despite these practices, Brazil lacks the educational infrastructure to fully support the APN role. Rezende et al. [95] note that while Brazil has a robust postgraduate nursing education system and an established Unified Health System (SUS), regulatory, political, and cultural barriers impede the formal adoption of APN. These include resistance from the medical profession, fragmented health policies, and the proliferation of private nursing schools with uneven quality of training, particularly through distance education models.

Nonetheless, regulatory efforts have begun. The Federal Nursing Council (COFEN) and the Pan American Health Organization (PAHO) have initiated discussions to align Brazilian nursing practice with the ICN's APN standards. COFEN's Technical Note 001/2023 outlines steps toward formalizing the APN role, particularly within PHC, emphasizing the need to expand nurses' scope of practice to improve health-care access and equity [93, 96].

Furthermore, there is growing interest among policymakers and academic institutions in aligning nursing practice in Brazil with international standards. Initiatives such as those led by the Pan American Health Organization (PAHO/WHO) have supported studies and policy recommendations to expand and formalize advanced nursing roles in Latin America, including Brazil [97].

Conclusion

Brazilian nurses are currently practicing as APNs in many contexts, particularly in PHC, where they provide autonomous, complex, and often protocol-driven care. Collaboration between professions continues for the benefit of improved healthcare. There are also collaborative efforts with APNs across the globe to acknowledge APNs in Brazil. However, the lack of formal recognition and standardized competencies limits the visibility and effectiveness of these roles. To bridge this gap, Brazil must address regulatory, educational, and systemic barriers, and recognize the advanced practices that are already being performed by nurses within the health system.

References

United States

1. State Practice Environment. American Association of Nurse Practitioners. 2024. https://www.aanp.org/advocacy/state/state-practice-environment. Accessed 18 Jul 2025.
2. Dunbar-Jacob J, Rohay JM. State health and the level of practice authority for nurse practitioners. Nurs Outlook. 2025;73(1):102319.
3. World Health Organization. Framework for action on interprofessional education and collaborative practice. Geneva. 2010.
4. Melek SP, Norris DT, Paulus J, Matthews K, Weaver A, Davenport S. Potential economic impact of integrated medical-behavioral healthcare. Seattle: Milliman; 2018.
5. Committee on Quality of Health Care in America. Crossing the quality chasm: a new health system for the 21st century. National Academies Press; 2001.
6. Wakefield K, Williams DR, Le Menestrel S, Lalitha J. The future of nursing 2020–2030: charting a path to achieve health equity. National Academy of Sciences; 2021.
7. American Association of Colleges of Nursing. The Essentials: Core competencies for professional nursing education. 2021.
8. Team-Based Care. American Association of Nurse Practitioners. https://www.aanp.org/advocacy/advocacy-resource/position-statements/team-based-care. 2023. Accessed 18 Jul 2025.

9. Comunale MJ, Lerch W, Reynolds B. Integrating advanced practice providers into value-based care strategies: one organization's journey to achieve success through interprofessional collaboration. J Interprofessional Educ Pract. 2021;22:100384.
10. Dunlap E, Fitzpatrick S, Nagarsheth K. Collaboration with advanced practice registered nurses to improve patient satisfaction in outpatient clinic. J Nurse Pract. 2022;18(9):1009–12.
11. Posey K, Prol L. Nurse practitioner faculty attitudes about interprofessional education. J Am Assoc Nurse Pract. 2024;36(8):446–54.
12. Karam M, Brault I, Van Durme T, Macq J. Comparing interprofessional and interorganizational collaboration in healthcare: a systematic review of the qualitative research. Int J Nurs Stud. 2018;79:70–83.
13. Kleinpell R, Kapu A, Abraham L, Alexander C, Andrews TD, Booth S, et al. The use of national collaborative to promote advanced practice registered nurse-led high-value care initiatives. Nurs Outlook. 2020;68(5):626–36.
14. Ferguson LA, Arnold C, Morris J, Rademaker A, Davis T. The nurse practitioner as a bridge to interprofessional research team collaboration in rural community clinics. J Am Assoc Nurse Pract. 2021;33(5):409–13.
15. Heath B, Wise RP, Reynolds K. A standard framework for levels of integrated healthcare. SAMHSA-HRSA Center for Integrated Health Solutions; 2013.
16. Reist C, Petiwala I, Latimer J, Raffaelli SB, Chiang M, Eisenberg D, Campbell S. Collaborative mental health care: a narrative review. Medicine. 2022;101(52):e32554.
17. Cook LK, Burge SA, Mathews TL, Kupzyk KA, Houfek JF. Implementing an APRN-Led integrated behavioral health clinic in a rural community. J Am Psychiatr Nurses Assoc. 2024;30(3):669–76.
18. Emerson MR, Huber M, Mathews TL, Kupzyk K, Walsh M, Walker J. Improving integrated mental health care through an advanced practice registered nurse–led program: challenges and successes. Public Health Rep. 2023;138(1 suppl):22S–8S.
19. Reising V, Diegel-Vacek L, Dadabo L, Corbridge S. Collaborative care: integrating behavioral health into the primary care setting. J Am Psychiatr Nurses Assoc. 2023;29(4):344–51.
20. Weber M, Stalder S, Techau A, Centi S, McNair B, Barton AJ. Behavioral health integration in a nurse-led federally qualified health center: outcomes of care. J Am Assoc Nurse Pract. 2021;33(12):1166–72.
21. Karam M, Chouinard MC, Poitras ME, Couturier Y, Vedel I, Grgurevic N, Hudon C. Nursing care coordination for patients with complex needs in primary healthcare: a scoping review. Int J Integr Care. 2021;21(1):16.
22. Brown M, Moore CA, MacGregor J, Lucey JR. Primary care and mental health: overview of integrated care models. J Nurse Pract. 2021;17(1):10–4.
23. Lieberman JA, Olfson M. Meeting the mental health challenge of the COVID-19 pandemic. Psychiatr Times. 2020;24
24. Judge-Ellis T, Hamm B, Wittman J, Dirks MS, Gentil-Archer A, Watson CA, Buckwalter KC. Leadership for an innovative practice role: the dually certified nurse practitioner. Nurse Lead. 2023;21(6):623–31.
25. Nurse Anesthetists, Nurse Midwives, and Nurse Practitioners. US department of labor. 2023. Retrieved from https://www.bls.gov/ooh/healthcare/nurse-anesthetists-nurse-midwives-and-nurse-practitioners.htm. Accessed 18 Jul 2025.
26. Crumley D, Matulis R, Brykman K, Lee B, Conway M. Integrating behavioral health care into primary care: advancing primary care innovation in Medicaid managed care, vol. 1, issue 14. enter for Health Care Strategies, Inc.; 2019.
27. Hooker RS, Curry K, Tracy C. Specialization of physician associates and nurse practitioners as reflected in workforce projections. Cureus. 2024;16(11)
28. Area health Resources File. Health Resources & Services Administration. 2023. https://data.hrsa.gov/topics/health-workforce/ahrf. Accessed 18 Jul 2025.
29. American Nurses Association. Psychiatric-mental health nursing: scope and standards of practice. 3rd Ed. 2023. ISBN: 9781947800977.

30. Jørgensen K, Juhl R, Hansen M, Lerbæk B, Frederiksen J, Watson E, Bjerrum M, Karlsson B. Perspectives of healthcare professionals on cross-sectoral collaboration between mental health centers and municipalities: a qualitative study. Int J Soc Psychiatry. 2025;71(4):694–704.
31. Jørgensen K, Hansen MS, Hansen M, Karlsson B. Health professionals' perceptions of user involvement in a mental health centre: a critical discourse analysis. Int J Ment Health Nurs. 2024;33(4):937–48.
32. DeSalvo KB, Wang YC, Harris A, Auerbach J, Koo D, O'Carroll P. Public health 3.0: a call to action for public health to meet the challenges of the 21st century. Prev Chronic Dis. 2017;14:E78.
33. Kimberly T. Bridging the gap to health care access: The role of the nurse practitioner. Int Achieves Pub Health Community Med. 2023;7(1):91.

United Kingdom

34. Stones AJ. The ACP–GP relationship. Br J Gen Pract. 2019;69(684):348.
35. Dyer C. BMA loses case over GMC's use of "medical professional" to describe associates. BMJ. 2025;389:r800.
36. Glasper A. The Government response to the consultation on nursing associates. Br J Nurs. 2018;27(11):646–7.
37. Haslam MB. The erosion of mental health nursing: the implications of the move towards genericism. Br J Ment Health Nurs. 2023;12(1):1–6.
38. Tatterton MJ, Carey MC, Hyde R, Hewitt C. Don't throw the baby out with the bathwater: Preserving children's undergraduate nurse education in the move towards genericism in nursing. J Child Health Care. 2024;28(1):3–7.
39. Warrender D, Ramsay M, Hurley J. Mental health nurse education: a contemporary view in the debate between generic and specialist approaches. Ment Health Pract. 2023;26(5):20–5.
40. Nursing and Midwifery Council. Standards of proficiency for registered nurses [Internet]. London: NMC; 2018 [cited 2025 Jul 10].
41. Royal Pharmaceutical Society. A competency framework for all prescribers [Internet]. London: RPharmS; 2021 [cited 2025 Jul 10]. Available from: https://www.rpharms.com/resources/frameworks/prescribing-competency-framework/competency-framework
42. Palmer W, Julian S, Vaughan L. Independent report on the regulation of advanced practice in nursing and midwifery [Internet]. London: The Nuffield Trust; 2023 [cited 2025 Jul 10]. Available from: https://www.nuffieldtrust.org.uk/research/independent-report-on-the-regulation-of-advanced-practice-in-nursing-and-midwifery
43. King R, Todd A, Sanders T. Development and regulation of advanced nurse practitioners in the UK and internationally. Nurs Stand. 2017;32(14):43–50.
44. Rise Associates. The nursing and midwifery council: independent culture review [Internet]. London: NMC; 2024 [cited 2025 Jul 10]. Available from: https://www.nmc.org.uk/globalassets/sitedocuments/independent-reviews/2024/nmc-independent-culture-review-july-2024.pdf
45. NHS England. NHS long term workforce plan [Internet]. London: NHS England; 2023 [cited 2025 Jul 10]. Available from: https://www.england.nhs.uk/wp-content/uploads/2023/06/nhs-long-term-workforce-plan-v1.21.pdf
46. NHS England: Centre for Advancing Practice. Digital Badges [Internet]. no date [cited 2025 Jul 10]. Available from: https://advanced-practice.hee.nhs.uk/our-work/digital-badges/
47. Royal College of Nursing. RCN Credentialling [Internet]. no date [cited 2025 Jul 10]. Available from: https://www.rcn.org.uk/Professional-Development/Professional-services/Credentialing
48. Hardy M. Advanced Practice: Research Report [Internet]. Bradford/London: University of Bradford/HCPC; 2021 [cited 2025 Jul 10]. Available from: https://www.hcpc-uk.org/globalassets/resources/policy/independent-research-report-advanced-practice-27th-january-2021.pdf

49. Leary A, Maclaine K, Trevatt P, Radford M, Punshon G. Variation in job titles within the nursing workforce. J Clin Nurs. 2017;26(23–24):4945–50.
50. International Council of Nurses. Guidelines on Advanced Nursing Practice [Internet]. Geneva: ICN; 2020 [cited 2025 Jul 10]. Available from: https://www.icn.ch/system/files/documents/2020-04/ICN_APN%20Report_EN_WEB.pdf
51. NHS England: Centre for Advancing Practice. Multi-professional framework for advanced practice in England [Internet]. London: NHS England; 2025 [cited 2025 Jul 10]. Available from: https://advanced-practice.hee.nhs.uk/mpf2025/downloads/
52. Joint Formulary Committee. British National Formulary (BNF) [Internet]. 2025 [cited 2025 Jul 10]. Available from: https://bnf.nice.org.uk/
53. Nursing and Midwifery Council. Advanced practice review [Internet]. 2025 [cited 2025 Jul 10]. Available from: https://www.nmc.org.uk/standards/future-standards/advanced-practice-review/
54. Health and Social Care Professions Council. Updates on advanced practice [Internet]. 2024 [cited 2025 Jul 10]. Available from: https://www.hcpc-uk.org/news-and-events/blog/2024/updates-on-advanced-practice/
55. Nursing and Midwifery Council. Principles for advanced practice [Internet]. 2025 [cited 2025 Jul 10]. Available from: https://www.nmc.org.uk/globalassets/sitedocuments/advanced-practice-review/principles-for-advanced-practice-english.pdf
56. PricewaterhouseCoopers. UK higher education financial sustainability report [Internet]. London: PwC; 2024 [cited 2025 Jul 10]. Available from: https://www.universitiesuk.ac.uk/sites/default/files/field/downloads/2024-01/pwc-uk-higher-education-financial-sustainability-report-january-2024.pdf
57. Crawford-Lee M. Higher and degree apprenticeships: the middle-class land grab? In: Baldwin J, Raven N, Webber-Jones R, editors. The future of technical education: ending england's long running saga. Cham: Palgrave Macmillan; 2024. p. 113–37.
58. Royal College of Nursing. State of the profession report: RCN employment survey 2023 [Internet]. London: RCN; 2024 [cited 2025 Jul 10]. Available from: https://www.rcn.org.uk/Professional-Development/publications/rcn-employment-survey-2023-uk-pub-011-484
59. Evans N. Advanced practice and why it still has its critics. Nurs Stand. 2024;39(6):19–22.

Brazil

60. ICN – International Council of Nurses. Guidelines on advanced practice nursing 2020. Geneva: ICN. 2020. Retrieved from https://www.icn.ch/system/files/documents/2020-04/ICN_APN%20Report_EN_WEB.pdf
61. Paim J, Travassos C, Almeida C, Bahia L, Macinko J. The Brazilian health system: history, advances, and challenges. Lancet. 2011;377(9779):1778–97. https://doi.org/10.1016/S0140-6736(11)60054-8.
62. Macinko J, Harris MJ. Brazil's family health strategy – delivering community-based primary care in a universal health system. N Engl J Med. 2015;372(23):2177–81. https://doi.org/10.1056/NEJMp1501140.
63. Castro MC, Massuda A, Almeida G, Menezes-Filho NA, Andrade MV, Noronha KVMS, Rocha R, Macinko J, Hone T, Tasca R, Giovanella L, Malik AM, Werneck H, Atun R. Brazil's unified health system: the first 30 years and prospects for the future. Lancet. 2019;394(10195):345–56. https://doi.org/10.1016/S0140-6736(19)31243-7.
64. Agência Nacional de Saúde Suplementar (ANS). Dados e Indicadores do Setor de Saúde Suplementar. 2024. https://www.gov.br/ans/
65. SUS: avaliação da eficiência do gasto público em saúde / Organização de Carlos Octávio Ocké-Reis. Alexandre Marinho, Francisco Rózsa Funcia... [et. al]. – Brasília : Ipea, CONASS, OPAS. 2022. Available from: https://repositorio.ipea.gov.br/server/api/core/bitstreams/66617a31-8608-4ed5-be21-3a2409146fb3/content

66. Macinko J, Harris MJ, Rocha MG. Brazil's national health system: progress and challenges. Lancet. 2017;377(9779):1778–97. https://doi.org/10.1016/S0140-6736(11)60054-8.
67. Terre BBF, Toso BRGO, Reis LF, Johann JA. Analysis of public policies to combat COVID-19 in the state of Paraná, Brazil. Front Public Health. 2024;2:1384561. https://doi.org/10.3389/fpubh.2024.1384561.
68. Giovanella L, Franco CM, Almeida PF, Mendonça MHM. Universal healthcare system resilience: the Brazilian SUS during the COVID-19 pandemic. Rev Panam Salud Publica. 2020;44:e135. https://doi.org/10.26633/RPSP.2020.135.
69. Brasil. Ministério da Educação. iretrizes Curriculares Nacionais do Curso de Graduação em Enfermagem. Resolução CNE/CES n.° 3/2001. Brasília: MEC; 2001.
70. Lima RBD, Miranda ES, da Silva ALA, de Freitas SEAP. Interprofessionality in Brazilian national curricular guidelines for health courses. Avaliação (Campinas) [Internet]. 2024;29:e024020. https://doi.org/10.1590/1982-57652024v29id27937920.
71. Ximenes Neto FRG, Lopes Neto D, Cunha ICKO, Ribeiro MA, Freire NP, Kalinowski CE, Oliveira EN, Albuquerque IMN. Reflections on Brazilian nursing education from the regulation of the Unified Health System. Cien Saude Colet. 2020;25(1):37–46. Portuguese, English. https://doi.org/10.1590/1413-81232020251.27702019. Epub 2019 Sep 20. PMID: 31859853.
72. MEC – Ministério da Educação. Educação Superior: panorama dos cursos de enfermagem. 2024. http://portal.mec.gov.br/
73. Dantas AC, Araújo MG, Araújo JNM, Medeiros ABM, Santos PHA, Borges BEC, Tinôco JDS, Bezerra HS. Advanced practice nursing in Brazil: bibliometric analysis of dissertations and theses. Rev Esc Enferm USP. 2024;58:e20240253. https://doi.org/10.1590/1980-220X-REEUSP-2024-0253en.
74. CAPES – Coordenação de Aperfeiçoamento de Pessoal de Nível Superior. Dados abertos sobre cursos e programas de pós-graduação em enfermagem. 2023. https://www.gov.br/capes/
75. Carregal FADS, dos Santos BM, de Souza HP, Santos FBO, Peres MADA, Padilha MICDS. Historicity of nursing graduate studies in Brazil: an analysis of the Sociology of the Professions. Rev Bras Enferm [Internet]. 2021;74(6):e20190827. https://doi.org/10.1590/0034-7167-2019-0827.
76. Toso BRGO, Peres EM. More advances than setbacks in implementing the advanced nursing practice in Brazil. Online Braz J Nurs. 2023;22(Suppl. 2):e20236694. https://doi.org/10.17665/1676-4285.20236694.
77. Brasil. Lei n° 5.905, de 12 de julho de 1973. Dispõe sobre a criação dos Conselhos Federal e Regionais de Enfermagem e dá outras providências. 1973. Retrieved from https://www.planalto.gov.br/ccivil_03/leis/l5905.htm
78. Brasil. Lei n° 7.498, de 25 de junho de 1986. Dispõe sobre a regulamentação do exercício da Enfermagem e dá outras providências. 1986. Retrieved from https://www.planalto.gov.br/ccivil_03/leis/l7498.htm
79. Brasil. Decreto n° 94.406, de 8 de junho de 1987. Regulamenta a Lei n° 7.498/1986. 1987. Retrieved from https://www.planalto.gov.br/ccivil_03/decreto/1980-1989/D94406.htm
80. Conselho Federal de Enfermagem (Cofen). Resolução Cofen n° 564/2017. Aprova o novo Código de Ética dos Profissionais de Enfermagem. 2017. Retrieved from http://www.cofen.gov.br/resolucao-cofen-564-2017_59145.html
81. Conselho Federal de Enfermagem (Cofen). Resolução Cofen n° 640/2020. Dispõe sobre a atuação da Enfermagem em práticas avançadas. 2020. Retrieved from http://www.cofen.gov.br/resolucao-cofen-no-640-2020_80344.html
82. Cassiani SH, Aguirre-Boza F, Hoyos MC, Barreto MF, Morán L, Cerón MC, et al. Competencies for training advanced practice nurses in primary health care. Acta Paul Enferm. 2018;31(6):572–84. https://doi.org/10.1590/1982-0194201800080.
83. Toso BRGO, Fungueto L, Maraschin MS, Tonini NS. Atuação do enfermeiro em distintos modelos de Atenção Primária à Saúde no Brasil. Saúde debate [Internet]. 2021;45(130):666–80. https://doi.org/10.1590/0103-1104202113008.
84. Cassiani SHB, Silva FAM. Expanding the role of nurses in primary health care: the case of Brazil. Rev Latino Am Enfermagem. 2019;27:e3245. https://doi.org/10.1590/1518-8345.0000.3245.

85. Brasil.Portarian°2.488,de21deoutubrode2011.AprovaaPolíticaNacionaldeAtençãoBásica.2011. Retrieved from https://bvsms.saude.gov.br/bvs/saudelegis/gm/2011/prt2488_21_10_2011.html
86. Ferraz CMLC, Vilela GS, Dionízio ACS, Caram CS, Rezende LC, Brito MJM. Collaborative practice in the family health strategy: expressions, possibilities and challenges for the production of care. REME Rev Min Enferm. [Internet]. 2022 [cited 2025 Aug. 2];26. Available from: https://periodicos.ufmg.br/index.php/reme/article/view/40294
87. Peduzzi M, Agreli HF. Trabalho em equipe e prática colaborativa na Atenção Primária à Saúde. Interface (Botucatu) [Internet]. 2018;22:1525–34. https://doi.org/10.1590/1807-57622017.0827.
88. Toso BRGO. Práticas avançadas de enfermagem em atenção primária: estratégias para implantação no Brasil. Enferm Foco [online]. 2016; 7(3/4), [cited 2025-08-02], 36–40. https://enfermfoco.org/article/praticas-avancadas-de-enfermagem-em-atencao-primaria-estrategias-para-implantacao-no-brasil/. ISSN 2177–4285.
89. Chagas LN, Nahum BAP, Freitas RJR, Martins APM. Competences of nurses in the Family Health Strategy: an integrative literature review (J. N. do Lago, Trans.). Int J Innov Educ Res. 2023;11(3):93–108. https://doi.org/10.31686/ijier.vol11.iss3.4103.
90. Brasil. Ministério da Saúde. Protocolos de Enfermagem na Atenção Primária à Saúde. Brasília: Ministério da Saúde; 2022. Retrieved from https://aps.saude.gov.br/ape/protocolos
91. Miranda Neto MV, Rewa T, Leonello VM, Oliveira MAC. Advanced practice nursing: a possibility for primary health care? Rev Bras Enferm [Internet]. 2018;71(Supl 1):716–21. Issue edition: contributions and challenges of practices in collective health nursing. https://doi.org/10.1590/0034-7167-2017-0672.
92. Minosso KC, Santos MB, Toso BRGO. Validation of the Brazilian Version of the Modified Scale for Delineating Advanced Practice Nursing Roles. Rev Bras Enferm. 2024;77(2):e20230211. https://doi.org/10.1590/0034-7167-2023-0211.
93. Freire BSM, Fracaroli YR, Nascimento FC, Costa ACB, Braga CG, Costa ICP. Advanced practice nursing and the actions performed by nurses: an analytical study. Revista de Pesquisa: Cuidado é Fundamental. 2025;17:e13580. Disponível em: https://seer.unirio.br/cuidadofundamental/article/view/13580
94. Carrer MO, Almeida LY, Vesga-Varela AL, Bonfim D, Almeida PA, Barreto CP, Serranegra NVF, Reis KGL, Martiniano CS, Miranda Neto MV. Acute events in primary health care settings: an analysis of advanced practice competencies in nursing consultations in Brazil. Nurs Open. 2025;12:e70247. https://doi.org/10.1002/nop2.70247.
95. Rezende LDA, Funabashi LMS, Ciscotto VMS, Freitas PSS, Fiorin BH, Nascimento DHRS. Perspectivas para a Prática Avançada de Enfermagem no Brasil. Rev Nurs. 2025;29(324):10932–41. https://doi.org/10.36489/nursing.2025v29i324p10932-10941.
96. Conselho Federal de Enfermagem (COFEN). Nota Técnica 001/2023: Enfermagem de Prática Avançada no Brasil: contexto, conceitos, ações empreendidas, implementação e regulamentação. Brasília: COFEN; 2023.
97. PAHO – Pan American Health Organization. Expanding the roles of nurses in primary health care. Washington, DC: PAHO; 2018. Retrieved from https://iris.paho.org/handle/10665.2/34958

Understanding the Difference: Collaboration Versus Autonomous Practice Across Different Health-Care Systems

Jennifer Manning

Introduction

The global health-care landscape faces unprecedented demands from aging populations, the rising tide of chronic disease, and persistent health disparities. In response, the World Health Organization (WHO) and other international bodies have called for the expansion and optimization of all nursing roles, particularly Advanced Practice Registered Nurses (APRNs)—a group typically comprising Clinical Nurse Specialists (CNSs), Nurse Practitioners (NPs), Certified Registered Nurse Anesthetists (CRNAs), and Certified Nurse-Midwives (CNMs) [7].

However, the successful integration and maximization of APRN potential hinges on a fundamental regulatory and philosophical distinction: the degree to which they practice autonomously versus collaboratively. This chapter explores these critical differences across varied global health-care systems, examining how legal frameworks, professional identity, and system needs dictate where an APRN falls on the spectrum between independent practice and physician-led collaboration [15].

Defining the Core Concepts: Autonomy Versus Collaboration

Autonomy in Advanced Practice Registered Nurse (APRN) practice refers to the independent authority to practice to the full extent of one's education and certification, including diagnosing, treating, prescribing, and managing patient care without mandated oversight or cosignature from another health-care professional, particularly a physician. This concept hinges on the APRN's professional accountability

J. Manning (✉)
Louisiana State University Health Sciences Center School of Nursing,
New Orleans, LA, USA
e-mail: jmanni@lsuhsc.edu

A. Kapu et al. (eds.), *A Global View on Clinical Autonomy for Advanced Practice Nurses*, Advanced Practice in Nursing,
https://doi.org/10.1007/978-3-032-21458-4_6

and their capacity to function as a primary and specialty care provider within their scope of practice, which is defined by state or national regulatory boards. High levels of autonomy are often associated with Full Practice Authority (FPA) models, which are supported by evidence demonstrating APRNs' ability to deliver safe, effective, and high-quality care, especially in underserved areas. Fundamentally, autonomy is about the power and legal right of the APRN to make and execute clinical decisions independently [17].

In contrast, collaboration describes a mutually respectful relationship between APRNs and other health-care providers (such as physicians, pharmacists, and physical therapists) to optimize patient outcomes, recognizing the specialized knowledge each member brings to the care team [8]. While collaboration is a professional imperative that enhances care quality and complexity management across all practice models, it is distinct from mandated supervision or required physician oversight, which are often regulatory barriers misrepresented as "collaboration." True professional collaboration is voluntary, dynamic, and patient-centered, focusing on shared decision-making and coordinated care, and should not be conflated with regulatory requirements that restrict APRN autonomy by requiring a formal agreement or cosignatory for routine practice [10].

Autonomous Practice: Licensed Independent Practitioner Status

Autonomous practice, frequently codified as Full Practice Authority (FPA), represents the highest level of professional independence for the Advanced Practice Registered Nurse (APRN). At its core, FPA recognizes the APRN as a licensed independent practitioner within their governing jurisdiction, a status earned through rigorous advanced education, clinical training, and board certification. This recognition is vital as it legally affirms the APRN's competence and right to act as a primary provider, aligning with the critical health-care recommendation from the National Academy of Medicine that nurses should be permitted to practice to the full extent of their education and skills to optimize care delivery [9].

This autonomous status is characterized by several key operational components that eliminate regulatory hurdles and optimize access to care. The first is that there are no oversight requirements. Under FPA, the APRN's licensure and ability to perform core clinical activities—including comprehensive assessment, diagnosing illnesses, establishing treatment plans, and prescribing medications—are not contingent on mandated contracts, physician supervision, delegation, or cosignature. The APRN functions as a fully self-governing clinician [18].

A second key component of the operation is the APRN's independent functioning. APRNs with FPA have the legal authority to establish and operate their own clinical practices, providing flexibility in health-care service delivery. They can bill for services rendered using their own provider identification number, securing equitable reimbursement, and are authorized to initiate and manage the full spectrum of evidence-based care appropriate for their specialty and population focus without external sign-off [3]. In a Full Practice Authority (FPA) environment, a Family Nurse Practitioner (FNP) provides a clear example of this independent functioning by establishing an autonomous primary care clinic in a rural community. Because the FNP is recognized as a licensed independent practitioner, they can perform comprehensive physical exams, diagnose chronic conditions like hypertension, and initiate a complete pharmacological treatment plan without a physician's cosignature or a mandated collaborative contract. Furthermore, the FNP uses their own National Provider Identifier (NPI) number to bill insurance and Medicare directly for these services, ensuring the clinic remains financially viable while providing essential health-care access to an underserved population without administrative delays.

The third key component is the provider's accountability. This independence is paired with direct professional responsibility for APRNs. In this model, accountability rests solely with the APRN and is managed by their governing body, which is typically the Board of Nursing. This structure ensures that the quality of care is overseen by the regulatory board explicitly tasked with maintaining nursing standards, rather than requiring oversight from a separate medical board. The global trend toward granting APRN Full Practice Authority is a direct response to increasing demands for efficient, accessible, and high-quality primary and specialty care, especially in areas facing provider shortages [12]. In a Full Practice Authority (FPA) setting, a Certified Registered Nurse Anesthetist (CRNA) practicing in a rural critical access hospital serves as a prime example of this direct professional accountability. When the CRNA independently develops and executes an anesthesia plan for a surgical patient, they assume sole responsibility for the clinical outcomes and safety of that care. If a practice concern arises, the CRNA is held accountable by the State Board of Nursing, which evaluates their actions against established advanced nursing standards rather than through a medical board. This streamlined oversight model eliminates the need for a supervising anesthesiologist to assume legal liability for the CRNA's independent decisions, directly supporting the global trend toward more efficient and accessible specialty care in regions where physician specialists may be unavailable.

Collaborative Practice: Interprofessional Interdependence

Collaborative practice defines a standard model of operation where the APRN functions in a structured state of interdependence with another provider, typically a physician (MD or DO). Unlike autonomous practice, where the APRN is the sole independent authority, this model requires a formal, often legally mandated, relationship with a physician to fulfill the APRN's full scope of practice. This collaborative structure is currently the default regulatory framework in many regions, establishing precise legal mechanisms that define the extent and limits of APRNs' roles, despite the high level of education and clinical experience they possess [4].

The interdependence inherent in this model is structured through specific regulatory requirements that limit the APRN's authority, often manifesting as supervision or delegation. In these frameworks, the APRN's ability to perform specific advanced tasks, particularly those involving prescribing controlled substances, ordering complex diagnostics, or managing specific patient populations, is explicitly delegated by the collaborating physician. This means the APRN's scope of practice is not inherent to their license but is instead conditional on the physician's explicit permission. This delegation structure ensures the physician retains a formal level of control over the types and complexity of services the APRN can legally provide [15].

A key operational component of this collaborative model involves contractual agreements. These frequently take the form of a written collaborative agreement or joint practice agreement that is mandated by state or regional licensing boards. This legal document formally outlines crucial elements of the relationship, including the specific scope of the APRN's practice, the defined frequency of supervision or consultation, and the allocation of shared responsibilities. While these agreements are intended to facilitate effective teamwork, they fundamentally tether the APRN's licensure continuity to the maintenance of the contractual relationship, creating an external dependency that is absent in autonomous practice [4].

One example in a collaborative practice model, a Clinical Nurse Specialist (CNS) specializing in oncology provides a clear example of this contractual dependency when they are required to maintain a written joint practice agreement with a lead oncologist. While the CNS utilizes their advanced expertise to independently design evidence-based protocols for chemotherapy symptom management, their legal authority to implement these system-wide changes—or to consult on complex patient cases—is often tethered to this mandated document. This formal agreement outlines the specific frequency of medical consultation and requires the oncologist to review a percentage of the CNS's clinical recommendations or prescriptive logs. Because the CNS's functional scope is conditional on this physician's explicit permission rather than being inherent to their license, any change or termination in the contractual relationship could immediately interrupt the CNS's ability to practice, illustrating the structural interdependence and external dependency that defines this model.

Ultimately, in collaborative practice, a system of shared responsibility is established, which legally shifts the ultimate burden of patient care. While the APRN may make highly sophisticated and independent clinical decisions daily, the legal and financial responsibility for the patient's overall medical management may be legally required to reside with the collaborating physician. This often necessitates burdensome administrative requirements, such as the physician reviewing patient charts, signing off on a certain percentage of records, or approving prescriptive logs. In essence, the collaborative model implies a professional relationship in which the APRN's legal authority is derived from or contingent upon the physician's oversight, thereby defining a relationship of professional interdependence rather than full independence [15].

The Global Spectrum: Where Systems Fall?

The global implementation of Advanced Practice Registered Nurse (APRN) roles reveals a complex spectrum of practice models rather than a simple binary choice between full autonomy and mandated collaboration. This variation is primarily a function of two powerful drivers: the national workforce needs—especially in primary care and underserved regions—and the historical professional dynamics between nursing and medicine within a country's existing regulatory structure. Nations like the United States, Canada, Australia, and New Zealand have varying degrees of Full Practice Authority (FPA), allowing APRNs to act as Licensed Independent Practitioners, particularly in primary care. This trend is often accelerated by population demands and clear evidence showing APRNs provide safe, high-quality care, pushing policy to remove restrictions that limit the workforce's full potential [11].

Conversely, many other systems—and even a subset of states within countries like the USA—maintain models where the APRN operates in a more interdependent capacity, requiring formal collaborative agreements, physician supervision, or chart review for prescriptive authority and other core functions. These restrictions are frequently a result of established medical practice acts and a conservative regulatory environment rooted in older, non–evidence-based notions about the quality of APRN care. The location of a country or region on this autonomy-collaboration spectrum thus determines more than just professional freedom; it directly impacts health-care access (especially in rural settings), economic efficiency, and the APRN's ability to seamlessly integrate and contribute to the interprofessional health-care team without administrative delay [4].

Full Practice Authority (FPA) Contexts

Systems that have adopted Full Practice Authority (FPA) for Advanced Practice Registered Nurses (APRNs), prevalent in many U.S. states and reflected in progressive models in Canada and Australia, primarily emphasize maximizing health-care efficiency and access. By removing regulatory hurdles such as mandated physician oversight or collaborative agreements, FPA allows APRNs to use their full scope of training immediately upon licensure. This regulatory freedom acts as a powerful access driver, particularly in areas struggling with provider shortages. Empirical evidence consistently shows that states and regions with FPA experience higher rates of APRNs choosing to practice in rural and underserved areas. This direct deployment of highly qualified providers is crucial for addressing primary care gaps, reducing patient wait times, and improving health outcomes without the administrative friction caused by unnecessary supervision mandates [15].

Although the general term FPA applies to all APRNs, the specific authorities granted often vary by role, creating nuances within the autonomous framework. While Nurse Practitioners (NPs) are typically the primary focus of FPA legislation regarding independent diagnosing, treatment, and prescribing rights (including controlled substances), other APRN roles face different challenges [13]. Clinical Nurse Specialists (CNSs) in the same FPA jurisdictions often enjoy de facto autonomy in their core specialty functions, such as leading complex care pathway development, performing advanced diagnosis in acute settings, and implementing evidence-based practice changes. However, their ability to independently prescribe medications may still be limited or absent if that authority was not explicitly legislated for the CNS role designation, highlighting that even in FPA systems, legislative consistency across all four APRN roles (Nurse Practitioner, Clinical Nurse Specialist, Certified Nurse-Midwife, and Certified Registered Nurse Anesthetist) remains an ongoing policy goal [18].

Reduced/Restricted Authority Contexts

The majority of global health-care systems, particularly across Europe and parts of Asia, operate under Reduced or Restricted Authority models for Advanced Practice Registered Nurses (APRNs), which mandate a specific form of physician involvement and misrepresent it as professional collaboration. These constraints are often rooted in protecting traditional medical domains, leading to a structure in which APRNs are authorized to perform high-level functions such as diagnosis and care management but face significant prescriptive barriers. For instance, an APRN may be required to obtain a physician's cosignature for every prescription, regardless of the drug's complexity or the APRN's training. This systemic friction creates administrative delays, compromises efficient patient care, and legally subordinates the APRN's practice to the physician's authority [14].

The primary constraints driving these restrictive models are frequently cultural resistance and medical dominance, which manifest as professional closure. Physicians often argue that their more extensive medical training entitles them to exclusive rights to core medical functions, such as prescribing, even though APRNs possess graduate-level education and specialized training in their areas of practice. In these restrictive systems, the APRN is commonly labeled a "physician extender," a term that fundamentally contradicts the concept of professional autonomy. This designation implies that the APRN's role is merely a subordinate complement to the physician's, rather than that of a fully accountable, independent practitioner. This regulatory and cultural environment ultimately prevents the full utilization of the APRN workforce [17].

Task-Shifting and Crisis Contexts

In numerous developing economies and crisis contexts, the acute need to address critical health-care workforce shortages compels an immediate and often unstructured practice of task-shifting—the delegation of tasks traditionally performed by physicians to qualified nurses and Advanced Practice Registered Nurses (APRNs). In these settings, autonomy is frequently gained out of necessity, overriding formal regulatory barriers. An APRN on the front lines in a rural clinic or disaster zone may be functioning as the sole autonomous provider, making diagnoses, initiating complex treatments, and prescribing essential medications simply because no physician is physically available. While this pragmatic approach ensures care is delivered, it often leaves APRN practice in a legal gray area, where de facto clinical autonomy is acknowledged but not fully codified or protected by outdated regulations [13].

The international path toward defining the APRN role is highly varied, demonstrating that even sophisticated systems require iterative adaptation. Countries like Australia and Hong Kong, for example, have effectively adapted elements of the U.S. full practice authority (FPA) model while meticulously tailoring them to their unique legislative frameworks, health-care funding mechanisms, and professional cultures. This underscores that implementing advanced practice nursing roles is rarely a seamless, single-step process. Instead, it evolves, with policymakers and professional bodies constantly negotiating the precise boundaries between granting full professional autonomy and defining the parameters for necessary interprofessional consultation to ensure high-quality, comprehensive patient care [11].

Role Differentiators: CNS and NP Within the Autonomy/Collaboration Framework

The distinction between the Clinical Nurse Specialist (CNS) and Nurse Practitioner (NP) roles profoundly affects how the concepts of autonomy and collaboration are manifested and regulated in practice, despite both roles being foundational under the Advanced Practice Registered Nurse (APRN) umbrella. While both share the core mandate of leveraging graduate-level expertise to improve health outcomes, their traditional spheres of influence—the NP focusing on the patient and the CNS focusing on the patient, staff, and system—create divergent regulatory and professional trajectories concerning independent authority [13].

The Nurse Practitioner (NP) is generally positioned to seek and achieve service-based professional autonomy primarily in the domain of direct patient care. The core of their advanced practice centers focuses on the patient/client sphere: performing advanced assessments, establishing diagnoses, formulating treatment plans, and managing acute and chronic conditions within their specialized population. Because their practice mirrors the direct provision of primary or specialty medical care, achieving prescriptive authority is a common and critical goal for NP practice optimization, making full practice authority (FPA) the preferred regulatory model for their clinical efficacy [15].

For the NP, collaboration often manifests as referrals and consultations. This occurs when a patient's clinical needs exceed the NP's defined scope of practice, or when the law explicitly mandates consultation, as in restrictive regulatory environments. In autonomous practice models, this relationship is typically a respectful, provider-to-provider dynamic in which the NP serves as the primary clinician seeking specialized input. In restrictive models, however, this "collaboration" is often a mandatory, supervisory tether that legally limits the NP's autonomy, even though their day-to-day clinical work is highly independent [7].

Conversely, the Clinical Nurse Specialist (CNS) is traditionally focused on three intertwined spheres of influence: the patient, the nurse, and the organization. Their practice, therefore, leans heavily on expert consultation and leadership across all three areas, making their role inherently one of intradisciplinary and interdisciplinary expertise synthesis. Their professional identity is defined by the ability to apply advanced knowledge to indirectly improve care quality, often by influencing others and modifying systems, rather than exclusively through direct patient panel management [16].

CNS's practice is defined by core collaboration. They collaborate with frontline staff nurses to elevate unit-level practice standards, work with managers and administrators to implement large-scale system change, and consult with physicians to synthesize the latest research and evidence into actionable clinical protocols. Their authority is less about the final medical prescription and more about autonomy in evidence translation. A CNS might autonomously design and implement a new, evidence-based sepsis treatment bundle. However, the physician or NP retains the legal authority to write the specific medication order within that protocol, depending on local jurisdiction [10].

In summary, the fundamental difference lies in independence. The NP generally strives for autonomy in clinical decision-making concerning an individual patient panel—the freedom to manage a caseload without mandated oversight. CNS, however, demonstrates its independence through leadership and systems innovation, often operating through expert collaboration and consultation across multiple teams. Their goal is to influence the system to empower the bedside nurse's autonomy and improve the quality of care delivered by the organization as a whole [5].

Regulatory Mechanisms: The Global Tools of Control

Health-care systems worldwide utilize specific regulatory mechanisms to deliberately either grant or restrict the scope of Advanced Practice Registered Nurse (APRN) practice. These tools directly define the legally permitted balance between professional autonomy and mandated collaboration. Understanding these mechanisms is crucial, as they determine the functional limits of the APRN role far more than their education or training alone. The most fundamental barriers often relate to the provider's legal recognition and control over pharmaceutical agents [12].

Title Protection and Credentialing

A crucial baseline for granting independence is Title Protection and Credentialing. In many countries, the lack of title protection means a practitioner may use a title such as "Specialist" or "Advanced Practitioner" without meeting a standardized graduate-level education or national certification requirements. To counter this ambiguity, mandatory national certification—often achieved through robust national nursing councils or bodies—is an essential enabler of autonomy. This certification signifies recognized competence beyond basic Registered Nurse licensure, providing standardized proof of readiness required for legislative action toward FPA [11].

The Prescribing Hurdle

Prescriptive authority is arguably the most significant regulatory gatekeeper defining the functional autonomy of the APRN role. Its scope varies across three primary models: Independent Prescribing, which is granted in FPA systems, allowing the APRN full, unsupervised control over the pharmacological aspect of the treatment plan. Collaborative Prescribing requires a documented, often contractual, relationship with a physician. While the APRN may write the vast majority of prescriptions, this mechanism maintains a legally collaborative structure and may impose administrative review requirements [6]. Finally, the No Prescribing Authority model is the most restrictive, limiting the APRN to ordering non-pharmacological diagnostics or treatments and forcing near-constant reliance on physician collaboration for medical management.

Institutional Versus Legislative Authority

A key global tension in APRN regulation lies between the authority granted by legislative authority (a macrolevel law) and that granted by institutional policy (a mesolevel hospital bylaw). In systems where state or national law restricts practice, a hospital can sometimes grant privileges that expand the APRN's scope within its walls (e.g., admitting patients or performing advanced procedures). However, this authority is nonportable; it dissolves if the APRN attempts to work outside that specific institution or establish a private practice. True, portable autonomy, which is essential for increasing access in diverse settings, requires definitive legislative backing [10].

Enhancing Access and Efficiency

The choice to foster autonomy rather than mandate collaboration has immediate, tangible implications for health system performance. FPA and High Autonomy models consistently demonstrate improvements in both access to care and care delivery efficiency. Removing bureaucratic requirements for physician sign-offs on routine orders dramatically streamlines the patient journey, reduces waiting times, and optimizes the full utilization of the highly trained APRN workforce, allowing resources to be deployed where they are needed most without administrative lag [2].

Quality-of-Care Parity

The foundation for removing restrictions rests on the robust evidence of Quality-of-Care Parity. Research consistently and overwhelmingly shows that the care delivered by APRNs, whether autonomously or collaboratively, is equal to or superior to usual care across numerous clinical indicators, particularly in areas such as chronic disease management and adherence to clinical best practices. This evidence strongly supports granting greater autonomy, as many regulatory restrictions are rooted in historical or political concerns about quality that are not supported by contemporary data [3].

Professional Identity and Workforce Retention

The impact extends to workforce stability. Mandated collaboration, particularly when it is perceived as unnecessary and purely administrative supervision, can be a significant professional stressor. This friction contributes to higher burnout rates, lower job satisfaction, and reduced professional efficacy compared to APRNs who practice in FPA environments [2]. When high-performing APRNs are systematically prevented from practicing to their full potential due to bureaucratic barriers, the health-care system loses their unique, specialty-focused contributions, ultimately weakening the overall nursing and clinical leadership pipeline.

The necessity for well-defined roles is critical not just for legal clarity but for system efficacy. By clarifying regulatory tools, systems can move past outdated restrictions and fully integrate APRNs to meet pressing global health challenges.

Conclusion

The difference between mandated collaboration and autonomous practice for Advanced Practice Registered Nurses (APRNs) globally is primarily a function of historical regulatory design and entrenched professional power dynamics, rather than a reflection of demonstrated clinical capability. Extensive evidence confirms that highly educated APRNs—whether they focus on direct patient care as a Nurse Practitioner (NP) or on organizational and systems improvement as a Clinical Nurse Specialist (CNS)—provide high-quality, cost-effective care that is equal or superior to traditional care models [6]. Mandated physician oversight, often misrepresented as necessary "collaboration," introduces administrative friction and restricts access without a corresponding benefit in quality, especially in underserved populations [1].

The ideal global model requires moving away from the zero-sum notion that autonomy must be gained at the expense of collaboration. Instead, successful health-care systems are those that foster a framework of earned autonomy within a culture of interprofessional respect. This means legislators should grant Full Practice Authority (FPA) where appropriate for their system's needs, clearly differentiating the roles of the NP as an independent primary provider and the CNS as an expert system consultant. Crucially, regulations should mandate formal mechanisms for consultation and referral (collaboration) based on genuine patient complexity, rather than requiring unnecessary supervision based merely on the provider's title (restricting autonomy). By aligning legal frameworks with clinical evidence, systems can unlock the full potential of their APRN workforce, ensuring more equitable, efficient, and high-quality care delivery worldwide.

References

1. Akintade B, Indenbaum-Bates K, Idzik S. Sustainable academic-clinical alliance: a model to improve academic-practice partnerships. J Dr Nurs Pract. 2024;17(2):77–85. https://doi.org/10.1891/JDNP-2023-0027.
2. Bryant-Lukosius D, Spichiger E, Martin J, Stoll H, Kellerhals SD, Fliedner M, Grossmann F, Henry M, Herrmann L, Koller A, Schwendimann R, Ulrich A, Weibel L, Callens B, De Geest S. Framework for evaluating the impact of advanced practice nursing roles. J Nurs Scholarsh. 2016;48(2):201–9. https://doi.org/10.1111/jnu.12199.
3. Davis W, Stanley J, Buck M, Walters E, DeGarmo S. LACE and the APRN consensus model: implications for advancing nursing practice. AACN Adv Crit Care. 2024;35(1):20–8. https://doi.org/10.4037/aacnacc2024956.
4. Fedel PR, Pennington G. Clinical nurse specialist collaboration with a community-based palliative care program: an evidence-based practice project. Clin Nurse Spec. 2021;35(2):88–95. https://doi.org/10.1097/NUR.0000000000000581.
5. Gabbard ER, Klein D, Vollman K, Chamblee TB, Soltis LM, Zellinger M. Clinical nurse specialist: a critical member of the ICU Team. Crit Care Med. 2021;49(6):e634–41. https://doi.org/10.1097/CCM.0000000000005004.
6. Harwood KJ, Pines JM, Andrilla CHA, Frogner BK. Where to start? A two-stage residual inclusion approach to estimating the influence of the initial provider on health care utilization and costs for low back pain in the US. BMC Health Serv Res. 2022;22(1):694. https://doi.org/10.1186/s12913-022-08092-1.
7. Kleinpell R, Scanlon A, Hibbert D, DeKeyser Ganz F, East L, Fraser D, Kam Yuet Wong F, Beauchesne M. Addressing issues impacting advanced nursing practice worldwide. Online J Issues Nurs. 2014;19(2):5.
8. Lucciola ME, Nelson NM, Rea JM, Boudreaux AJ, Fedderson DJ, Hodge NS. Clinical nurse specialist impact on COVID-19 preparation at a military treatment facility. Clin Nurse Spec. 2021;35(3):138–46. https://doi.org/10.1097/NUR.0000000000000593.
9. Manning JM. Implications of the future of nursing report on clinical nurse specialists. Clin Nurse Spec. 2022;36(4):179–80. https://doi.org/10.1097/NUR.0000000000000684.
10. Mayo AM, Ray MM, Chamblee TB, Urden LD, Moody R. The advanced practice clinical nurse specialist. Nurs Adm Q. 2017;41(1):70–6. https://doi.org/10.1097/NAQ.0000000000000201.
11. McCleery E, Christensen V, Peterson K, Humphrey L, Helfand M. Evidence brief: the quality of care provided by advanced practice nurses. Department of Veterans Affairs (US); 2014.
12. Meadows AL, Strickland JC, Qalbani S, Conner KL, Su A, Rush CR. Comparing changes in controlled substance prescribing trends by provider type. Am J Addict. 2020;29(1):35–42. https://doi.org/10.1111/ajad.12962.
13. Mohr LD, Coke LA. Distinguishing the clinical nurse specialist from other graduate nursing roles. Clin Nurse Spec. 2018;32(3):139–51. https://doi.org/10.1097/NUR.0000000000000373.
14. Murphy S, Ehritz C. Clinical nurse specialist practice strategies for children with medical complexity. Clin Nurse Spec. 2021;35(1):38–43. https://doi.org/10.1097/NUR.0000000000000567.
15. Petersen PA, Keller T, Way SM, Borges WJ. Autonomy and empowerment in advanced practice registered nurses: lessons from New Mexico. J Am Assoc Nurse Pract. 2015;27(7):363–70. https://doi.org/10.1002/2327-6924.12202.
16. Rice J, Hildebrand A, Waslo CS, Cameron MH, Jones KD. Cannabis for medical purposes: a cross-sectional analysis of health care professionals' knowledge. J Am Assoc Nurse Pract. 2021;34(1):100–6. https://doi.org/10.1097/JXX.0000000000000590.
17. Schirle L, Norful AA, Rudner N, Poghosyan L. Organizational facilitators and barriers to optimal APRN practice: an integrative review. Health Care Manag Rev. 2020;45(4):311–20. https://doi.org/10.1097/HMR.0000000000000229.
18. Schorn MN, Myers C, Barroso J, Hande K, Hudson T, Kim J, Kleinpell R. Results of a national survey: ongoing barriers to APRN practice in the United States. Policy Polit Nurs Pract. 2022;23(2):118–29. https://doi.org/10.1177/15271544221076524.

Is True Clinical Nursing Autonomy Possible?

Demetrius J. Porche

Posing the question "Is true clinical nursing autonomy possible?" is timely. The United States Department of Education (USDOE) has initiated policy statements that could have not only a national but eventually global impact on nursing. The USDOE has proposed the reclassification of nursing with nursing no longer listed as a professional degree educational program. The USDOE uses professional degree programs as a classification system to distinguish among educational programs that qualify for higher financial aid limits. Even though this move was to reclassify educational financial aid loan funding levels, this designation has the potential to impact the public perception of nursing as a professional discipline. This could also serve as a potential distractor of nursing as an acceptable professional discipline for a health-care career [1].

Nursing, Nursing Profession, and Societal Commitment

The International for Nurses (ICN) recognizes nursing as a profession. ICN defines a nurse as "a professional who is educated in the scientific knowledge, skills and philosophy of nursing, and regulated to practice nursing based on established standards of practice and ethical codes." [2] ICN further asserts that a nurse's scope of practice is defined by their educational level, experience, competency, professional standards, and lawful authority in the coordination, supervision of, and delegation to others who may assist in the provision of health-care services [2]. According to the ICN, nurses work autonomously and collaboratively across settings to improve health through advocacy, evidence-based practice, informed decision making, and a

D. J. Porche (✉)
School of Nursing, Louisiana State University Health Sciences Center – New Orleans, New Orleans, LA, USA
e-mail: DPorch@lsuhsc.edu

A. Kapu et al. (eds.), *A Global View on Clinical Autonomy for Advanced Practice Nurses*, Advanced Practice in Nursing,
https://doi.org/10.1007/978-3-032-21458-4_7

culturally safe, therapeutic relationship with the patient, family, and/or community [2].

To further approach this chapter's question, nursing needs to be explored as a professional discipline and nurses as professionals as ICN states. A profession is a specific career identified by a specific body of knowledge. Having a specific body of knowledge in higher education classifies the specific content area as a discipline. As nursing has a specific body of nursing science and knowledge, it should be a considered professional discipline. A professional refers to the individual within and representative of the profession. Professionalism is considered the conduct, attitude, and behaviors associated with a specific profession such as nursing. Higher levels of professionalism can improve a nurses' autonomy, empowerment, increase their recognition, and facilitate organizational citizenship behaviors [3]. A profession has several key defining characteristics that have embedded attitudes, values, and behaviors. These defining key characteristics are as follows:

- Specialized body of knowledge and advanced education and training. A profession is based on specialized theoretical body of knowledge specific to that discipline. Nursing science integrates knowledge from biological, social, behavioral, and ethical sciences through formal educational collegiate programs.
- Authority and autonomy over practice: Nursing as a profession should have the authority to make clinical judgments about nursing practice. Autonomy is considered a distinguishing factor of a profession from a mere occupation. Autonomy is rooted in accountable and self-regulated practice through professional standards and ethics codes.
- Ethical codes and professional standards: A profession maintains a formal ethical code representative of the discipline with the ability to self-regulate and enforce the ethical and professional standards.
- Professional identity and commitment to lifelong learning: Nursing identity is established through professional values and image representation of the discipline.
- Distinct professional role with societal recognition: The public continues to recognize nursing as a distinct profession through established licenses, certification credentials, and a defined legal scope of practice.
- Commitment to public good and society with a service orientation and altruistic commitment: Nursing is grounded in meeting societal needs through the promotion, prevention, treatment, and rehabilitation of health-care alterations [3].

Other authors have identified other defining criteria or standards for nursing professionalism. Miller et al. identified nine standards criteria for professionalism that include educational background; adherence to the code of ethics; participation in a professional organization; continuing education and competency; communication and publication; autonomy and self-regulation; community service; theory use, development, and evaluation, and research involvement [4]. Yuen et al. described nurses professionalism as consisting of five themes—self-concept of the profession, social awareness, professionalism of nursing, roles of nursing services, and originality of nursing [5]. Additionally, Yoder described six components of nursing professionalism. These six components are acting in the patient's best interest, showing humanism, practicing social responsibility, demonstrating sensitivity to people's cultures, values, and beliefs, having high standards of competence and knowledge, and demonstrating high ethical standards [6].

The American Nurses Association's (ANA) Social Policy Statement proposes that there is a social contract between the nursing profession and society. Through this social contract, society grants the nursing profession the authority for the practice of nursing. This social contract proposes what society expects of nursing as well as what society can expect to receive from nursing practice in return. ANA's social contract is the basis of and provides relevance for nursing practice as it outlines the mutual expectations, obligations, and trust that exist between the nursing profession and members of society. There is a synergistic and reciprocal relationship [7].

Several foundational tenets provide the framework for this mutual covenant grounding nursing practice. Foundational tenets are authority over professional standards and practice, a recognized body of knowledge, independent clinical judgment, public accountability, self-regulation, advocacy, and collaboration without subordination [7]. Through this mutual covenant, nursing is expected to create, maintain, and update professional nursing standards of practice and codes of ethics. Nursing is also expected to utilize and discover a scientific body of nursing knowledge that uses nursing theory, research, and clinical evidence to guide the practice of nursing, representing the profession's true praxis. This scientific body of nursing knowledge is used to guide independent clinical judgment [7].

Autonomy Defined

Before approaching the question of "Is true clinical autonomy possible?," we must have a mutual understanding of the meaning of autonomy. According to the Merriam-Webster dictionary, autonomy is defined as a state of being self-governing, having self-directed freedom, or the will of one's actions [8]. Likewise, the ANA's Scope and Standards of Practice describes autonomy as the nurse's ability to act independently and to make appropriate decisions as it relates to control over their own nursing practice [9]. These definitions embrace some aspect of self-control, self-governance, or self-will to act based on independence.

ANA's concept of autonomous practice can further be delineated into professional nursing autonomy and clinical nursing autonomy. In the nursing literature, the words autonomy, professional nursing autonomy and clinical nursing autonomy are frequently used interchangeably. For the purpose of this chapter, these terms will be differentiated. Throughout this chapter, clinical nursing autonomy is considered as a key component of professional nursing practice.

Professional nursing autonomy is essential to empower nursing to have greater decision-making authority over their practice [10]. Professional nursing autonomy enables nurses to make timely decisions regarding a patient's care. These decisions are based on expert judgement from access to a unique body of knowledge coupled with an ethical commitment to patients [11]. Professional nursing autonomy is affected by various factors such as organizational, political, and sociocultural influences. Nurses with professional autonomy exhibit leadership and management skills in the delivery of quality nursing services through clinical reasoning, decision making, and effective professional interactions with other health-care providers/ professionals, patients, and families. Balasi, Hazrati, Ashouri, Ebadi, and Elahi identified that nurses with professional nursing autonomy scored high in all seven dimensions of professional autonomy—professional care, professional mutual respect, professional decision making, leadership role, professional discipline, clinical skills, and critical thinking, except professional mutual respect. These authors state that medical dominance in the clinical setting may have negatively impacted nurses scoring high on the professional autonomy dimension of professional mutual respect [10].

Professional nursing autonomy is concerned with the freedom for action or freedom of will. This practice of professional nursing autonomy requires the nurse to have the capacity for critical analysis that enables them to influence nursing practice [12]. This critical analysis is frequently referred to as critical thinking or clinical reasoning.

Clinical nursing autonomy is grounded in the nurse's ability to make independent decisions directly related to patient care. Essential elements of clinical nursing autonomy are based on the use of clinical judgment or clinical reasoning in an independent manner for the enactment of the nursing process—assessment, planning, implementation/interventions, and evaluation—to improve patient and health-care outcomes.

Other terms identified in the literature associated with autonomous nursing practice are decisional autonomy, prescriptive autonomy, and organizational autonomy. Decisional autonomy is generally directly considered independent clinical judgement in the assessment, diagnosis, and management of health conditions. Prescriptive autonomy is the ability of the nurse, generally an advanced practice nurse, who within their scope of practice has the ability to prescribe medications and other treatments and therapies inclusive of the ordering and interpretation of diagnostic test. Organizational autonomy is more aligned with professional autonomy and refers to the nurse's ability to engage in decision making such a s peer review, work scheduling, and organizational workflow or other processes in the work environment [10, 11].

Determinants of Clinical Nursing Autonomy

The determinants of clinical nursing autonomy are factors known to influence clinical nursing autonomy. Determinants of clinical nursing autonomy are regulatory and licensure-related factors, scope of practice factors, and educational and experiential factors. Regulatory and licensure factors provide a clear statutory guidance through nurse practice acts and protected nursing licensure titles. Scope of practice factors is delineated through professional nursing standards of practice along with the regulatory statutory professional boundaries identified in the respective protected nursing licensure titles through the nurse practice act or other appropriate statutory laws. Lastly, educational factors delineate along with nursing experience, the educational background, and level of nursing knowledge gained through both formal and experiential education. These determinants provide the initial professional boundaries that guide the extent to which the nurse can engage in clinical nursing autonomy [12–14].

Clinical Nursing Autonomy and Independent Nursing Practice: Similarities and Differences

Clinical nursing autonomy has common elements that intersects with independent nursing practice. Independent nursing decision making is frequently considered clinical nursing autonomy as related to direct patient care. However, independent nursing practice is generally referred to in reference to advanced practice nurses as related to their ability to have full practice authority within their respective advanced practice role's scope of practice. When the phrase "independent nursing practice" is used in nursing referring to advanced practice nurses, it refers to the advanced scope of practice that includes independent decision making and clinical reasoning for advanced nursing practice. This advanced nursing practice consists of advanced physical and diagnostic assessment, ordering and interpretation of diagnostic test, prescriptive authority, development, management, and evaluation of treatment plans for acute, chronic, and some complex health conditions, care coordination, collaboration and referral management, and leadership and clinical consultation [14–16].

Independent nursing practice for advanced practice nurses implies limited or no supervision by other health-care professionals such as requiring physician supervision, physician collaborative practice agreements, or contracts as a required component for advanced nursing practice. It also references the nurse or advanced practice nursing's ability to independently own and operate a health-care business practice. Clinical nursing autonomy is frequently subsumed within the concept of independent nursing practice as it is a prerequisite for independent nursing practice. However, there are situations in which clinical nursing authority to practice autonomously and independent nursing practice intersect but are not the same. For example, a nurse may have the legal authority within their scope of practice to perform specific nursing actions (clinical autonomous practice), but institutional policy does not permit the specific actions or restricts that level of autonomous decision making (limited independent practice). Additionally, a nurse may have a high level of perceived clinical nursing autonomy, but the state practice act may limit independent assessment, prescribing, diagnosing, ordering of test, and clinical management.

In summary, some similarities between clinical autonomous practice and independent nursing practice are as follows: both involve independent nursing-driven decision making, require accountability and professional responsibility, support high-level patient-centered care, and grounded in nursing knowledge, science, and the nursing process. A major difference in the use of the terminology clinical autonomous practice and independent nursing practice is that independent nursing practice generally refers to the advanced practice nurse's ability to practice to the fullest scope of authority for their respective role [13, 14].

Models Encompassing Autonomy

A model is a representation of an object, process, systems, or conceptual framework that is used to facilitate a visualization or understanding of theory and/or science. A nursing model is a conceptual or theoretical representation that organizes, guides, and provides a framework for nursing practice. The model defines and explains the interrelationships between the elements of the respective model. In nursing, we utilize models as structured frameworks from which to organize, explain, guide, and teach nursing concepts, principles, theories, and nursing praxis. Nursing models provide a unique perspective or nursing lens from which to view the nursing discipline, including nursing practice. Nursing models can be classified as descriptive in nature, prescriptive or predictive depending on whether the model explains, directs, or forecast into the future nursing actions or patient outcomes [17].

Nursing theorist and academicians developed nursing models as a means to further define nursing as a discipline and develop a theoretical and scientific basis for nursing practice. This foundation of nursing models paved the way for the inclusion of the concept of autonomy into nursing models. The primary purposes of nursing models are as follows:

- To guide clinical practice, inclusive of nursing leadership and management; Nursing models provide a systematic approach that standardizes nursing practice. As a guide, nursing models provide a consistent framework from which to approach nursing practice.
- Defines nursing as a discipline and profession: The nursing perspective and lens articulates the philosophical and theoretical nursing foundations as a unique discipline.
- Support pedagogical perspectives of nursing education and knowledge development: Nursing models serve as a communication and educational tool.
- Advances the discipline through nursing research: Nursing models provide a theoretical or conceptual perspective to guide nursing knowledge development through evidence-based practice or research. Nursing models identify core concepts and relationships among these concepts that support variable selection, research question generation, hypothesis development, and guide methodological designs to advance nursing knowledge, which formulates the scientific discipline of nursing.
- Guide and inform nursing leadership and policy: Nursing models guide leadership decision making and influence the perspectives that influence and frame health policy agendas and policy solutions for nursing practice [17].

Several theoretical and empirical nursing models have been developed to describe autonomous nursing practice. The Professional Practice Model of Autonomy (PPM) conceptualizes nursing autonomy as a structural and cultural component of nursing practice. Within the PPM, nursing autonomy is embedded in governance structures, decision-making processes, professional nursing standards, and relationships within the health-care environment. Key and major concepts of PPMs are independent clinical decision making, shared governance for nursing decision making and empowerment, accountability based on professional nursing standards of practice, interdisciplinary collaboration with the coexistence of autonomy, and professional identity [18].

The Kanter Theory-Based Structural Empowerment Model is not unique to nursing practice but demonstrates how structural conditions can support or restrict clinical autonomy. Major concepts of this model are access to information and knowledge needed to inform decision-making; access to managerial and peer support to facilitate autonomous practice, access to resources that permit independent clinical action, and access to opportunities that enhance a nurses confidence and feeling of empowerment to engage in autonomous practice. This model describes the concept of empowerment which is considered to result in clinically autonomous practice [19].

The Decisional Involvement Model describes how nursing input into decision-making at the unit level and organizational level correlates with greater perceived autonomy of nursing practice and improved patient outcomes. Major concepts of this model are nursing participation in clinical decision-making, participation in administrative decisions, a shared decision-making organizational climate, and nurse-leader partnership. The Decisional Involvement Model categorizes decisions into unit level clinical decisions, unit level operational decisions, and organizational level decisions. These autonomous decisions are rendered through three typical patterns of involvement—traditional, shared, and staff driven. Traditional involvement patterns are decisions rendered by management with low levels of nursing autonomy. Shared involvement patterns exhibit high autonomy with nurses and leaders sharing decision making. Lastly, staff-driven involvement patters have the highest level of autonomy with nurses leading decision making independently [20].

The Autonomy and Accountability Model (AAM) focuses on autonomy as a combination of clinical independence and professional accountability. Autonomous nursing practice is enabled through internal (competence driven) and external (structural and legal) conditions. The three major concepts of this model are clinical independence in the assessment, planning, implementation, and evaluation of nursing care without direct oversight and supervision; professional accountability as an obligation to provide evidenced-based ethical care; clinical expertise and competence through specialized nursing knowledge; and trust provided to nurses by other health-care providers, patients, families, and the organization [21].

Nurses are considered the most trusted health-care professional. This trust granted by society is a result of nursing being considered an ethical profession. The Ethical Autonomy Model conceptualizes autonomy not only as a form of independent practice but as an ethical duty. In this model, nurses are expected to act independently to ensure the health, welfare, and safety of patients. Major concepts of this model are patient advocacy through autonomous nursing actions, moral agency that informs independent ethical reasoning, and professional nursing values of respect for human dignity, justice, and beneficence. These professional nursing values influence and guide autonomous nursing practice decisions and choices of action [22].

The Magnet Model developed by the American Nurses Credentialing Center considers autonomy as a central force of magnetism. Other major concepts of magnetism are transformational leadership, empowered structural environment, exemplary professional practice, and new knowledge and innovations. Research on the forces of magnetism, which includes autonomous nursing practice is associated with higher patient satisfaction, lower mortality rates, and improved nursing retention [23].

Nursing Shared Governance Model (SGM) is a collaborative decision-making model that grants the opportunity for frontline practicing nurses along with nursing leaders and managers to partner to manage nursing practice, quality of care, and patient care outcomes. The SGM is considered a practice model in which nurses "have voice" and are considered to "own" their practice. In the SGM, nurses share authority to develop, implement, and evaluate policies, practice standards, evidence-based practice, translate research findings, and provide leadership oversight for continued nursing professional development. [23, 24] Health-care environments that adopt an SGM of practice typically align with the nursing core values of autonomy, accountability, empowerment, collaboration, and respect.

In an SGM practice model, organizational structures support and facilitate the empowerment of autonomous nursing decision making. Organizational structures vary but frequently have unit-based councils, central or organizational level councils, and executive level councils. Unit-based councils (e.g., intensive care unit, medical-surgical nursing) engage frontline nurses in shared decision-making processes that impact patient care, which is representative of clinical nursing autonomous practice. Unit based councils not only develop and implement unit-based policies but also identify policies to be considered for institution wide implementation. The central or organizational level council is frequently referred to as a Professional Practice and Quality Council. This level of council promotes representation of the other unit-based councils into policies and procedures that impact institutional wide policy. The central or organizational level council develops system-wide policy. The executive council includes nurses with formal leadership and management titles along with front-line nurses from the unit-based and central or organizational level council into one executive decision-making council [23–25]. SGM embraces shared principles of partnership, equity, ownership, accountability, and democratic decision making. Within SGM, there is a commitment to evidence-based practice, nursing research, quality improvement, and professional nursing development.

Autonomy Measurement

Clinical nursing autonomy as a nursing concept or nursing practice phenomenon can be further explicated through nursing measurement. Nursing phenomena and concepts of practice with a well-defined psychometrically sound research instrument have the potential to advance the discipline of nursing and document clinical autonomy's contribution to high-quality nursing care. Nursing measurement instruments provide a systematic and objective method to capture conceptual domains and subdomains to identify the contribution of phenomena such as clinical autonomy and builds a robust empirical foundation for nursing practice. Further, instruments that measure the phenomena of clinical autonomy presents empirical evidence to answer the question posed in this chapter, "Is true clinical nursing autonomy possible?" Utilization of reliable and valid instruments measuring clinical autonomy provide data to document the existence of clinical autonomy and also provides a consistent and stable measure to detect changes in clinical autonomy over time, as well as determine the relationship of clinical autonomy to patient outcomes [26].

The following are instruments or tools that can be utilized to measure various dimensions of autonomy. A brief summary of these instruments is provided:

- Dempster Practice Behaviors Scale (DPBS): The Dempster practice behavior scale measures professional autonomy through behaviors that reflect independent decision making, advocacy, and practice ownership. This is a 30-item instrument with Likert-type scales. The instrument measures domains of professional advocacy, collegial relationships, decision-making authority, patient advocacy, and self-regulation. The instrument has been valid with Registered Nurses and Advanced Practice Nurses in the United States with a Cronbach alpha of 0.89 and subscales ranging from 0.74 to 0.86. [27]
- Schutzenofer Professional Nursing Autonomy Scale (SPNAS): The Schutzenhofer Professional Nursing Autonomy Scale measures a nurse's perceived autonomy in clinical practice. This is a 30-item instrument with Likert-type scales. The instrument measures the domains of autonomy in clinical decision making, control over practice, and influence in professional nursing issues. The instrument has been used in multiple countries with a Cronbach's alpha of 0.89–0.85. [28]
- Kramer and Schmalenberg's Autonomy Subscale of the Essentials of Magnetism Instrument (EOM II): The Essentials of Magnetism Instrument is designed to examine the Magnet hospital environment. Within this instrument, there is a subscale that measures clinical autonomy. This clinical autonomy subscale focuses on clinical decision making without physician oversight, scope of independent practice, and organizational support for autonomy. The subscale consists of 8 items within the 58-item instrument. The Cronbach alpha for the autonomy subscale is between 0.85 and 0.88. [29]
- Blegen's Autonomy Scale: The Blegen's Autonomy Scale measures the nurses' perception of autonomy within their respective role. The instrument consists of 12 Likert-type items that measures the domains of practice independence, policy influence, and control over work schedule. The Cronbach alpha is 0.82. [30]

- Decisional Involvement Scale (DIS): The Decisional Involvement Scale measures the nurse's participation in decision making at the unit and organizational level. This is a 30-item Likert scale validated in multiple nursing settings and internationally. The instrument measures the domains of clinical decision making, quality improvement, strategic/organizational planning, and professional standards. The Cronbach alpha is 0.91. [31]
- Autonomy Scale of the Revised Nursing Work Index (NWI-R). The Revised Nursing Work Index has 57 items, of which 15 measure the subscale of autonomy. The instrument measures the autonomy domains of freedom in decision making, authority over nursing care processes, and collaboration with medical staff. The instrument has been validated internationally with a Cronbach alpha of 0.78–084 for the autonomy scale [32];
- Autonomy Items of the Casey-Fink Nurse Retention Survey: The Casey-Fink Nurse Retention Survey has about 5 items that measure autonomy. The autonomy scale has predictive autonomy scale of retention. These items focus on the autonomy domains of decision-making authority, professional independence, and confidence in practice. The autonomy items have a Cronbach alpha of about 0.80. [33]
- Job Autonomy Scale of the Work Design Questionnaire: The Job Autonomy Scale is not specific to nursing practice. This scale measures general job autonomy and has been applied in nursing research studies. It consists of a 3-item scale with a Cronbach alpha reliability of 0.91–0.93 [34].

The measurement of clinical autonomy can be captured through the autonomy of practice with regulatory indices, practice surveys, and organizational metrics. The measurement of the nursing phenomenon of clinical nursing autonomy is necessary to empirically document findings to support a positive response to the generative question of this chapter, "Is true clinical nursing autonomy possible?"

Autonomy, Nursing Practice, and Magnet Health-Care Environments

Clinical nursing autonomy is consistently reported as an essential cornerstone of excellent magnet health-care environments [35]. Nurses who work in magnet-designated hospitals consistently report healthier work environments, which include the opportunity and support for autonomous clinical practice. In these work environments, nurses are provided the freedom to make decisions about their patient's health-care needs. In the clinical setting, autonomous clinical decision making consists of both independent and interdependent decision making, depending on one's professional scope of practice.

True clinical autonomy is afforded in the clinical setting when the nurse has the ability to and support to practice to the highest scope of their licensure as regulated by their respective licensing board, both at the Registered Nurse (RN) and Advanced Practice Nursing (APN) level. Nursing competence has been associated with autonomous decision making [35]. Nursing can still maintain clinical autonomy through interdependent decision making that is out of their scope of practice through the practice of clinical collaboration while maintaining their respective decision-making boundary for their own practice within their legal scope. It is also important to note that clinical nursing autonomy may be permitted by the state regulatory board, but institutional policy can further limit this scope of practice, thereby diminishing the level of clinical nursing autonomy. The Institute of Medicine (IOM) support higher levels of clinical nursing autonomy. The IOM recommends that higher levels of clinical nursing autonomy be given to nurses so that nurses are trusted and supported in using evidence-based practice initiatives to make patient care decisions [36].

Nursing Autonomy, Patient, and Health-Care Outcomes

There is a growing body of empirical knowledge generated through research that demonstrates the consistent relationship between clinical nursing autonomy and improved nursing, patient, and health-care outcomes. Rao, Kumar, and Mc Hugh conducted a large cross-sectional multihospital secondary data analysis demonstrating the relationship between hospital-level nurse autonomy and patient outcomes from 570 United States hospitals and inpatient surgical discharge records. These authors reported greater nurse autonomy was associated with substantially lower odds of a 30-day mortality and failure-to-rescue. This emphasizes that increased nursing autonomy is directly related to improved patient survival outcomes [37]. Similarly, another multisite study reported that the nursing practice environment, which included autonomy and control over nursing practice, was associated with better outcomes. In this study, Aiken, Clarke, Sloan, Lake, and Cheney reported that better practice environments with greater nursing input and autonomy was associated with lower patient mortality and failure-to-rescue, and better nursing job outcomes of less burnout and lower intent to leave the institution [38].

The impact of autonomous nursing practice and nurse practice environment has also been associated with patient safety. Olds et al. in a cross-sectional study of 600 hospitals and about 853,000 surgical patients reported that predictive roles of nurse work environment and patient safety climate impacted patient mortality. This study demonstrated that a nurse practice environment with nursing autonomy and a patient safety climate was associated with about an 8% reduction in the odds of patient mortality. This study emphasized the importance of organizational environments to support nursing autonomy with a culture toward patient safety as a means to influence patient survival [39]. Similarly, Yuk and Yu conducted a cross-sectional study of nursing working in Magnet hospitals. This study reported that professional autonomy was the strongest predictor of nurses' engagement in patient safety activities with the work environment also being a significant predictor of patient safety [40].

In summary, the investment in nursing autonomy has been directly associated with improved patient and health-care outcomes. In addition, this investment in nursing autonomy is also associated with improved nursing satisfaction at work, nursing retention, and improved intent to stay in the current employment arrangement. The implementation of organizational structural changes that promote nursing autonomy warrants the attention of health-care leaders.

Prerequisites to True Clinical Nursing Autonomy

Nursing leadership and management support and sanctioning of clinical autonomy is necessary for autonomous nursing practice. However, nursing competence is a necessary prerequisite for clinical nursing autonomy. Nursing leaders and managers provide the opportunities for nurses to maintain and advance their knowledge base. In addition to providing opportunities for nurses to gain exquisite competence through knowledge, nursing leaders and managers must communicate a culture and climate of trust that empowers nurses to function in an autonomous manner. The practice of clinically autonomous nursing must have established organizational rewards systems in place that perpetuate the culture and climate of a trusted environment toward patient safety through clinically autonomous practice [18].

An Italian study of newly licensed nurses identified that self-confidence positively influences nursing performance. A newly licensed nurse's confident attitude was also reported to reduce stress and anxiety, leading to better mental health and job satisfaction among nursing workers. The nurse's self-perceived confidence is directly associated with the nurse's perceived clinical autonomy [41].

Nurse's clinical autonomy is also based on a prerequisite skill of clinical reasoning. Clinical reasoning is considered a cognitive process used to collect and interpret clinical data related to a patient's condition, thereby rendering a clinical decision. Clinical reasoning is thought to be based on critical thinking influences. Communication skills are a critical element of clinical reasoning. A nurse's communication competence is a vital skill directly linked to their clinical reasoning. A nurse's clinical reasoning ability and communication competence are related to the nurse's professional autonomy. In summary, communication competence, clinical reasoning, and professional nursing autonomy are crucial competencies for nursing practice. Communication competence is also associated with higher job satisfaction, and higher job satisfaction is associated with higher professional nursing autonomy [42].

Advanced Practice Nursing and Clinical Nursing Autonomy

Advanced practice nursing roles with nursing title protection are nurse practitioner, certified registered nurse anesthetist, certified nurse midwife, and clinical nurse specialist [15]. The United States accounts for over half a million advanced practice nurses. Globally, about 62% of the countries report the existence of advanced practice nursing roles. There is no global reporting system that documents the number of title-protected advance practice nurses in the world. However, there appears to be a global policy trend with more countries adopting advanced practice nursing roles and expanding clinical nursing autonomy [43].

As an advanced practice nurse, the APN clinical nursing autonomy consists of advanced education, knowledge, and experience that has a differentiated clinical responsibility within the realm of clinical diagnosis and treatment using interventions within the medical realm. Specifically, APN must develop a deeper level of clinical decision making and clinical autonomy. Lockwood & Schober reported that intrinsic motivators that supported nurse practitioners in providing innovative healthcare consisted of competence, relatedness, and clinical nursing autonomy [44]. Additionally, Lockwood, Lehwaldt, Sweeney, and Matthew's reported that an advanced practice nurse's ability to bounce back from clinical challenges could impact their ability to practice clinical nursing autonomy [45].

The International Council of Nurses (ICN) reports that throughout history, there has been the continued evolution of the nursing profession as a means to address the health, societal, and person-centered challenges [46]. ICN recognizes that advanced practice nursing refers to "enhanced and expanded healthcare services and interventions provided by nurses who, in an advanced capacity, influence clinical healthcare outcomes and provide direct services to individuals, families, and communities (pg. 9) [46]. Further, ICN recognizes that the "degree and range of judgement, skill, knowledge, responsibility, autonomy, and accountability broadens and takes on additionally extensive range between the preparation of a generalist nurse and that of the APN" (pg. 9) [46].

ICN identifies similarities that exist between the clinical nurse specialists and nurse practitioner advanced practice nursing roles. These similarities consist of

- Minimum of a master's educational degree.
- Autonomous and accountable practice at an advanced level.
- Provision of safe and competent patient care within their respective role.
- Hold a generalized nursing qualification as their foundation.
- Have measurable roles at an increased level of clinical competence.
- Acquired an ability to apply theoretical and clinical skills at an advanced practice nursing level using research, education, leadership, and diagnostic clinical skills.
- Have definite competencies and standards of practice.
- Influenced by global, social, political, economic, and technological advancements.
- Recognize their limitations and maintain clinical competence through continued nursing professional development.
- Have and adhere to an ethical code of conduct.
- Provide holistic care.
- Are recognized through a system of credentialing [46].

Conclusion

Autonomy enabling organizational and professional structures along with leadership and management best practices are necessary to promote clinical nursing autonomy. Clinical nursing autonomy should be considered contextual in nature, political, and relational. There will continue to be organizational polices, structures, practices, and power hierarchies that impact clinical nursing autonomy. These can be mitigated through mutually respectful relationships among nursing colleagues, leaders/managers, physicians, and other health-care providers.

In conclusion, it is proposed that true clinical nursing autonomy is in existence and is possible to continue in the future. The continued existence of true clinical nursing autonomy can be supported by the following recommendations:

- Nursing research should continue to develop psychometrically sound instruments/tools that measure the concepts of professional nursing autonomy, clinical nursing autonomy, and independent nursing practice.
- Nursing research priorities should focus on demonstrating the relationships and impact of clinical nursing autonomy on health-care system and patient outcomes.
- Health-care organizations and institutions should develop leadership, management and operational organizational structures, and processes that support professional nursing practice models inclusive of a shared governance framework.
- Nurses must engage in continued professional nursing development to build their self-confidence and build their level of clinical competence.
- Nurses must be engaged in advocacy and policy making that supports structures and processes of clinical nursing autonomy at the institutional, local, state, and national levels.
- Nursing must refer to its specific body of knowledge as nursing knowledge and science.
- Nurse educators should differentiate nursing knowledge and science during the education of nursing students to inform students of our unique body of knowledge.
- Clinical competence, communication skills, and interprofessional collaboration are supportive and not limiting factors to maintaining clinical nursing autonomy.
- Nursing should continue to reference itself as a professional discipline regardless of the political and policy rhetoric emerging for financial reasoning.
- Nursing should continue to strive to be the most trusted profession as this provides our societal mandate for clinical nursing autonomy.

References

1. United States Department of Education. Myth vs fact: the definition of professional degrees. November 24, 2025. Accessed on November 29, 2025. https://www.ed.gov/about/news/press-release/myth-vs-fact-definition-of-professional-degrees.
2. International Council of Nurses (ICN). Current nursing definitions. 2025. Available from: https://www.icn.ch/resources/nursing-definitions/current-nursing-definitions.
3. Zhang Y, et al. What is nursing professionalism? A concept analysis. BMC Nurs. 2023;22:34.
4. Miller B, Adams D, Beck L. A behavioral inventory for professionalism in nursing. J Prof Nurs. 1993;9:5.
5. Yeun E, Kwon Y, Ahn O. Development of a nursing professional values scale. Raegan Kanho Hakhoe Chi. 2005;35(6):1091. https://doi.org/10.4040/jkan.2005.35.6.1091.
6. Yoder L. Professionalism in nursing. Med-Surg Nurses. 2017;26:5.

7. American Nurses Association (ANA). Guide to nursing' social policy statement: understanding the profession from social contact to social covenant. American Nurses Association; 2015.
8. Merriam-Webster. Autonomy. Merriam-Webster.com Dictionary. HTTPS://www.merriam-Webster.com/dictionary/autonomy. Accessed 27 Nov 2025.
9. American Nurses Association (ANA). Nursing: scope and standards of practice. 4th ed. American Nurses Association; 2021.
10. Balasi L, Hazrati M, Ashouri A, Ebadi A, Elahi N. The status of professional autonomy and its predictors in clinical nursing in Iran. Nurs Open. 2023;11:e700.11. https://doi.org/10.1002/nop2.70011.
11. Traynor M, Boland M, Buus N. Professional autonomy in 21st century healthcare: nurses' accounts of clinical decision-making. Soc Sci Med. 2010;71:1506–12.
12. Laperriere H. Developing professional autonomy in advanced nursing practice: the critical analysis of sociopolitical variables. Int J Nurs Pract. 2008;14:391–7. https://doi.org/10.1111/j.1440-172X.2008.00700.x.
13. American Association of Nurse Practitioners (AANP). Nurse practitioner scope of practice. 2023.
14. National Council of State Boards of Nursing (NCSBN). APRN consensus model. Chicago: NCSBN; 2020.
15. National Council of State Boards of Nursing (NCSBN). Legal/regulatory authority for independent practice. In: NCSBN APRN consensus model for APRN regulation: licensure, accreditation, certification & education. Chicago: NCSBN; 2008.
16. American Academy of Nurse Practitioners. Issues at a glance: full practice authority. Washington, DC: AANP; 2023.
17. Alligood MR. Nursing theorists and their work (10). 2021. St. Louis: Elsevier.
18. Kramer M, Schmalenberg C. Development and evaluation of a professional practice model. Nurs Adm Q. 2008;32(4):264–73.
19. Laschinger H, Finegan J, Shamian J, Wilk P. Impact of structural and psychological empowerment on job strain in nursing work settings. J Nurs Adm. 2001;31(5):260–72.
20. Havens D, Warshawksy N, Vasey J. The nursing practice environment in rural hospitals: practice environment scale of the nursing work index. Nurs Res. 2012;61(1):18–25.
21. Skar R. The meaning of autonomy in nursing practice. J Clin Nurs. 2010;19(15–16):2226–34.
22. Rodney P, Varcoe C, Storch J. Ethics in health care: a Canadian focus. In: Toward a moral horizon. 2nd ed. Toronto: Pearson; 2013.
23. American Nurses Credentialing Center (ANCC). Magnet recognition program manual. Silver Spring, MD: ANCC; 2023.
24. Graystone R. The value of magnet® recognition. J Nurs Adm. 2019 Oct;49(10S Suppl):S1–3.
25. O'May F, Buchanan J. Shared governance: a literature review. Int J Nurs Stud. 1999;36(4):281–300.
26. Waltz C, Strickland O, Lenz E. Measurement in nursing and health research. Springer Publishing Company; 2016.
27. Dempster, J. A study of the relationship between professional autonomy and selected characteristics of BSN and ADN graduates. Dissertation: George Mason University.
28. Schutzenhofer K. The measurement of professional autonomy. J Prof Nurs. 1983;1(4):230–7.
29. Kramer M, Schmalenberg C. Magnet hospital staff nurse describe clinical autonomy. Nurs Outlook. 2003;51(1):13–9.
30. Blegen M, Mueller C. Nurses' job satisfaction: a longitudinal study analysis. Res Nurs Health. 1987;10(3):227–37.
31. Havens D, Vasey J. Measuring staff nurse decisional involvement: the decisional involvement scale. J Nurs Adm. 2003;33(6):331–6.
32. Aiken L, Patrician P. Measuring organizational traits of hospitals: the revised nursing work index. Nurs Res. 2000;49(3):146–53.
33. Casey K, Fink R, Krugman M, Propst J. The graduate nurse experience. J Nurs Adm. 2004;34(6):303–11.
34. Breaugh J. The measurement of work autonomy. Hum Relat. 1985;38(6):551–70.

35. Schmalenberg C, Kramer M, Brewer B, et al. Clinically competent peers and support for education: structures and practices that work. Crit Care Nurse. 2008;28(4):54–65.
36. Institute of Medicine of the National Academies. Keeping patients safe: transforming the work environment of nurses. Washington, DC: National Academies Press; 2004.
37. Rao A, Kumar A, Mc Hugh M. Better nurse autonomy decreases the odds of 30-day mortality and failure-to-rescue. J Nurs Scholarsh. 2017;49(1):73–9. https://doi.org/10.1111/jnu.12267.
38. Aiken L, Clarke S, Sloan D, Lake E, Cheney T. Effects of hospital care environment on patient mortality and nurse outcomes. J Nurs Adm. 2008;38(5):223–9.
39. Olds D, Aiken L, Cimiotti J, Lake E. Association of nurse work environment and safety climate on patient mortality: a cross-sectional study. Int Nurs Stud. 2017;74:155–61. https://doi.org/10.1016/j.ijnurstu.2017.06.004.
40. Yuk S, Yu S. The effect of professional autonomy and nursing work environment on nurses' patient safety activities: a perspective on magnet hospitals. J Nurs Manag. 2023; https://doi.org/10.1155/2023/55875.01.
41. Stirparo G, Di Fronzo P, Sulla D, Bottignole D, Gambolo L. Are Italian newly licensed nurses ready? A study on self-perceived clinical autonomy in critical care scenarios. Healthcare. 2024;12:809. https://doi.org/10.3390/healthcare12080809.
42. Noh S, Kang Y. The relationships among communication competence, professional autonomy and clinical reasoning competence in oncology nurses. Nurs Open. 2024;11:e70003. https://doi.org/10.1002/nop2.70003.
43. World Health Organization (WHO). State of the world's nursing 2025. WHO News Release, May 12, 2025.
44. Lockwood E, Schober M. Factors influencing the impact of nurse practitioner's clinical autonomy: a self determining perspective. Int Nurs Rev. 2024;71:375–95. https://doi.org/10.1111/inr.12948.
45. Lockwood E, Lehwaldt D, Sweeney M, Matthew's A. An exploration of the levels of clinical autonomy of advanced nurse practitioners: a narrative literature review. Int J Nurs Pract. 2022;28:e12978. https://doi.org/10.1111/ijn.12978.
46. International Council for Nurses (ICN). Guidelines on advanced practice nursing. Geneva: ICN; 2020.

Enhancing Patient Care Through Clinical Autonomy: Evidence from International Studies

Emma Clark

Introduction and Setting the Context

Advanced Practice Nurses (APNs), including nurse practitioners (NPs), nurse-midwives (NMs), clinical nurse specialists (CNSs), and nurse anesthetists, are increasingly recognized as critical contributors to patient care and health system performance globally. Health systems in low-, middle-, and high-income countries alike continue to grapple with workforce shortages, rising chronic disease burdens, including mental health needs, and persistent inequities in who can access care and the quality of care they receive. APNs offer a scalable, cost-effective, globally applicable solution for these challenges by expanding access to comprehensive, patient-centered care [1]. Interest in APNs has been further accelerated by global health movements such as Universal Health Coverage (UHC) [2] and the Sustainable Development Goals (SDGs) [3]. Acute system shocks such as the COVID-19 pandemic, epidemics such as Ebola and Mpox, and humanitarian disasters have been accompanied by calls to "build back better," [2] including investing in cadres of APNs who are equipped to facilitate an improved health system response [4].

The World Health Organization's *State of the World's Nursing 2025* publication reported a total of 104 countries (62% of those providing a response to the 2024 National Health Workforce Accounts) having advanced practice roles for nurses. The report recommended that APN roles be further developed to increase access to high-quality health services, including addressing an identified need for the APN role, gaining acceptance by ministries of health, and fostering collaboration between ministries of health, educational institutions, regulators, and employers [5]. Despite this growing recognition of how APNs can advance patient, system, and global goals, APN roles vary widely across countries. Significant differences exist in

E. Clark (✉)
Georgetown University, Washington, DC, USA
e-mail: evc8@georgetown.edu

A. Kapu et al. (eds.), *A Global View on Clinical Autonomy for Advanced Practice Nurses*, Advanced Practice in Nursing,
https://doi.org/10.1007/978-3-032-21458-4_8

educational preparation, regulatory frameworks, scopes of practice, and degree of integration into health systems [6]. While some nations have long-established, strong, independent APN cadres, others are still in nascent stages of role definition and/or have restrictive policies limiting independent practice in place. Inconsistent global support and guidance on the APN role are likely contributing factors to the significant variation in the APN role worldwide.

Clinical autonomy, or the authority to independently perform clinical tasks such as assessment, diagnosis, ordering tests, prescribing medications, and managing treatment plans across full episodes of evidence-based patient care, is fundamental for APNs to fully leverage their advanced training and expertise [7]. The global evidence base increasingly demonstrates that higher levels of clinical autonomy for APNs correlate with improved health service delivery outcomes, including enhanced access to care, better chronic disease management, increased patient satisfaction, and fewer unnecessary hospitalizations [7–9]. However, like the APN role definition more broadly, clinical autonomy varies widely between countries. Legal and regulatory restrictions, or limited or absent regulation, may constrain APNs' ability to autonomously practice to the full scope of their training [10]. Even in countries with enabling legislation, APN autonomy faces challenges, including hierarchical health systems, institutional policies, sociocultural norms, and interprofessional tensions that may curtail autonomy. These factors can undermine workforce morale and retention while limiting the health system's capacity to expand APN roles [11, 12].

Countries considering reforms to support APN clinical autonomy as part of role development can draw valuable lessons from diverse international experiences. High-income countries (HICs) such as the United States (U.S.), Canada, Australia, and the United Kingdom (UK) have APNs working with varying degrees of autonomy across levels of care (e.g., primary, secondary, specialty) and settings (e.g., rural, urban) [13–15]. This includes the U.S., where a patchwork of state-level regulations ranges from full practice authority to highly restricted practice. This provides a natural experiment for assessing how autonomy influences care quality and workforce outcomes, and research on this topic has consistently demonstrated a positive correlation between full-scope practice (which generally includes substantial clinical autonomy) and patient outcomes [16–18]. Meanwhile, in recent years, the UK and Australia have implemented legislative reforms in recent years, expanding prescribing rights and autonomous decision-making for APNs with demonstrable benefits for maternal and child health and chronic disease management [19–21]. However, in some settings, such as rural Australia, evidence for the benefits of APNs is limited [22]; this is discussed in additional detail in the section on barriers below.

In other HICs, such as the Netherlands and Scandinavian countries, some autonomous APN roles, particularly midwifery, have long been relatively well-integrated into health system structures. This is associated with favorable patient outcomes and efficient service delivery. In the Netherlands, midwifery-led care is embedded in a tiered maternity system, and population-based studies report comparable or better outcomes; low-risk women receiving midwife-led intrapartum care versus obstetrician-led care at the onset of labor, with no excess in severe maternal morbidity or perinatal mortality, and with lower intervention rates that support efficient resource use [23, 24]. Dutch primary care increasingly utilizes APNs, and research has shown clinically appropriate case management and high stakeholder acceptance, evidence that clinical autonomous APN roles can maintain quality while addressing workforce pressures [25]. In Sweden, recent studies have linked midwifery care and expanded midwifery responsibilities to positive experiences of care, practical support for complex social and mental health needs, and enhanced trust and engagement among patients and their families [26–28]. Evidence from these mature systems highlights regulated prescriptive authority, advanced decision-making, and defined accountability as key design features of APN integration. As such, these systems provide excellent models for introducing or expanding APN roles in primary and specialized fields, such as mental health nursing, with a focus on system efficiency, interdisciplinary collaboration, and patient-centered care [6].

In low- and middle-income countries (LMICs), the APN role is more nascent, with ongoing efforts to develop autonomous APN cadres in countries such as Kenya, South Africa, Eswatini, India, Thailand, the Philippines, Jamaica, Haiti, Indonesia, and Botswana [1, 29–31]. The relationship between clinical autonomy and patient outcomes in resource-limited settings is particularly crucial. Many of these settings emphasize task shifting and role expansion to address critical gaps in maternal and child health, emergency care, and primary care in underserved rural areas with low physician density [32–34]. Despite limited formal regulatory frameworks, these APNs often operate with a high degree of de facto autonomy, making their experiences relevant for resource-constrained health systems [35, 36]. For example, midwife-led autonomous care models have demonstrated reductions in maternal and neonatal mortality, lower cesarean section rates, and enhanced respectful maternity care, supporting global efforts to improve maternal and newborn health outcomes [37, 38].

This chapter synthesizes international evidence on how clinical autonomy among APNs impacts patient care outcomes. Ultimately, clinical autonomy is not simply a guaranteed professional privilege. Instead, it is a structural enabler of high-quality, equitable, and resilient health systems that drive improved patient outcomes. As countries aim to optimize health workforce strategies, fostering and sustaining APN autonomy must be a priority to ensure accessible, effective care for diverse populations. The international evidence discussed below provides a wealth of insights into how countries can learn from the successes–and challenges–of other countries.

Relevant Conceptual Frameworks for Understanding Autonomy and Patient Care Outcomes

Several commonly used health system frameworks can be used to understand the relationship between clinical autonomy and patient outcomes, which can be useful for interpreting international evidence for clinical autonomy. These include Donabedian's structure–process–outcome model [39], the WHO's health system building blocks [40], and the Institute of Medicine's (IOM) six domains of healthcare quality [41]. These frameworks provide distinct yet complementary lenses for considering the complex interplay between provider authority and health system performance.

- The Donabedian model looks at how relationships between underlying structures and care processes affect outcomes and the pathways through which autonomy as a structural attribute translates into clinical actions and patient health [39].
- The WHO framework situates clinical autonomy within the broader health system, emphasizing the blocks that can enable or constrain the authority of APNs [40].
- The IOM domains focus on the qualitative attributes of care influenced by autonomy (safety, effectiveness, patient-centeredness, timeliness, efficiency, and equity), linking provider scope-of-practice directly to care quality [41].

Together, these frameworks highlight that APN autonomy is not simply a regulatory or professional scope-of-practice issue but an integral component of health system functionality and equity.

The Donabedian Structure–Process–Outcome Model

The Donabedian model uses a triad of constructs to conceptualize health care quality: structure, process, and outcome [39]. The structural construct describes the overall care context. Actual care delivery occurs under the processes construct and includes diagnosis, treatment, and patient management. The outcomes construct refers to the measurable effects of healthcare, such as morbidity, mortality, and patient satisfaction. In this model, the structural measures influence process measures, which in turn affect outcome measures. While Avedis Donabedian himself was the first to admit that the quality of care is far from simplistic, his model nonetheless provides a valuable, straightforward, and long-lasting framework to consider diverse healthcare performance topics [42].

In the case of clinical autonomy, the Donabedian model links the regulatory frameworks and organizational policies that define the degree of APN authority, determining whether APNs may diagnose, prescribe, and manage care independently or under supervision. These structural factors influence care processes by enabling or limiting timely clinical decisions, diagnostic testing, and treatment initiation, all of which have notable effects on patient outcomes. Kenya provides an excellent example of how this framework can be applied. Under the 2010 constitution, devolution, or the process of delegating more power from the Kenyan central government to county governments, created new county-level governance structures [43]. These new structures substantially changed the "structure" components of healthcare delivery by enabling organizational adaptations in workforce capacity and regulation. Counties were able to expand clinical duties and informal task-shifting in response to workforce shortage and resource constraints. This, in turn, allowed nurses and midwives, often in senior or shift-leader roles, to exercise greater autonomy in clinical tasks such as triage, diagnosis, and care initiation, key "process" mechanisms that bypassed centralized bottlenecks and navigated constrained work environments. Examples of functions provided outside traditional roles include nutritional counselling or even limited prescribing in the absence of physicians [44]. One qualitative study among critical care nurses in rural Kenya confirmed that autonomy enables them to deploy professional knowledge effectively, increasing provider agency and responsiveness [45]. These "structural" and "process" changes have corresponded with measurable "outcomes". For example, nurse-led HIV care services at Kenyan health facilities were significantly associated with quality of care, including a considerably higher comprehensive patient retention rate 12 months after enrollment in care [46]. Kenya is also using a stakeholder-driven process to develop nurse-sensitive indicators, which will better demonstrate the unique contributions of nurses to patient outcomes [47]. In this example, the Donabedian model clarifies how shifts in governance and institutional structure in Kenya unlocked new processes of autonomy, which in turn have begun to translate into improved care continuity, responsiveness, and overall quality.

WHO Health System Building Blocks

The WHO health system building blocks framework is a widely used tool for understanding how six core components or "building blocks" of health systems interact to shape service delivery and outcomes: service delivery, health workforce, health information systems, access to essential medicines and technologies, financing, and leadership/governance [40]. This framework highlights that clinical autonomy is not just an individual professional attribute but a function of all system blocks and adjustments across multiple building blocks are likely necessary to lead to a degree of change sufficient to influence processes of care and ultimately patient outcomes.

- **Service delivery:** Autonomy for APNs to manage clinics, initiate treatment, and provide continuity of care, improving efficiency and patient-centeredness.
- **Health workforce:** Scope of practice reforms to expand decision-making authority, allowing APNs to substitute or complement physician roles in underserved settings.
- **Health information systems:** Independent use of patient data and decision-support tools allowing APNs to act without waiting for supervisory approval, reducing delays in care.
- **Access to medicines and technologies:** Prescribing rights for APNs, or authority to initiate diagnostic tests, to ensure timely initiation of therapy.
- **Financing:** Reimbursement mechanisms that recognize nurse-led services to create incentives for autonomous practice and sustainability of expanded roles.
- **Leadership and governance:** National regulations granting prescribing authority or clinical independence to formally institutionalize clinical autonomy across the health system.

Ghana has been implementing its Community-based Health Planning and Services (CHPS) strategy as national policy since 1999, following a successful pilot that promoted universal health coverage, even in remote areas. Rural CHPS compounds rely heavily on trained nurses and midwives as frontline providers and often serve as the sole clinical contact for remote populations where physician density is lowest [48]. In many CHPS zones, clinicians exercise substantial day-to-day clinical independence (e.g., assessment, syndromic diagnosis, protocol-guided prescribing/dispensing from the essential medicines list, and management of uncomplicated deliveries). This pattern functions as de facto autonomy even where formal role definitions lag codification in health policy. This model maximizes the health workforce's capacity, broadens the scope of accessible services, and addresses critical shortages in physician availability, aligning with WHO's workforce and service delivery blocks. However, regulatory frameworks often lag behind practice realities, representing a governance gap that limits formal recognition and institutional support for nurse and midwife autonomy, even as they function autonomously [49]. In districts where CHPS has been scaled with strong frontline discretion, studies report higher immunization coverage and improved uptake of maternal/newborn services; community-based nurse-led chronic disease programs also show clinically meaningful improvements (e.g., blood pressure control) when nurses are authorized to titrate therapy per protocol [50].

IOM Six Domains of Health Care Quality

The Institute of Medicine (IOM, now the National Academy of Medicine) defines high-quality healthcare as care that is safe, effective, patient-centered, timely, efficient, and equitable [41]. Clinical autonomy among APNs influences each domain in critical ways, as demonstrated by growing international evidence.

Australia's experience with using clinical autonomous APNs in emergency departments (EDs) provides a clear example of how autonomy influences patient outcomes when viewed through the IOM domains of quality. This example also highlights that clinical autonomy for APNs is not a trade-off between different domains of care. Instead, all domains are maintained or enhanced. Safety is maintained or improved as studies confirm comparable or better clinical outcomes and appropriate decision-making for APNs [51]. Timeliness improves because NPs reduce wait times, shorten time to analgesia, and expedite treatment pathways, which are critical in overcrowded EDs [52]. Effectiveness is evident in the delivery of evidence-based care, including the appropriate use of prescribing and diagnostic ordering [53]. Efficiency is also maintained, with no significant differences in median waiting times, treatment times, or length of stay for APN-managed patients compared to traditional ED care [54]. In rural areas, the APN model was particularly valued for reducing the burden on general practitioners while improving access to care [55]. Consistently high patient satisfaction and positive experiences of communication and care demonstrate patient-satisfaction [56, 57]. And equity is enhanced as APNs help extend services to patients who might otherwise experience delays or lower-quality care due to ED overcrowding or staffing shortages [55]. Using the IOM framework to consider these studies helps demonstrate that APN clinical autonomy at the point of care translates role expansion into measurable process improvements and better patient outcomes through strengthened ED performance.

Integrating the Frameworks

These frameworks demonstrate that APN autonomy is a complex construct with multiple influencing and potential paths to improved outcomes. Improving autonomy requires strengthening the multiple foundational structures and system functions that underpin high-performing health systems. These frameworks can help researchers, policymakers, and practitioners to identify leverage points for optimizing APN autonomy. Throughout the rest of the chapter, we will explore how a diverse set of countries and health systems have used (or, in some cases, failed to use) these leverage points as they build and adapt APN cadres to attempt to address system needs.

Current Landscape: Where We Are Now—International Overview of Clinical Autonomy among Advanced Practice Nurses

Though APNs work in more than 104 countries globally, their roles and degree of clinical autonomy vary dramatically [5]. This is shaped by differences in the legal scope of practice, prescriptive authority, institutional regulations, professional recognition, and health system integration. These differences influence workforce dynamics, patient outcomes, and health system capacity.

Regulatory and Policy Environments

Strong regulation and policy are foundational for APN clinical autonomy, as they typically provide a framework for related issues such as registration, certification, licensure, and a defined scope of practice, authorized clinical tasks, and entry requirements. Collectively, this provides role clarity, credibility, and consistency [58]. In countries with strong regulatory systems, APNs are substantially more likely to practice at full clinical autonomy, allowing health systems and patients to reap the rewards of that autonomy. However, complex practice and titling issues can make APN regulation difficult to track. At the same time, limited regulation (and global evidence for regulation, including unique factors that affect APN regulation) can make it more challenging for countries to justify and develop regulations that support consistent practice and titling [10]. This presents a challenging cycle for countries to break and speaks to the value of strong regulation from the outset of

APN cadre development. The ICN has attempted to strengthen nursing regulation globally, but significant country-level variation in APN regulation persists. The regulatory landscape for APNs continues to range from strong national regulation with regular review and updates to a patchwork by jurisdiction, to relying on registered nursing regulation, to being totally absent [58].

In OECD countries with relatively mature APN cadres (e.g., Australia, Canada, the Netherlands, New Zealand), regulation is largely in place to support broad clinical autonomy, generally reinforced by robust education and credentialing standards and institutions, though models of regulation vary [59]. For example, in Ireland, Australia, and New Zealand, national boards of nursing and midwifery carry out many tasks of regulating APNs, while in Norway, the Ministry of Education and Research regulates APN roles [60]. However, experiences in these countries demonstrate that while strong APN regulation is essential, it is insufficient to ensure clinical autonomy. Institutional policies, regulatory inconsistencies between health system components, and interprofessional dynamics can still create practical barriers to clinical autonomy, requiring ongoing efforts to clarify roles, responsibilities, and collaborative frameworks. These are discussed further in the challenges section below. ICN continues to advocate for global dialogue and research on how APN regulation can evolve to address these issues globally [58].

In LMICs, APN regulation and policy are more likely to be absent or in an early stage of development, though notably, HIC countries such as Finland, Spain, and a number of other European countries with relatively new APN cadres also fall into this category [60]. Many countries rely on task-shifting policies endorsed by WHO and other global agencies to expand access to care while mitigating workforce shortages [61]. While task-shifting and APN clinical autonomy should not be conflated, there are areas of overlap. In some LMICs, de facto autonomy may be high due to resource constraints, but legal frameworks lag behind, creating regulatory uncertainty and potential medico-legal risks for practitioners. Nonetheless, this regulatory variability creates both opportunities and challenges for scaling APN roles in ways that ensure safety, quality, and sustainability. In Kenya, most nurses, by default, perform at an advanced level, despite lacking advanced training. This is due to an overwhelming shortage of healthcare workers, as well as the fact that nurses and midwives outnumber physicians eight to one and the concentration of physicians in urban areas. Even as more nurses and midwives obtain graduate-level training, the training is not standardized and has not been accompanied by clear role documentation. Despite this scenario, regulation is limited and does not reflect the expanding role of nurses and midwives. Transformational change is necessary to integrate truly autonomous APNs with safeguarded practice into Kenya's healthcare system. This begins with developing legislation that includes clear standards, ethical codes, educational preparation, and entry requirements, and an autonomous scope of practice for APNs. However, it must also be accompanied by efforts to determine aspects of the autonomous APN role, such as rational remuneration, stakeholder understanding of the role, and ongoing investments in developing strong and aligned APN educational programs [29].

Scope of Practice and Diagnostic, Treatment, and Prescriptive Authority

One of the areas where regulation and clinical autonomy are most closely linked is through the scope of practice. Unsurprisingly, given the state of regulation globally, the APN scope of practice falls on a continuum across countries and may vary substantially sub-nationally, depending on how practice authority is structured or the degree of decentralization in a country.

- Full practice authority (FPA) allows independent diagnosis, treatment, and prescribing to the fullest extent of an individual's education and training. In some countries, this includes APN authority to operate their own practices. In Canada, the scope of practice is largely provincially regulated within a national framework, but it is generally broad. APNs are authorized to independently diagnose and prescribe a wide range of medications, including controlled substances, subject to jurisdictional guidelines [62]. Despite ongoing efforts to create additional APN-specific regulation, APNs in the UK practice at one of the fullest scopes globally and "are doing more work traditionally conducted by physicians than nurses in most other countries." [60], pg. 31.
- Reduced or restricted practice authority, where there are varying degrees of limitations on diagnosis, treatment, and prescribing, and these may require collaboration or supervision with another health care provider to some extent (typically a significant extent, in the case of restricted practice authority) to fully practice to the extent of their education and training. One of the challenges practitioners in countries with reduced/restricted practice authorities and significant workload shortages faced was an expectation that they would work beyond the designated scope of practice to meet patient needs [58].
- Absent or very limited formal practice authority designations, where APN tasks have been adopted informally or by default without policy and regulation to support the role. Many LMICs maintain limited formal recognition of APN roles, relying on task-shifting policies that allow nurses to perform select physician tasks under supervision rather than fully autonomous practice [6]. Because of this, in many countries, particularly LMICs, formal scope of practice authority also has a less straightforward relationship with day-to-day clinical autonomy than might be expected. As we saw above, many of Kenya's rural nurses are working at an expanded scope of practice without formal APN education and varying degrees of education to support their role [29]. The Netherlands specifically introduced additional regulations to combat informal practice [6].

Notably, acknowledging the intertwined nature of health system components discussed in the frameworks section, it is not unusual for an APN cadre to legally have one degree of practice authority while facing another health system component that prevents them from fully embracing the role. For example, Australian APNs enjoy broad clinical autonomy, including prescriptive authority and diagnostic ordering, but in some circumstances, they have limited access to financial reimbursement for their services. As a result, they often require formal collaboration with medical practitioners. This represents an economic barrier to complete autonomy despite legal clinical autonomy [63].

Effects of Autonomy on Workforce Development

Workforce well-being has become an increasingly discussed topic, particularly after the significant burdens placed on health workers during the COVID-19 pandemic. Global evidence consistently links higher autonomy and improved job satisfaction, professional role legitimacy, and positive interprofessional collaboration. Multiple studies of Swedish [64, 65], Australian [66, 67], and Czech [68] midwives, who have varying degrees of clinical autonomy, have demonstrated that clinical autonomy is vital for job satisfaction. In contrast, low autonomy is associated with poor job satisfaction. A Malaysian study found that empowering nurses through transformational leadership, including shared decision-making and enhanced autonomy, reduces feelings of powerlessness and job burnout and increases job satisfaction. Some of this arises from allowing nursing staff to respond to patient needs through rapid decision-making, increasing their autonomy while also ensuring patients get prompt care [69]. Job satisfaction has critical implications for workforce retention, preventing health worker burnout, and ensuring the delivery of high-quality care. Burnout is associated with increased medical errors, compromised patient safety, and poorer patient satisfaction [70]. Building on this, the WHO states that investing in midwives' health and well-being is associated with better outcomes for mothers and newborns in terms of both physical and psychological health [71].

Impacts on Patient Care

Though patient outcome data are more abundant in HICs, international evidence supports the conclusion that autonomous NP practice maintains or improves care quality without increasing adverse events. The literature abounds with examples of positive APN impacts on patient care in a diverse array of international contexts and specializations, particularly when the NP role possesses the requisite scope and autonomy to be evaluated [1]. These include:

- Canadian patients with diabetes admitted to inpatient cardiology units who had significantly decreased HbA1c and LDL values and improved quality of life under APN care [72];
- English patients with lung cancer who had a 17% lower risk of death and fewer unplanned cancer-related admissions compared to those not assessed by APNs [73];
- Australian patients with mental health needs in emergency departments who had streamlined access to care and expedited access to follow-up under APN care [74].

Even in countries such as Norway, where APN cadres are still relatively new, evidence is accumulating that APN care is as safe as physician care for various types of care, including orthopedic care [75]. Additional examples of the impacts of autonomous APN care on patient outcomes are discussed throughout this chapter.

Data from LMICs remains limited but emerging. Modeling studies show that if the coverage of midwives were scaled up substantially, 41% of maternal deaths, 39% of neonatal deaths, and 26% of stillbirths could be averted—a total of 2.2 million deaths averted per year by 2035, mostly in LMICs. Universal coverage would enable the saving of 4.3 million lives per year by 2035 [38]. This requires midwifery to be recognized as a skilled, autonomous profession, both to ensure midwives can deliver services at their full scope of practice and to attract sufficient individuals to the profession.

In South Africa, following 2011 policy reforms, nurses assumed an increasing role in coordinating and supporting the management of patients with multi-drug-resistant TB (MDR-TB), a task previously undertaken only by physicians and medical officers. In 2019, additional policy shifts allowed clinical nurse practitioners (CNPs) to manage sub-district treatment initiation sites, shifting nurses from a support role to an overall leadership role [76]. These structural shifts enabled significant process-level changes where independent APNs conducted diagnostic follow-up and treatment adjustments without physician oversight. Nurse-Initiated Management of MDR-TB was officially incorporated into policy in 2023, citing data that showed that patients who initiated MDR-TB treatment with a nurse had comparable outcomes to those who initiated with a physician [76]. A retrospective cohort study from the KwaZulu–Natal province found that treatment success rates for CNP-led MDR-TB care were comparable to or better than those for physician-led care, with a 61% treatment success rate for CNPs and a 52.7% treatment success rate for physicians. However, the difference was not statistically significant. Notably, the overall MDR-TB treatment success rate was 57.9%, significantly higher than the South African national average during the same time period. Looking back to the Donabedian framework, this also exemplifies how granting clinical autonomy at the structural level can enable process shifts that catalyze improved efficiency and patient outcomes [77].

Using Case Studies in Understanding Clinical Autonomy and Patient Outcomes

Case studies serve as illustrations of how clinical autonomy among APNs influences patient outcomes within varied and complex health systems, revealing how local regulatory environments, health system structures, and socio-cultural contexts shape care delivery. We selected cases from Canada and India to represent two very different health system models: a single-payer universal care with a well-established APN cadre and a mixed public/private system with free but underfunded public services implementing a new APN model of care.

Case Study: Nurse Practitioners in Rural Canada—Enhancing Healthcare Through Clinical Autonomy

Background and Context

Canada's healthcare system is a publicly funded, single-payer model administered at the provincial and territorial levels, providing universal coverage for medically necessary services. Canada, like many countries, faces an expanding gap in health workforce supply and demand [78]. This gap drives delays in care, missed follow-ups, and overburdened hospitals, all of which contribute to poor patient outcomes. While the gap may be worsening, access to high-quality healthcare and workforce distribution have long been challenges for Canada, particularly in rural and remote communities, including many First Nation and Inuit communities. These communities face long travel distances to care and limited access to specialist care, both of which create significant additional barriers to timely and equitable healthcare [78].

Additionally, First Nation and Inuit populations require culturally safe care that integrates local health beliefs and traditional practices, which can be challenging to provide without autonomous decision-making [79]. This has significant health implications for Indigenous populations as compared to the general population; First Nation [80] and Inuit people [81] have a shorter life expectancy than the non-Indigenous population [80], and only 44% of First Nations people living on-reserve report very good/excellent health as compared to 60% of non-Indigenous people [82]. Overall, First Nations in Canada have disproportionately higher rates of chronic disease compared to the general population and chronic diseases are now the major causes of morbidity, mortality, and disability among First Nations people [83].

Overall, Canada has an increasingly diverse population and rising rates of mental illness, addiction, and chronic diseases alongside persistent access to care issues and rising health care costs, all of which have been identified as major policy levers for implementing nurses in advanced roles in primary care [84]. Two APN roles exist in Canada: CNSs and NPs. While CNSs were introduced in the 1970s to focus on complex client care, their use declined in the 1980s and 1990s due to budget cuts. NPs originated from the work of nurses who worked in rural and remote areas to provide care that was otherwise unavailable, sometimes beyond their scope of practice. NPs were formally recognized in the 1970s to provide care to isolated populations, though formal legislation and regulation did not begin until 1998 [85]. As of 2022, there were 7,523 NPs in Canada and 46,145 family physicians [86].

The following case study examines Canada's slow start in implementing the APN role, as well as its strategic and relatively rapid formalization of the role. It closely examines how the inclusion of clinical autonomy across regulatory and implementation components is particularly critical in rural and remote communities, and how it has helped drive culturally responsive, patient-centered care and improve health outcomes, despite some persistent challenges.

Key Challenges or Barriers

Despite recognizing that rural and remote areas were desperately in need of improved healthcare access and that an APN cadre would be well-placed to meet these needs, efforts to expand and formalize the APN role were limited for several decades after their initial introduction in the 1970s [85]. APN education programs were initiated, but the APN role lacked enabling legislation and there were remuneration-related issues as well as a perceived oversupply of physicians. The 1990s witnessed a resurgence of interest in NPs as part of larger health reforms and an increasing recognition of the need for improved access to primary care, integrated care, and culturally appropriate care for diverse populations, including First Nation and Inuit populations [85].

However, even with increased recognition of their potential role in improving primary care access, APNs have historically been underutilized, partly due to limited training seats. This has limited their impact on reducing the need for other primary care providers, such as family physicians [87, 88].

Strategy/Intervention Implemented

With the resurgence of interest in APNs in the 1990s, several key initiatives were undertaken to formalize and support the role of APNs. First, the NP role was formally legislated and regulated starting in 1998, and all Canadian provinces now have NP-related legislation and regulation. Critical components of this include the publication of a national framework for advanced practice nursing, first published in 2000, which defines advanced practice nursing, the necessary education, domains of practice, and roles, and regulation. Notably, this framework is intentionally broad to ensure the role can evolve and jurisdictions can adapt to meet their own specific needs. In 2002, a graduate degree was adopted as the minimal educational requirement for advanced nursing practice [85].

Since then, numerous adjustments and updates have been made to the NP framework to update and expand scopes of practice, ensuring that competencies are consistent across jurisdictions but flexible enough to ensure substantial clinical autonomy to NPs to meet client population needs and the context of practice. However, there are differences in the scope of practice for APNs across Canadian provinces and territories and provincial and/or institutional variations impact the ability of some APNs to practice to the full extent of their education and training. Overall, the Canadian regulatory environment allows NPs to operate autonomously, positioning them to fill critical workforce shortages, improve access, and enhance care equity in underserved areas. APNs have been granted the authority to assess patients, order and interpret diagnostic tests, prescribe medications, and manage complex chronic and acute conditions [85]. For example, NPs managing diabetes in these communities initiate insulin therapy promptly, adjust doses in response to blood glucose fluctuations, and manage comorbidities such as hypertension without physician intervention [72].

Second, the number of training seats was increased to ensure an adequate supply. The number of NP graduates increased by 13% between 2018 and 2023. NPs and physiotherapists are the only groups of health professionals in Canada today slated to have additional capacity in the coming years, primarily due to these concerted efforts to increase educational and training seats. While there is a projected need for 2700 more NPs in Canada (a 35% increase), the rise in training seats could help meet demand by 2031, based on the current projections [86].

Third, significant efforts have been made to strategically position APNs as autonomous primary care leaders in rural clinics. They independently manage chronic conditions such as diabetes, hypertension, and cardiovascular disease, initiating and adjusting medications according to patient needs. NPs also order and interpret laboratory and imaging studies without mandatory physician oversight, enabling timely diagnosis and treatment [89]. Cultural tailoring of care is emphasized, with NPs collaborating closely with Indigenous elders, using local languages, and integrating traditional health practices to foster trust and enhance patient adherence [90]. Additionally, NPs lead local quality improvement initiatives, conduct community health education, and serve as the first point of contact for acute care, reducing reliance on distant hospitals and emergency departments [91].

Outcomes and Impact

Overall, Canada has demonstrated improved patient outcomes and strong integration of APNs into the health system; approximately three million Canadians receive care from an APN [92]. Autonomy is critical because it allows NPs to act swiftly without the delays often caused by requiring physician approval, which is logistically challenging in remote areas. Autonomous APN care has increased access to care by reducing appointment wait times, enhancing continuity of care, and improving comprehensiveness and convenience of care [89]. And clinical outcomes demonstrate that autonomous NP-led management of chronic conditions achieves measurable improvements. For example, patients under NP care had a 55% reduction in the use of multiple medications to manage chronic conditions [93]. Other patients exercised more, made dietary changes, and understood the reasons for their medication prescriptions better [94].

One area with particularly substantial evidence is the role of NPs in reducing pressure on emergency departments (EDs), including a 20% reduction in emergency department admissions from long-term care facilities. One of these is managing exacerbations of chronic conditions locally in communities. A study of NP-led clinics across Ontario found that these clinics facilitated access to services, fostered patient self-management, and were overall a successful alternative model to care that could reduce reliance on emergency departments to manage their chronic conditions [95]. Another study, conducted in Edmonton, Alberta, found reduced patient return visits, decreased wait times, and fewer patients leaving without treatment, along with high patient satisfaction, following the implementation of NPs in the emergency department. This included an NP-led transition clinic for urgent or emergency follow-up patients from the ED, as well as an NP-led Intravenous Therapy Clinic [96]. Another Canadian emergency department found that adding a broad-scope NP to the emergency department decreased the number of patients who left without treatment and reduced the proportion of low-acuity patients seen by physicians, thereby expediting care [97]. Patient satisfaction in ED settings was also high, with patients feeling that sufficient time was spent with them and that their concerns were taken seriously [98]. These findings underscore how autonomous NP practice enhances equity, quality, and system efficiency in resource-constrained rural and urban settings, mitigating the impact of physician shortages and geographical isolation.

Beyond clinical metrics, autonomous NP practice has a positive impact on patient-reported outcomes, including a 24% increase in family satisfaction with the quality of care [93]. Patients report strong coordination of care, which is associated with increased patient satisfaction and improvements in mental health as well as enhanced physical and social functioning, due to NP education and counseling [99]. This has translated into trust and respect for APNs, and 93% of Canadians are confident that NPs can meet their day-to-day needs [100]. NP autonomy enables tailored, culturally safe care that integrates Indigenous health beliefs and community values, which are critical for enhancing patient trust, adherence, and outcomes. In Nunavut, for example, healthcare providers emphasized the importance of respecting Inuit culture, including involving Elders and medical interpreters, recognizing family roles, and acknowledging a strong sense of community connection ("sense of home") in delivering end-of-life care. These adaptations reflect a culturally competent approach that aligns care with patients' holistic needs and improves responsiveness to social determinants of health [101].

Discussion and Lessons Learned

The Canadian experience highlights that APNs have tremendous actual and potential value in both urban and rural settings. APN clinical autonomy is a critical part of this, including helping overcome geographic and workforce barriers in rural regions. In both rural and urban settings, independent decision-making enables NPs to rapidly apply clinical knowledge, tailor care to meet patient needs, and address social determinants of health along with biomedical concerns. Autonomous practice not only improves clinical and patient-centered outcomes but also enhances system efficiency by reducing unnecessary transfers and hospitalizations. Integration with cultural frameworks demonstrates that autonomy can foster trust, engagement, and adherence in diverse populations, highlighting its value beyond purely clinical metrics.

However, this case study also highlights some areas where additional effort could likely continue to expand clinical autonomy for APNs and how APNs can maximize outcomes in their role. Even where APNs are in practice, system constraints, including limited local infrastructure and referral pathways, necessitate NPs' ability to make independent clinical decisions to maintain continuity of care. Despite overall strong system and regulatory support for the APN role, diverse practice settings pose barriers to the successful implementation of the role, including a lack of physician and/or administrative support, an unclear understanding of how the APN role works with other healthcare team members, and isolation of NPs. Additional efforts are necessary to ensure administrative support and an APN champion, patient satisfaction with NPs, building staff familiarity with the NP role, and preparing the NP to facilitate their own implementation [14]. Attracting and retaining APNs from rural and remote areas remains a challenge, as the majority of NP educational and training programs are predominantly located in urban settings (27/30 programs) [86]. This may limit the number of rural students who can access NP education and serve as providers in their communities, which is crucial for health worker retention and the provision of culturally congruent care [102].

Conclusion and Future Considerations

Canada's experience demonstrates that NP clinical autonomy is crucial for delivering high-quality, equitable, and efficient care in rural and underserved areas. Autonomous NP care achieves clinical outcomes comparable to or better than specialist care, including the effective management of chronic diseases and a reduction in emergency visits and hospitalizations. Beyond these clinical outcomes, personalized, timely care by autonomous NPs leads to high patient satisfaction and trust. Notably, the cultural tailoring enabled by NP autonomy improved patient engagement in Indigenous communities. Policies supporting autonomous APN practice, as seen in Canada, enhance overall workforce capacity, improve patient outcomes, and strengthen system resilience.

Case Study: India's Midwifery Initiative and the Introduction of Nurse Practitioners in Midwifery

Background and Context

In 2015, the Sustainable Development Goals (SDGs) set a lofty target: by 2030, the maternal mortality ratio (MMR) would be reduced to fewer than 70 maternal deaths per 100,000 live births, a 68% reduction from the 216 maternal deaths per 100,000 live births in 2015 [3]. In India, where maternal mortality remains a pressing challenge despite recent progress, achieving this goal requires targeted investments in workforce solutions capable of delivering high-quality maternal and newborn care. Midwives are increasingly recognized globally as a cost-effective solution because of their ability to provide comprehensive reproductive, maternal, and newborn health services, including antenatal, intrapartum, and postpartum care [38].

However, global evidence demonstrates that midwives only achieve their full impact when supported by appropriate education, regulation, professional recognition, and enabling work environments [38]. In December 2018, driven by the Lancet Series and commitments to the SDGs as well as learning from countries such as Nigeria and Indonesia, India announced its Midwifery Initiative. The initiative includes the introduction of a new cadre of Nurse Practitioners in Midwifery (NPMs) trained to International Confederation of Midwives (ICM) standards, the creation of midwifery-led care units (MLCUs) at public healthcare facilities, and the development of an enabling policy environment for the practice of midwifery. It is essential to acknowledge that there are skilled birth attendants in India who currently use the term "midwife" but do not meet the standards of the International

Confederation Midwives for midwifery training and competencies. There are also some "traditional midwives" in practice [103].

While implementation is not yet complete, the comprehensive approach outlined in the *Guidelines on Midwifery Services in India* [104] represents a groundbreaking opportunity to consider how clinically autonomous midwives, fully integrated into a health system, can improve maternal health outcomes in an LMIC context.

Key Challenges or Barriers

Historically, India has faced systemic barriers in establishing a robust and autonomous midwifery workforce. Earlier large-scale programs in other LMICs offer cautionary lessons. Until the mid-2010s, the focus of many interventions was almost entirely on physical access, and many countries conducted a significant scale-up of the midwifery workforce with limited investment in role definition and regulation, including ensuring sufficient clinical autonomy for midwives to work at their full scope of practice [105–107]. For instance, Indonesia's village midwife program and Nigeria's midwives services scheme expanded coverage of midwives but failed to achieve sustained reductions in maternal mortality. When evaluating the situation in Indonesia after their rapid scale-up of midwifery training, the Joint Committee on Reducing Maternal and Neonatal Mortality in Indonesia (2013) found evidence that system-level efforts to expand the midwifery workforce must be preceded or accompanied by improvements in the regulatory environment to achieve meaningful and sustained outcomes [108]. A 2015 evaluation of the job satisfaction of midwives in Nigeria's Midwife Service Scheme found that retention was very poor due to factors such as lack of career structure and inadequate supervision. They suggested that improving job satisfaction, such as through clinical autonomy, will enhance retention and, in turn, maternal health, but noted that this requires updates to the regulatory system at a higher level [109]. Within India, previous small-scale efforts to introduce midwifery faced similar structural challenges with inconsistent training quality that did not prepare midwives to practice at their full scope, nurses and midwives had low professional recognition, and maternal health systems remained overly physician-centric. Persistent gender inequities within India's health workforce also constrained midwifery's development, with nurses and midwives often positioned as subordinate to physicians rather than autonomous practitioners; 90% of midwives globally are female and subject to significant gendered disparities in pay rates, career pathways, and decision-making power [110].

Social determinants further compound these barriers. Women in India continue to encounter the "three delays" in accessing the care they need to prevent and manage complications: first, a delay in identifying a need for healthcare, then a delay in reaching healthcare, and finally a delay in receiving appropriate services once healthcare is reached [111]. This model incorporates the reality that complications in childbirth can arise quickly and unexpectedly in otherwise healthy women and that having an autonomous skilled birth attendant—someone with specialized birth training and skills who is empowered to work at their full scope of practice—is essential to quickly recognize and appropriately manage complications [112].

Strategy/Intervention Implemented

A central component of India's Midwifery Initiative is the creation of midwifery-led care units (MLCUs) situated within maternal health facilities. MLCUs will include Labor Room Quality Improvement Initiative (LaQshya)-certified labor rooms. The LaQshya-certified labor rooms in MLCUs promote clinical autonomy by creating physically separate spaces led by NPMs, which promotes scope-appropriate task-shifting and physiologically normal birth while still allowing for prompt access to specialists should complications occur [113]. This set-up also ensures that spaces have essential equipment, adequate human resources, and capacity-building and quality-improvement processes, all of which are essential for full-scope, clinically autonomous practice [114]. By co-locating MLCUs in these quality-assured settings, NPMs gained environments conducive to safe, respectful, and effective perinatal care.

Education is prioritized through the creation of national and regional midwifery training institutes, with curricula aligned to the gold standard International Confederation of Midwives standards [115]. As of 2022, six out of 14 planned national midwifery training institutes have been established, and the goal is to train 90,000 NPMs. As midwifery researcher Saraswathi Vedam and her team eloquently point out, meeting global standards for midwifery education is essential to ensure NPMs are prepared to competently and autonomously provide care at their full scope of practice guided by a midwifery philosophy of care. However, a strong foundational education is also critical for developing midwifery leadership in clinical and broader health system settings, and promoting the professional as an independent practitioner [103].

While midwifery in India has yet to be approved as a separate profession from nursing, both technically and by society [116], in 2018, the Ministry of Health and Family Welfare (MoHFW) did publish guidelines on midwifery services in India that included direction for midwifery education, training, and quality assurance of and the methods by which to integrate midwives into the existing health system [117]. Policy and regulatory frameworks were revised to define NPMs' scope of practice, granting them authority to independently provide antenatal, intrapartum, and postnatal care, prescribe medications, and manage complications within defined protocols. These documents also emphasize the importance of supportive supervision, career pathways, and integration into interdisciplinary teams, aiming to foster an enabling environment.

Outcomes and Impact

The Government of India designed the Midwifery Initiative as a comprehensive, systems-oriented reform that signaled India's intent to move beyond traditional nursing roles into full professional autonomy within integrated health services. Evidence from global systematic reviews and meta-analyses strongly suggests that midwife-led continuity models improve maternal and newborn health, reduce unnecessary interventions, and enhance women's experiences of care. India's initiative has the potential to generate large-scale, concrete, context-specific proof of how integrated, autonomous midwives can impact maternal health outcomes in an LMIC [38, 118]. Although still in the implementation phase, India's midwifery initiative has attracted many researchers who are engaged in evaluating both components and the overall approach. Outcomes of interest include increased uptake of antenatal care (particularly early initiation and four or more visits), improved institutional delivery rates, reductions in preventable complications such as postpartum hemorrhage and eclampsia, and declines in maternal mortality and stillbirths. Routine monitoring and data collection should be used to track maternal and newborn outcomes, including person-centered quality metrics such as respect, patient autonomy, and mistreatment [103].

Discussion and Lessons Learned

The India Midwifery Initiative demonstrates that scaling up midwifery requires more than just increasing the number of providers; it requires investment in the whole ecosystem that enables midwives to thrive. Integrating NPMs into LaQshya-certified facilities ensures a foundation of quality and accountability, while embedding research and evaluation ensures continuous learning and improvement. Notably, India's approach has the potential to contrast with previous programs that failed to improve maternal outcomes due to inadequate training, a lack of regulation, and insufficient professional support.

There is substantial work left to be done, including a demand for care provided by NPMs through community awareness, mass media, motivated local political leaders, and midwifery champions. This includes a clear understanding of NPMs as autonomous providers and what birthing people and their families can expect from this role [119]. Like Canada, India will need to revisit their initial frameworks and continuously update and evolve them, including supporting them with formal legal and regulatory frameworks, to enable midwives to provide full-scope practice in line with both midwifery philosophy and global standards [113]. The development of midwifery leadership to safeguard and advance the midwifery profession across the health system, including addressing misconceptions about autonomous roles and expertise, is also critical [103].

Conclusion and Future Directions

India's Midwifery Initiative represents a landmark experiment in health workforce development, with the potential for global impact. By creating a new cadre of autonomous NPMs trained to international standards and supported by enabling policies, India will both address key maternal health challenges and contribute to the global midwifery evidence base. If successful, the program could serve as a model for other LMICs, demonstrating that strategic investment in autonomous, well-integrated midwives can accelerate progress toward SDG 3 and substantially reduce maternal mortality. Sustained investment, robust monitoring, and political commitment will be essential to adapting, scaling, and fully institutionalizing these reforms over the coming decade.

Challenges and Barriers to Clinical Autonomy

While the value of autonomous APNs is supported by robust evidence, the international case studies above reveal persistent, multifaceted challenges to autonomy that must be addressed to realize the full potential of APN roles. These challenges span regulatory, professional, institutional, cultural, educational, and community domains, underscoring the complex ecosystem in which clinical autonomy is situated. They also reiterate the usefulness of using health system frameworks in considering clinical autonomy, as few of these challenges and barriers fall cleanly into one category but are instead influenced by a diverse mix of factors.

Regulatory Fragmentation and Lack of Full Practice Authority

Globally, the regulatory environment governing APNs remains highly heterogeneous, often characterized by fragmented policies that restrict full practice authority and limit autonomous clinical decision-making. This is true both within and between countries. For instance, as discussed at length previously, in Canada, APN scope of practice varies significantly by province; some provinces grant full prescribing rights and diagnostic autonomy, while others maintain requirements for physician oversight for particular medications or clinical decisions [120]. This patchwork regulatory landscape creates inequities in patient access to care and frustrates efforts toward standardization. ITo address this issue, the European Union has issued directives aimed at harmonizing midwifery regulation across its member states. Yet disparate country-level adoption and interpretation continue to restrict autonomous practice—particularly in emergent obstetric care—due to differing training requirements and legal frameworks [121, 122]. In many African countries, midwifery remains regulated under broader nursing councils, resulting in inconsistent recognition of advanced scopes of practice and fragmented governance; APN practice regulation lags even behind this [31, 123]. This lack of unified regulatory frameworks undermines workforce development and contributes to variable maternal and neonatal outcomes, particularly in resource-limited settings. Regulation also has important implications for credibility, which is critical for a profession beset by misunderstandings of its scope of practice [124], something that has significant implications for physician and community resistance, as discussed below.
Non-nursing-focused global health agencies such as the WHO readily acknowledge health workforce shortages but have been inconsistent in advancing the APN role and providing guidance to support it. For example, the WHO's most recent global strategy on human resources for health does not mention APNs a single time; instead; an undefined "mid-level practitioner" is mentioned a handful of times [125]. However, the WHO European Region has an extensive technical brief on advancing roles for nurses [9].

Physician Resistance, Interprofessional Tensions, and Weak Collaboration

Interprofessional dynamics represent a significant barrier to APN autonomy worldwide. In a review of the APN role in 12 Organization for Economic Co-operation and Development (OECD) countries, opposition from the medical profession was identified as one of the main barriers to the development of APN roles [59]. Such resistance is often rooted in entrenched professional hierarchies and concerns about clinical accountability and quality of care. The OECD findings attribute this to overlapping scopes of practice and fears APNs will cause a loss of activity and/or income; legal liability concerns if malpractice occurs under teamwork arrangements; and concerns about the skills and expertise of APNs in relation to their degree of autonomy and independence [59]. Similarly, within the UK's National Health Service (NHS), some general practitioners (GPs) have expressed concerns regarding potential role overlap with autonomous APNs, which can generate professional tensions and impede the integration of APNs into expanded roles [126]. However, beyond simply complicating APN role development, APN/physician relationships have significant potential consequences for patient outcomes. Interprofessional collaboration is required both to ensure access to the full range of essential interventions and to improve the safety, timeliness, and effectiveness of care, ultimately enhancing its overall quality. One study in Indonesia found that seven out of 30 maternal deaths were related to poor communication between midwives at the primary level and physicians at the tertiary level [127]. Barriers to interprofessional collaboration identified in providing collaborative maternity care in Australia include contested scope of practice, professional role boundaries, and philosophical differences about maternity care [128]. The persistence of such resistance highlights the importance of fostering interprofessional education and collaborative practice environments. It also speaks to the need for inclusive policy-making processes that engage all stakeholders in defining APN roles to enhance acceptance and support for autonomous practice. Australia, the Netherlands, and the United Kingdom, which all demonstrate low rates of maternal mortality, low birthweight, and newborn death, all have health systems that emphasize midwifery care and interprofessional collaboration, and specific guidelines around the need for midwives who can practice autonomously at full scope [38].

Limited Institutional Support and Role Ambiguity

Legislative or regulatory authority for APNs often fails to translate fully into practice without supportive institutional policies and clear role definitions. Two decades ago, an ICN study in 18 countries highlighted 13 different APN titles and noted role ambiguity as a primary concern [129]. As of 2024, the issue remained a significant concern, driven by a lack of standardized titles and definitions which hindered the integration of APNs into teams and muddled the clarity of APN responsibilities [130]. In Australia, despite progressive legislative reforms granting APNs advanced scopes of practice, studies show organizational policies and workplace cultures lag behind, leaving APNs without clear guidance or institutional endorsement to exercise autonomy fully [63]. In particular, in the context of Canadian aged care by APNs, researchers found that the impact of APN care on patient outcomes varied substantially across three sites with varying physician presence and APN roles [131]. This disconnect can result in role ambiguity, reduced job satisfaction, and underutilization of APN skills. APNs in Thailand, which has a relatively new APN cadre, reported very mixed levels of autonomy they reported in their roles as well as general confusion about role development and career progression [30]. In Kenya, which is early in its APN journey, private practice nurses report considerable uncertainty about the extent of their legal authority, leading to hesitancy in making independent clinical decisions and diminishing the potential benefits of their expanded roles [44]. Strengthening institutional frameworks, clarifying role expectations, and embedding supportive clinical governance mechanisms are therefore essential to operationalize legislative reforms and empower APNs to practice autonomously [12]. However, it is acknowledged that incorporating "substantially repurposed occupational groups" such as APNs into very complex and hierarchical organizations (e.g., the UK's NHS) is poorly understood [132].

Gender Norms

Gender dynamics deeply influence APN autonomy, particularly for midwives in many LMICs. While a broad discussion of patriarchy, gender, and power is beyond the scope of this chapter, there is ample evidence globally to suggest that gender and gender norms are significant barriers to APN clinical autonomy [133]. APNs, particularly midwives, working in a female-dominated profession, frequently exist within male-dominated medical hierarchies that limit women's professional influence and opportunities for leadership [134]. In South Asia, cultural norms and gender biases systematically devalue midwives' clinical decision-making capabilities, despite evidence demonstrating that midwife-led care significantly improves maternal and neonatal outcomes [135, 136]. These entrenched gendered professional hierarchies create systemic barriers that undermine APN authority, inhibit career advancement, and perpetuate disparities in health workforce governance. Addressing these gender biases through policy reforms, leadership development programs, and gender equity initiatives is critical to advancing APN autonomy and optimizing maternal health services.

Inadequate Education, Training, and Mentorship

While a graduate degree in nursing is increasingly accepted as the global standard for becoming an APN, as with regulation, there is extensive variation in educational requirements across countries [59]. Educational preparation has significant implications for the definition of scope of practice, the ability to practice at full scope, and interprofessional credibility. It also has implications in terms of direct costs for potential APNs (e.g., cost of training programs) and indirect costs (e.g., time spent on education and training) [137]. Many countries have attempted to streamline certain aspects of education programs to reduce costs and expedite the availability of APNs in settings where the demand for the health workforce exceeds the supply. Unfortunately, this is often detrimental to patient outcomes. In an attempt to overcome a significant shortfall of midwives, Indonesia launched a Midwifery Education Rapid Training Program in 1989, aiming to substantially expand the number of schools offering a three-year midwifery curriculum. This initiative was successful in that Indonesia increased the number of midwifery training schools 15-fold and its midwives from 52,000 in 2006 to over 200,000 in 2012. However, the number of midwives graduated far exceeded the capacity of schools to offer hands-on childbirth training, and many graduated without ever having managed a labor or birth. It also incorporated midwives who had received only a one-year training program with limited hands-on experience for birth emergencies [138]. While numerous other system factors contributed as well, this education has not prepared most midwives in Indonesia to provide high-quality, autonomous care. Thus, the effects of this massive investment in education have not translated into the hoped-for reductions in maternal mortality [108].

Beyond direct education, the rapid scale-up of APN and midwifery education programs, particularly in regions like Latin America, has sometimes outpaced the availability of high-quality clinical training and mentorship [139]. This discrepancy leaves many new graduates inadequately prepared and less confident in making autonomous clinical decisions, which affects patient safety and care quality. It is reported that Japanese midwives are "unclear about their authority over midwifery care and lack awareness of such authority; hence, they often provide midwifery care under the direction of physicians," and attribute this to midwifery education that does not allow midwives to provide autonomous care [140, 141]. These findings underscore the critical role of rigorous education, robust clinical mentorship, and ongoing professional development in building APN competence and confidence necessary for safe autonomous practice.

Lack of Patient Awareness of APN Roles and Capabilities

Patient and community understanding of APN roles and capabilities remains limited in many settings, hindering acceptance of autonomous APN roles even in countries where these roles are well-established. Evidence from Canada [142] and the UK [143] reveals widespread patient confusion regarding the extent to which APNs can prescribe medications, order diagnostic tests, or manage chronic conditions independently. This type of confusion acts as a deterrent to integrating APNs into the workplace. In New Zealand, study participants reflected medical hierarchies, placing APNs "below" GPs, despite not being able to routinely articulate why they believed APNs operated at lower tiers [144]. A study looking at barriers to APN autonomy across sub-Saharan Africa noted that "society tends to be skeptical about extending the roles of nurses for diagnosis and prescription." [145] And a study in the Netherlands found that while in general patients were satisfied with primary care from a general practitioner or APN, patient preferences for the type of provider varied with the kind of care required and reflected standard physician/nurse work demarcations rather than expanded clinically autonomous roles APNs actually play [146]. Without adequate public awareness, patients may default to seeking physician care or express skepticism about APN-led services, believing that their care has been substandard or of a lower tier. The evidence from these countries, all of which have well-established APN cadres, may serve as a deterrent to countries considering expanding APN roles as it may lead them to believe that APNs will not be well tolerated or utilized by target populations. However, in Ethiopia, expansion of midwifery roles has been linked to community engagement campaigns designed to build trust, educate populations on midwives' competencies, and encourage utilization of services [147]. These findings highlight the importance of targeted patient and community education initiatives as part of broader strategies to support autonomous APN practice.

Strategies, Innovations, and Best Practices

Addressing regulatory, educational, institutional, cultural, and technological challenges requires coordinated strategies that operate at multiple levels of the health system. Effective initiatives combine policy and legislative reform with educational innovation that emphasizes clinical and leadership competencies, integrated team-based care models, the adoption of global standards, and the strategic use of telehealth and digital health tools. These approaches collectively promote the development, acceptance, and sustainability of autonomous APN practice across diverse healthcare contexts worldwide.

Policy and Legislative Reform: Full Practice Authority and Regulatory Harmonization

There is a growing body of evidence to support the overall approach of investment in regulatory work. When researchers assessed the impact on national regulations and organizational capacity of The African Health Professions Regulatory Collaborative's (ARC) program of technical assistance and grants to country teams of nursing and midwifery leaders to improve national HIV service delivery regulations, they found significant increases in leadership, collaboration, and organizational capacity and improved national nursing regulations. They posit that these changes helped ensure nurse-initiated and managed treatment for people living with HIV, but did not directly assess any clinical outcomes and were unable to establish a causal relationship [148].

The need for regulation increases with the expansion of nursing and midwifery functions, a fact well recognized by key stakeholders in the sub-Saharan African context. However, marked discrepancies exist between regulation, practice, and education, and insufficient capacity at the nursing and midwifery council level acts as a barrier to regulatory progress. They suggest strengthening the capacity of regulatory councils as an essential first step in regulatory reform, and that global initiatives and data supporting the expanded roles of nurses and midwives are helpful for regulatory advancement efforts [149]. Similarly, the Countdown Working Group on Health Policy and Health Systems found that a strong global and national commitment, adequate financial resources, and intensive technical support are necessary to reduce the gap between maternal health policy and implementation. An improved understanding of the effect of midwifery regulatory measures can also play a role achieving this goal [150].

A specific area of focus for regulatory work to promote clinical autonomy is full practice authority. While the United States provides much of the most compelling evidence of the effect of full practice authority, due to the state-by-state regulatory variations, international evidence is also available. Some of the evidence focuses on how the length of this process can be and offers suggestions for expediting it. For example, the Netherlands implemented time-limited laws combined with a nationwide evaluation to accelerate the reform process [151]. Australia has elected to implement self-regulation, where regulation is delegated to nursing regulatory bodies, allowing updates to practice authority to occur more quickly than through legislation [152].

Educational Models: Competency-Based Training for Clinical Reasoning and Leadership

While LMICs are sometimes perceived as the countries struggling with inconsistent educational preparation standards for APNs, the reality is that there is considerable variation across HICs as well. The ICN recommends a master's level preparation for APNs, but its minimum standards are limited. The development of a strong curricula framework for minimum levels of advanced practice could help set educational and practice requirements internationally. Quality assurance mechanisms for nursing education are in place in most countries, including faculty qualifications (90%), national accreditation mechanisms (88%), and coordination between education and regulation settings for accreditation standards (77%). While this quality assurance can help drive clinical autonomy by setting clear standards, ensuring APNs can provide high-quality care at a known scope, little is known about how much it is actually being implemented; therefore, this remains an area where additional research and innovation are required [5].

It is worth noting that some specific global professional organizations exist for distinct groups of APNs (e.g., midwives). These are typically competency-based education (CBE) models, which are increasingly recognized as foundational for preparing APNs for autonomous practice. By focusing on measurable competencies such as clinical reasoning, decision-making, evidence-based care, and leadership skills, CBE frameworks ensure that graduates possess the knowledge and capabilities required for independent clinical roles [153]. In Europe, midwifery education has adopted standardized competencies aligned with the International Confederation of Midwives (ICM) global standards, facilitating cross-border recognition and improving professional mobility [122].

These education reforms have been accompanied by innovations, including simulation-based training in Tanzania [154], interprofessional learning in the Middle East [155], and extended clinical placements that enhance practical readiness and confidence in Norway [156]. However, effective implementation demands investment in faculty development, clinical mentorship programs, and sufficient experiential learning sites. Leadership training embedded within curricula further equips APNs to navigate complex health systems, advocate for their roles and autonomy, and participate in policy development. For example, in Australia, a formal, structured mentoring program for APN candidates was successful in enhancing clinical leadership skills and self-reported leadership practices [157].

Integrated Care Teams: Enabling APN-Led Models of Care

Successful integration of APNs as leaders of multidisciplinary and/or collaborative teams has been shown to optimize care delivery, particularly in chronic disease management and primary care [126]. By fostering mutual respect, reducing interprofessional tensions, and creating environments where APN autonomy is protected while closely linked to care beyond the APN's scope of practice, well-designed APN-led care has a profound impact on job satisfaction and patient outcomes. Key enablers of such integration include clear role delineations, formalized collaborative practice agreements, well-defined communication methods and pathways, and institutional policies that support APN independent diagnostic and prescribing authority [10]. The success and safety of New Zealand's midwife-led freestanding birth units owes a great deal to significant efforts to develop mutually respectful formal relationships with obstetric colleagues along these lines [158]. In Canada, patients who received care from a collaborative team that included an NP saw improved chronic disease management across the full spectrum of the patient population [159]. However, educational preparation, including leadership training and mentorship, is critical to ensure that APNs are prepared to lead within collaborative teams and multidisciplinary models [160].

Use of Telehealth and Digital Tools: Supporting Autonomous Decision-Making in Remote Settings

Telehealth and digital health technologies have emerged as enablers of APN autonomy, particularly in remote, rural, and resource-constrained environments. Teleconsultation platforms enable APNs to maintain clinical authority while accessing specialist input, facilitating timely and autonomous clinical decision-making. For example, Australian rural APNs utilize telehealth to collaborate with urban specialists, thereby expanding access to specialty care without compromising their autonomous practice [161]. Rwanda implemented a hybrid telemedicine model where nurses and midwives were supported in providing first-trimester medication abortion by physicians who provided clinical guidance and reviewed client data. An evaluation found that this model was feasible, effective, safe, and accepted by clients while substantially expanding access to first-trimester abortion [162]. And apps such as the Indian "E-Midwife" mobile app are increasingly providing e-learning platforms that offer culturally relevant information on managing obstetric complications in a widely available and cost-effective format [163].

Effective telehealth implementation requires a basic digital infrastructure, standardized clinical protocols, secure patient data systems, and enabling legal frameworks that recognize telehealth encounters as valid clinical practice [164]. While these requirements have limited the spread of telehealth and digital technologies in some of the hardest-to-reach areas, scaling these technologies nonetheless offers a promising avenue to capitalize on APN autonomy, overcoming geographical and resource barriers and enhancing patient outcomes.

Future Considerations and Directions

This chapter has discussed numerous regulatory, policy, educational, and scope of practice issues that must be addressed to advance clinical autonomy for APNs. However, there are several specific opportunities that could be valuable in fully realizing autonomous APN practice and improving patient outcomes across diverse settings. Several of these are discussed below.

Need for Global Monitoring Frameworks on APN Regulation and Outcomes

ICN's recent 26-country survey showed significant variability in APN regulation and a paucity of standardized data on APN workforce characteristics, scopes of practice, and patient outcomes [10]. This fragmentation limits comparative analyses and data for evidence-based policymaking. Harmonized global monitoring frameworks that incorporate uniform regulatory indicators, workforce data, and patient outcome metrics would enable benchmarking, facilitate international comparisons, and support workforce planning that safeguards the clinical autonomy of APNs. Countries such as Australia have begun implementing comprehensive clinical quality registries linked to outcome monitoring [165]. These could be used to compare outcomes between provider types more systematically. However, they must be appropriately set up to capture provider type, which can be challenging with some collaborative care models [166]. A globally coordinated effort could leverage these approaches to establish universal standards as a path to regulatory coherence and policy responsiveness.

Strengthen Research on APN Clinical Autonomy

Ample evidence has been shared throughout this chapter to demonstrate that APN-led care is comparable or superior to physician-led care in terms of safety, effectiveness, and patient satisfaction across diverse clinical indicators such as chronic disease management, preventive care, and maternal-child health. However, substantial geographical gaps, particularly in LMICs, and methodological heterogeneity, including varied outcome measures and study designs, persist in the global APN autonomy evidence base. This can make it difficult to compare across countries or contexts. To address these gaps, research on APN clinical autonomy must deploy rigorous methodologies, including randomized controlled trials, prospective cohorts, mixed methods approaches that incorporate qualitative nuances of experience, and longitudinal studies that can track changes over time. These studies must also be conducted across varied health system contexts; as is evident from the evidence in the chapter, much of the global evidence base is skewed toward HICs. Incorporating standardized outcome metrics, including clinical outcomes, system-level efficiency, and cost-effectiveness, will clarify how degrees of APN autonomy influence patient and health system outcomes globally.

Expand Patient-Reported Outcomes and Experience Measures in Evaluating Autonomy

Incorporating patient-reported outcome measures (PROMs) and patient-reported experience measures (PREMs) is essential for evaluating the quality and person-centeredness of autonomous APN care [167]. These metrics capture patients' perspectives on symptom burden, functional status, satisfaction, and access, all of which are critical domains for comprehensive care assessment. Despite growing use in HICs, uptake of PROMs and PREMs remains limited in LMICs due to resource constraints and lack of validated tools adapted for local contexts [168]. Global efforts to develop culturally appropriate, validated PROMs and PREMs specific to APN care can enhance understanding of care quality from the patient viewpoint and support tailored role development responsive to community needs. Successful implementation in pain clinics in Canada, oncology clinics in Australia, pediatric/adult chronic condition clinics in the Netherlands, and Canadian primary care clinics demonstrates the feasibility and utility of PROMs/PREMs in APN evaluation frameworks [169].

Conclusion

International evidence confirms that clinical autonomy is vital for delivering high-quality, equitable, and efficient patient care by APNs. This body of research demonstrates that autonomy has a direct influence on workforce well-being, patient outcomes, and health system performance. Variations in the scope of practice and regulatory frameworks across countries profoundly shape the autonomy of APNs, thereby affecting their ability to deliver timely, culturally competent, and patient-centered care.

The Canada case study provides numerous examples of how autonomous APN practice translates into tangible health benefits. Empowered and autonomous APNs in Canada have been able to provide clinically effective care aligning with cultural norms and patient preferences. This care has driven significant advances in chronic disease management, emergency care, and patient satisfaction by fostering trust and engagement while simultaneously reducing costs and alleviating workforce strain. This demonstrates the dual role of autonomy as a catalyst for quality improvement and a mechanism to address workforce shortages. Meanwhile, the India case study demonstrates the concerted and coordinated effort required to build an autonomous APN cadre from the ground up. India's current experience in developing a highly autonomous, internationally recognized midwifery cadre also highlights the immense amount of country-to-country learning that most countries undertake in their efforts to position and support APNs.

Most countries globally fall somewhere between India and Canada on the spectrum of APN autonomy, as the evidence and examples shared throughout this chapter highlight. Regardless of a country's position on the spectrum of autonomous APN cadre development, as global health systems grapple with escalating workforce shortages, increasing care demands, and entrenched health inequities, expanding and protecting clinical autonomy for APNs should be a strategic priority for many. Policy initiatives that dismantle unnecessary legislative and regulatory barriers, harmonize practice standards, and clarify credentialing and liability frameworks can unlock the full potential of APNs to deliver comprehensive, efficient, and high-quality care. Furthermore, embedding autonomy within integrated health team models promotes collaborative yet independent practice, optimizing resource utilization and patient outcomes.

Importantly, international evidence also highlights significant disparities in APN autonomy, particularly between HICs and LMICs. Many LMICs face additional structural, educational, and cultural challenges that constrain APN practice. Future research must prioritize generating rigorous, comparable data from diverse settings, especially LMICs, to inform contextually appropriate autonomy reforms. This evidence will be vital to ensure that policy and educational interventions align with global standards while being effectively tailored to local realities. Harnessing international evidence enables health leaders, policymakers, educators, and clinicians to advocate for and/or develop strategies that maximize the APN capabilities. Through deliberate reforms and sustained investment in autonomy-enabling mechanisms, APNs can become agents of transformative, accessible, and patient-centered health care worldwide.

References

1. Poghosyan L, Maier CB. Advanced practice nurses globally: responding to health challenges, improving outcomes. Int J Nurs Stud. 2022;132:104262. https://doi.org/10.1016/j.ijnurstu.2022.104262.
2. World Health Organization. Universal health coverage (UHC). Geneva: WHO; 2019. [cited 2025 Aug 26]. Available from: https://www.who.int/news-room/fact-sheets/detail/universal-health-coverage-(UHC).
3. United Nations. Sustainable development goals. New York: UN. [cited 2025 Aug 26]. Available from: https://sdgs.un.org/goals.
4. Porat-Dahlerbruch J, Boyd J, Fighel H. Investing in the advanced practice nursing workforce to improve health system responses to armed conflict. Int Nurs Rev. 2025;72(3):e70074. https://doi.org/10.1111/inr.70074.
5. World Health Organization. State of the world's nursing 2025: investing in education, jobs, leadership and service delivery. Geneva: WHO; 2025. Licence: CC BY-NC-SA 3.0 IGO.
6. Maier CB, Aiken LH. Task shifting from physicians to nurses in primary care in 39 countries: a cross-country comparative study. Eur J Pub Health. 2016;26(6):927–34. https://doi.org/10.1093/eurpub/ckw098.
7. Lockwood EB, Schober M. Factors influencing the impact of nurse practitioners' clinical autonomy: a self-determining perspective. Int Nurs Rev. 2024;71(2):375–95. https://doi.org/10.1111/inr.12948.
8. Swan M, Ferguson S, Chang A, Larson E, Smaldone A. Quality of primary care by advanced practice nurses: a systematic review. Int J Qual Health Care. 2015;27(5):396–404. https://doi.org/10.1093/intqhc/mzv054.
9. World Health Organization regional Office for Europe. Technical brief on strengthening the nursing and midwifery workforce to improve health outcomes: what is known about advancing roles for nurses: evidence and lessons for implementation. Copenhagen: WHO; 2023. Licence: CC BY-NC-SA 3.0 IGO.
10. Wheeler KJ, Miller M, Pulcini J, Gray D, Ladd E, Rayens MK. Advanced practice nursing roles, regulation, education, and practice: a global study. Ann Glob Health. 2022;88(1):42. https://doi.org/10.5334/aogh.3698.
11. Poghosyan L, Liu J, Shang J, D'Aunno T. Practice environments and job satisfaction and turnover intentions of nurse practitioners: implications for primary care workforce capacity. Health Care Manag Rev. 2017;42(2):162–71. https://doi.org/10.1097/HMR.0000000000000094.
12. Schirle L, Norful AA, Rudner N, Poghosyan L. Organizational facilitators and barriers to optimal APRN practice: an integrative review. Health Care Manag Rev. 2020;45(4):311–20. https://doi.org/10.1097/HMR.0000000000000229.
13. Laurant M, van der Biezen M, Wijers N, Watananirun K, Kontopantelis E, van Vught AJ. Nurses as substitutes for doctors in primary care. Cochrane Database Syst Rev. 2018;7:CD001271. https://doi.org/10.1002/14651858.CD001271.pub3.
14. Sangster-Gormley E, Martin-Misener R, Downe-Wamboldt B, DiCenso A. Factors affecting nurse practitioner role implementation in Canadian practice settings: an integrative review. J Adv Nurs. 2011;67(6):1178–90. https://doi.org/10.1111/j.1365-2648.2010.05571.x.
15. Weeks G, George J, Maclure K, Stewart D. Non-medical prescribing versus medical prescribing for acute and chronic disease management in primary and secondary care. Cochrane Database Syst Rev. 2016;11:CD011227. https://doi.org/10.1002/14651858.CD011227.pub2.
16. Kuo YF, Loresto FL Jr, Rounds LR, Goodwin JS. States with the least restrictive regulations experienced the largest increase in patients seen by nurse practitioners. Health Aff (Millwood). 2013;32(7):1236–43. https://doi.org/10.1377/hlthaff.2013.0072.
17. Vedam S, Stoll K, MacDorman M, et al. Mapping integration of midwives across the United States: impact on access, equity, and outcomes. PLoS One. 2018;13(2):e0192523. https://doi.org/10.1371/journal.pone.0192523.
18. Federal Trade Commission. Policy perspectives: competition and the regulation of advanced practice nurses. Washington, DC: FTC; 2014. [cited 2025 Aug 18]. Available from: https://www.ftc.gov/reports/policy-perspectives-competition-regulation-advanced-practice-nurses.

19. Birthplace in England Collaborative Group, Brocklehurst P, Hardy P, et al. Perinatal and maternal outcomes by planned place of birth for healthy women with low risk pregnancies: the birthplace in England national prospective cohort study. BMJ. 2011;343:d7400. https://doi.org/10.1136/bmj.d7400.
20. Gardner G, Gardner A, Middleton S, Della P, Kain V, Doubrovsky A. The work of nurse practitioners. J Adv Nurs. 2010;66(10):2160–9. https://doi.org/10.1111/j.1365-2648.2010.05379.x.
21. Evans C, Poku B, Pearce R, et al. Characterising the outcomes, impacts and implementation challenges of advanced clinical practice roles in the UK: a scoping review. BMJ Open. 2021;11(8):e048171. https://doi.org/10.1136/bmjopen-2020-048171.
22. Rossiter R, Phillips R, Blanchard D, van Wissen K, Robinson T. Exploring nurse practitioner practice in Australian rural primary health care settings: a scoping review. Aust J Rural Health. 2023;31(4):617–30. https://doi.org/10.1111/ajr.13010.
23. de Jonge A, Mesman JA, Manniën J, et al. Severe adverse maternal outcomes among women in midwife-led versus obstetrician-led care at the onset of labour in The Netherlands: a nationwide cohort study. PLoS One. 2015;10(5):e0126266. https://doi.org/10.1371/journal.pone.0126266.
24. Wiegerinck MMJ, van der Goes BY, Ravelli ACJ, et al. Intrapartum and neonatal mortality among low-risk women in midwife-led versus obstetrician-led care in the Amsterdam region of The Netherlands: a propensity score matched study. BMJ Open. 2018;8(1):e018845. https://doi.org/10.1136/bmjopen-2017-018845.
25. van der Biezen M, Adang E, van der Burgt R, Wensing M, Laurant M. The impact of substituting general practitioners with nurse practitioners on resource use, production and healthcare costs during out-of-hours: a quasi-experimental study. BMC Fam Pract. 2016;17(1):132. https://doi.org/10.1186/s12875-016-0528-6.
26. Thies-Lagergren L, Johansson M. Intrapartum midwifery care impact Swedish couple's birth experiences: a cross-sectional study. Women Birth. 2019;32(3):213–20. https://doi.org/10.1016/j.wombi.2018.08.163.
27. Fahlbeck H, Johansson M, Hildingsson I, Larsson B. A longing for a sense of security': women's experiences of continuity of midwifery care in rural Sweden: a qualitative study. Sex Reprod Healthc. 2022;33:100759. https://doi.org/10.1016/j.srhc.2022.100759.
28. Hildingsson I, Karlström A, Larsson B. Childbirth experience in women participating in a continuity of midwifery care project. Women Birth. 2021;34(3):e255–61. https://doi.org/10.1016/j.wombi.2020.04.010.
29. Ndirangu-Mugo E, Kimani RW, Onyancha C, et al. Scopes of practice for advanced practice nursing and advanced practice midwifery in Kenya: a gap analysis. Int Nurs Rev. 2024;71(2):276–84. https://doi.org/10.1111/inr.12947.
30. Rakhab A, Jackson C, Nilmanat K, et al. Factors supporting career pathway development amongst advanced practice nurses in Thailand: a cross-sectional survey. Int J Nurs Stud. 2021;117:103882. https://doi.org/10.1016/j.ijnurstu.2021.103882.
31. Gray DC, Rogers M, Miller MK. Advanced practice nursing initiatives in Africa, moving towards the nurse practitioner role: experiences from the field. Int Nurs Rev. 2024;71(2):205–10. https://doi.org/10.1111/inr.12835.
32. Tamayo RLJ, Moncatar TJR. From task shifting to advanced practice nursing in primary care: a contextualized framework for LMICs informed by evidence from The Philippines. J Nurs Scholarsh. 2025; https://doi.org/10.1111/jnu.70041.
33. Coales K, Jennings H, Afaq S, et al. Perspectives of health workers engaging in task shifting to deliver health care in low- and middle-income countries: a qualitative evidence synthesis. Glob Health Action. 2023;16(1):2228112. https://doi.org/10.1080/16549716.2023.2228112.
34. Dawson AJ, Buchan J, Duffield C, Homer CS, Wijewardena K. Task shifting and sharing in maternal and reproductive health in low-income countries: a narrative synthesis of current evidence. Health Policy Plan. 2014;29(3):396–408. https://doi.org/10.1093/heapol/czt026.
35. Moulton JE, Botfield JR, Subasinghe AK, Withanage NN, Mazza D. Nurse and midwife involvement in task-sharing and telehealth service delivery models in primary care: a scoping review. J Clin Nurs. 2024;33(8):2971–3017. https://doi.org/10.1111/jocn.17106.

36. Scanlon A, Murphy M, Smolowitz J, Lewis V. Advanced nursing practice and advanced practice nursing roles within low- and lower-middle-income countries. J Nurs Scholarsh. 2023;55(2):484–93. https://doi.org/10.1111/jnu.12838.
37. Hailemeskel S, Alemu K, Christensson K, Tesfahun E, Lindgren H. Midwife-led continuity of care improved maternal and neonatal health outcomes in North Shoa Zone, Amhara Regional State, Ethiopia: a quasi-experimental study. Women Birth. 2022;35(4):340–8. https://doi.org/10.1016/j.wombi.2021.08.008.
38. Nove A, Friberg IK, de Bernis L, et al. Potential impact of midwives in preventing and reducing maternal and neonatal mortality and stillbirths: a Lives Saved Tool modelling study. Lancet Glob Health. 2021;9(1):e24–32. https://doi.org/10.1016/S2214-109X(20)30397-1.
39. Donabedian A. The quality of care. How can it be assessed? JAMA. 1988;260(12):1743–8. https://doi.org/10.1001/jama.260.12.1743.
40. World Health Organization. Monitoring the building blocks of health systems: a handbook of indicators and their measurement strategies. Geneva: World Health Organization; 2010. [cited 2025 Aug 27]. Available from: https://apps.who.int/iris/bitstream/handle/10665/258734/9789241564052-eng.pdf.
41. Institute of Medicine (US) Committee on quality of health care in America. Crossing the quality chasm: a new health system for the 21st century. Washington, DC: National Academies Press; 2001. https://doi.org/10.17226/10027.
42. Berwick D, Fox DM. "Evaluating the quality of medical care": Donabedian's classic article 50 years later. Milbank Q. 2016;94(2):237–41. https://doi.org/10.1111/1468-0009.12189.
43. Ministry of Health (Kenya). Kenya health policy 2014–2030 [Internet]. Nairobi: Ministry of Health; 2014. [cited 2025 Aug 18]. Available from: https://extranet.who.int/countryplanningcycles/sites/default/files/planning_cycle_repository/kenya/kenya_health_policy_2014_to_2030.pdf.
44. Mbuthia D, Brownie S, Jackson D, et al. Exploring the complex realities of nursing work in Kenya and how this shapes role enactment and practice: a qualitative study. Nurs Open. 2023;10(8):5670–81. https://doi.org/10.1002/nop2.1812.
45. Njoroge JK, Onsongo L, Githemo GG. Experiences of professional autonomy among critical care nurses in Kenya: a qualitative study. Ann Health Res. 2023;9(3):238–46. [cited 2025 Aug 20]. Available from: https://www.annalsofhealthresearch.com/index.php/ahr/article/view/510.
46. Rabkin M, Lamb M, Osakwe ZT, Mwangi PR, El-Sadr WM, Michaels-Strasser S. Nurse-led HIV services and quality of care at health facilities in Kenya, 2014–2016. Bull World Health Organ. 2017;95(5):353–61. https://doi.org/10.2471/BLT.16.180646.
47. Gathara D, Zosi M, Serem G, et al. Developing metrics for nursing quality of care for low- and middle-income countries: a scoping review linked to stakeholder engagement. Hum Resour Health. 2020;18(1):34. https://doi.org/10.1186/s12960-020-00470-2.
48. Adusei AB, Bour H, Amu H, Afriyie A. Community-based health planning and services programme in Ghana: a systematic review. Front Public Health. 2024;12:1337803. https://doi.org/10.3389/fpubh.2024.1337803.
49. Phillips JF, Awoonor-Williams JK, Bawah AA, et al. What do you do with success? The science of scaling up a health systems strengthening intervention in Ghana. BMC Health Serv Res. 2018;18(1):484. https://doi.org/10.1186/s12913-018-3250-3.
50. Elsey H, Abboah-Offei M, Vidyasagaran AL, et al. Implementation of the community-based health planning and services (CHPS) in rural and urban Ghana: a history and systematic review of what works, for whom and why. Front Public Health. 2023;11:1105495. https://doi.org/10.3389/fpubh.2023.1105495.
51. Dinh M, Walker A, Parameswaran A, Enright N. Evaluating the quality of care delivered by an emergency department fast track unit with both nurse practitioners and doctors. Australas Emerg Nurs J. 2012;15(4):188–94. https://doi.org/10.1016/j.aenj.2012.09.001.
52. Jennings N, O'Reilly G, Lee G, Cameron P, Free B, Bailey M. Evaluating outcomes of the emergency nurse practitioner role in a major urban emergency department, Melbourne,

Australia. J Clin Nurs. 2008;17(8):1044–50. https://doi.org/10.1111/j.1365-2702.2007.02038.x.
53. Roche TE, Gardner G, Jack L. The effectiveness of emergency nurse practitioner service in the management of patients presenting to rural hospitals with chest pain: a multisite prospective longitudinal nested cohort study. BMC Health Serv Res. 2017;17(1):445. https://doi.org/10.1186/s12913-017-2395-9.
54. Considine J, Martin R, Smit D, Winter C, Jenkins J. Emergency nurse practitioner care and emergency department patient flow: case-control study. Emerg Med Australas. 2006;18(4):385–90. https://doi.org/10.1111/j.1742-6723.2006.00870.x.
55. Wilson E, Hanson LC, Tori KE, Perrin BM. Nurse practitioner-led model of after-hours emergency care in an Australian rural urgent care centre: health service stakeholder perceptions. BMC Health Serv Res. 2021;21(1):819. https://doi.org/10.1186/s12913-021-06864-9.
56. Jennings N, Clifford S, Fox AR, O'Connell J, Gardner G. The impact of nurse practitioner services on cost, quality of care, satisfaction and waiting times in the emergency department: a systematic review. Int J Nurs Stud. 2015;52(1):421–35. https://doi.org/10.1016/j.ijnurstu.2014.07.006.
57. Dilworth S, Ball J, Giles M, et al. Patient acceptability and satisfaction with the rural emergency department nurse practitioner model of care (RED-NP MoC). Australas Emerg Care. 2025; https://doi.org/10.1016/j.auec.2025.05.002.
58. Heale R, Rieck Buckley C. An international perspective of advanced practice nursing regulation. Int Nurs Rev. 2015;62(3):421–9. https://doi.org/10.1111/inr.12193.
59. Delamaire ML, Lafortune G. Nurses in advanced roles: a description and evaluation of experiences in 12 developed countries, OECD Health Working Papers No. 54. Paris: OECD Publishing; 2010. https://doi.org/10.1787/18152015.
60. Nuffield Trust. Regulation of advanced practice in nursing and midwifery. London: Nuffield Trust; 2023. [cited 2025 Aug 25]. Available from: https://www.nuffieldtrust.org.uk/sites/default/files/2023-05/Advanced%20practice%20report%20FINAL%5B69%5D.pdf.
61. Anwar S. The global health workforce crisis: are task-shifting strategies sustainable? BMJ Glob Health. 2025;10(6):e019264. https://doi.org/10.1136/bmjgh-2025-019264.
62. Duff E, Golonka R, O'Rourke T, Alraja AA. The nurse practitioner workforce in western Canada: a cross-sectional practice analysis comparison. Policy Polit Nurs Pract. 2022;23(1):32–40. https://doi.org/10.1177/15271544211065432.
63. Peters MDJ, Marnie C, Helms C. Enablers and barriers to nurse practitioners working in Australian aged care: a scoping review. Int J Nurs Stud. 2024;158:104861. https://doi.org/10.1016/j.ijnurstu.2024.104861.
64. Hansson M, Lundgren I, Hensing G, Dencker A, Eriksson M, Carlsson IM. Professional courage to create a pathway within midwives' fields of work: a grounded theory study. BMC Health Serv Res. 2021;21(1):312. https://doi.org/10.1186/s12913-021-06264-y.
65. Hansson M, Lundgren I, Hensing G, Carlsson IM. Veiled midwifery in the baby factory: a grounded theory study. Women Birth. 2019;32(1):80–6. https://doi.org/10.1016/j.wombi.2018.01.003.
66. Catling C, Rossiter C. Midwifery workplace culture in Australia: a national survey of midwives. Women Birth. 2020;33(5):464–72. https://doi.org/10.1016/j.wombi.2019.08.004.
67. Sheehy DA, Smith MR, Gray PJ, Ao PCH. Understanding workforce experiences in the early career period of Australian midwives: insights into factors which strengthen job satisfaction. Midwifery. 2021;93:102880. https://doi.org/10.1016/j.midw.2020.102880.
68. Nedvědová D, Dušová B, Jarošová D. Job satisfaction of midwives: a literature review. Cent Eur J Nurs Midwifery. 2017;8(2):650–6. https://doi.org/10.15452/CEJNM.2017.08.0017.
69. Choi SL, Goh CF, Adam MBH, et al. Transformational leadership, empowerment, and job satisfaction: the mediating role of employee empowerment. Hum Resour Health. 2016;14:73. https://doi.org/10.1186/s12960-016-0171-2.
70. Hansson M, Dencker A, Lundgren I, Carlsson IM, Eriksson M, Hensing G. Job satisfaction in midwives and its association with organisational and psychosocial factors at work:

a nationwide, cross-sectional study. BMC Health Serv Res. 2022;22(1):436. https://doi.org/10.1186/s12913-022-07852-3.
71. World Health Organization. Year of the nurse and the midwife. Geneva: WHO; 2020. [cited 2025 Aug 26]. Available from: https://www.who.int/campaigns/year-of-the-nurse-and-the-midwife-2020.
72. Li S, Roschkov S, Alkhodair A, et al. The effect of nurse practitioner-led intervention in diabetes care for patients admitted to cardiology services. Can J Diabetes. 2017;41(1):10–6. https://doi.org/10.1016/j.jcjd.2016.06.008.
73. Stewart I, Leary A, Khakwani A, et al. Do working practices of cancer nurse specialists improve clinical outcomes? Retrospective cohort analysis from the English National Lung Cancer Audit. Int J Nurs Stud. 2021;118:103718. https://doi.org/10.1016/j.ijnurstu.2020.103718.
74. Wand T, White K, Patching J, Dixon J, Green T. An emergency department-based mental health nurse practitioner outpatient service: part 2, staff evaluation. Int J Ment Health Nurs. 2011;20(6):401–8. https://doi.org/10.1111/j.1447-0349.2011.00743.x.
75. Boman E, Duvaland E, Gaarde K, Leary A, Rauhala A, Fagerström L. Implementation of advanced practice nursing for minor orthopedic injuries in the emergency care context: a non-inferiority study. Int J Nurs Stud. 2021;118:103910. https://doi.org/10.1016/j.ijnurstu.2021.103910.
76. Davids LC, Crowley T. Policy analysis: key milestones in MDR-TB management over the past decade in South Africa. J Public Health Afr. 2024;15(1):703. https://doi.org/10.4102/jphia.v15i1.703.
77. Farley JE, Ndjeka N, Kelly AM, et al. Evaluation of a nurse practitioner-physician task-sharing model for multidrug-resistant tuberculosis in South Africa. PLoS One. 2017;12(8):e0182780. https://doi.org/10.1371/journal.pone.0182780.
78. Tikkanen R, Osborn R, Mossialos E, Djordjevic A, Wharton GA. Canada health care system profile. New York: The Commonwealth Fund; 2020. [cited 2025 Aug 26]. Available from: https://www.commonwealthfund.org/international-health-policy-center/countries/canada.
79. Nguyen NH, Subhan FB, Williams K, Chan CB. Barriers and mitigating strategies to healthcare access in indigenous communities of Canada: a narrative review. Healthcare (Basel). 2020;8(2):112. https://doi.org/10.3390/healthcare8020112.
80. First Nations Information Governance Centre. Our data, our stories, our future: the national report of the first nations regional early childhood, education and employment survey [internet]. Ottawa: FNIGC; 2016. [cited 2020 Mar 29]. Available from: https://fnigc.ca/sites/default/files/docs/fnigc_fnreees_national_report_2016_en_final.pdf.
81. Statistics Canada. Projections of the Aboriginal populations, Canada, provinces and territories. Cat. No. 91-547-X [Internet]. Ottawa: Statistics Canada; 2015. [cited 2020 Mar 27]. Available from: https://www150.statcan.gc.ca/n1/en/catalogue/91-547-X.
82. Wylie L, McConkey S. Insiders' insight: discrimination against indigenous peoples through the eyes of health care professionals. J Racial Ethn Health Disparities. 2019;6(1):37–45. https://doi.org/10.1007/s40615-018-0495-9.
83. Indigenous Services Canada. Preventing and managing chronic disease in first nations communities: a guidance framework, Cat. H34–313/1-2017E-PDF., ISBN 978-0-660-09257-7. Ottawa: Indigenous Services Canada; 2018.
84. Maier CB, Aiken LH, Busse R. Nurses in advanced roles in primary care: policy levers for implementation. OECD Health Working Papers, No. 98 [Internet]. Paris: OECD Publishing; 2017. [cited 2025 Aug 20]. Available from: https://doi.org/10.1787/a8756593-en.
85. Canadian Nurses Association. Advanced practice nursing: a Pan-Canadian framework [Internet]. Ottawa: CNA; 2019. [cited 2025 Aug 20]. Available from: https://hl-prod-ca-oc-download.s3-ca-central-1.amazonaws.com/CNA/2f975e7e-4a40-45ca-863c-5ebf0a138d5e/UploadedImages/documents/nursing/Advanced_Practice_Nursing_framework_e.pdf.
86. Health Canada. Caring for Canadians: Canada's future health workforce—the Canadian Health Workforce Education, Training and Distribution Study (executive summary) [Internet]. Ottawa: Health Canada; 2025. [cited 2025 Aug 20]. Available from: https://www.canada.ca/content/dam/hc-sc/documents/services/health-care-system/health-human-resources/

workforce-education-training-distribution-study/workforce-education-training-distribution-study.pdf.
87. Almost J. Regulated nursing in Canada: the landscape in 2021 [Internet]. Ottawa: Canadian Nurses Association; 2021. [cited 2024 July 10]. Available from: https://hl-prod-ca-oc-download.s3-ca-central-1.amazonaws.com/CNA/2f975e7e-4a40-45ca-863c-5ebf0a138d5e/UploadedImages/documents/Regulated-Nursing-in-Canada_e_Copy.pdf.
88. Canadian Federation of Nurses Unions. Fulfilling nurse practitioners' untapped potential in Canada's health care system: results from the CFNU pan-Canadian Nurse Practitioner Retention & Recruitment Study [Internet]. Ottawa: CFNU; 2018. [cited 2024 July 8]. Available from: https://nursesunions.ca/wp-content/uploads/2018/06/CFNU_UntappedPotentialFinal-EN.pdf.
89. Roots A, MacDonald M. Outcomes associated with nurse practitioners in collaborative practice with general practitioners in rural settings in Canada: a mixed methods study. Hum Resour Health. 2014;12:69. https://doi.org/10.1186/1478-4491-12-69.
90. Beaudry S, Duff E, Ziegler E. 2-Spirit indigenous health care and cultural humility. J Nurse Pract. 2024;20(2):104892. https://doi.org/10.1016/j.nurpra.2023.104892.
91. Wilson EC, Pammett R, McKenzie F, Bourque H. Engagement of nurse practitioners in primary health care in northern British Columbia: a mixed-methods study. CMAJ Open. 2021;9(1):E288–94. https://doi.org/10.9778/cmajo.20200075.
92. Martin-Misener R, Donald F, Kilpatrick K, Bryant-Lukosius D, Rayner J, Landry V, et al. Benchmarking for nurse practitioner patient panel size and comparative analysis of nurse practitioner pay scales: update of a scoping review. Hamilton (ON): Canadian Centre for Advanced Practice Nursing Research, McMaster University; 2015. Available from: https://fhs.mcmaster.ca/ccapnr/documents/np_panel_size_study_updated_scoping_review_report.pdf.
93. Klaasen K, Lamont L, Krishnan P. Setting a new standard of care in nursing homes. Can Nurse. 2009;105(9):24–30.
94. Sangster-Gormley E, Griffith J, Schreiber R, Feddema A, Boryki E, Thompson J. Nurse practitioners changing health behaviours: one patient at a time. Nurs Manag. 2015;22(6):26–31. https://doi.org/10.7748/nm.22.6.26.s29.
95. Floriancic N, Garnett A, Donelle L. Chronic disease management in a nurse practitioner-led clinic: an interpretive description study. SAGE Open Nurs. 2024;10:23779608241299292. https://doi.org/10.1177/23779608241299292.
96. Shand W, Klemmer D, Grubb S, Chesney S, Olsen B, So L. Research to action: nurse practitioners in the emergency department, emergency department transition clinic, and intravenous therapy clinic at Strathcona Community Hospital. Can J Emerg Nurs. 2020;43(1):23–7. https://doi.org/10.29173/cjen44.
97. Steiner IP, Nichols DN, Blitz S, et al. Impact of a nurse practitioner on patient care in a Canadian emergency department. CJEM. 2009;11(3):207–14. https://doi.org/10.1017/s1481803500011222.
98. Thrasher C, Purc-Stephenson R. Patient satisfaction with nurse practitioner care in emergency departments in Canada. J Am Acad Nurse Pract. 2008;20(5):231–7. https://doi.org/10.1111/j.1745-7599.2008.00318.x.
99. Sidani S, Doran D. Relationships between processes and outcomes of nurse practitioners in acute care: an exploration. J Nurs Care Qual. 2010;25(1):31–8. https://doi.org/10.1097/NCQ.0b013e3181af675c.
100. Nanos Research. Canadians' opinions on home healthcare and nurses: CNA research summary [Internet]. Ottawa: Canadian Nurses Association; 2016. [cited 2025 Aug 25]. Available from: https://hl-prod-ca-oc-download.s3-ca-central-1.amazonaws.com/CNA/2f975e7e-4a40-45ca-863c-5ebf0a138d5e/UploadedImages/documents/Canadians_opinions_on_home_healthcare_and_nurses.pdf.
101. Vincent D, Rice J, Chan J, Grassau P. Provision of comprehensive, culturally competent palliative care in the Qikiqtaaluk region of Nunavut: health care providers' perspectives. Can Fam Physician. 2019;65(4):e163–9.

102. MacLeod MLP, Stewart NJ, Kulig JC, et al. Nurses who work in rural and remote communities in Canada: a national survey. Hum Resour Health. 2017;15(1):34. https://doi.org/10.1186/s12960-017-0209-0.
103. Vedam S, Titoria R, Niles P, et al. Advancing quality and safety of perinatal services in India: opportunities for effective midwifery integration. Health Policy Plan. 2022;37(8):1042–63. https://doi.org/10.1093/heapol/czac032.
104. Ministry of Health and Family Welfare, Government of India. Guidelines on midwifery services in India [Internet]. New Delhi: MoHFW; 2018. [cited 2021 Oct 4]. Available from: https://nhm.gov.in/New_Updates_2018/NHM_Components/RMNCHA/MH/Guidelines/Guidelines_on_Midwifery_Services_in_India.pdf.
105. Abimbola S, Okoli U, Olubajo O, Abdullahi MJ, Pate MA. The midwives service scheme in Nigeria. PLoS Med. 2012;9(5):e1001211. https://doi.org/10.1371/journal.pmed.1001211.
106. Kruk ME, Gage AD, Joseph NT, Danaei G, García-Saisó S, Salomon JA. Mortality due to low-quality health systems in the universal health coverage era: a systematic analysis of amenable deaths in 137 countries. Lancet. 2018;392(10160):2203–12. https://doi.org/10.1016/S0140-6736(18)31668-4.
107. Shankar A, Sebayang S, Guarenti L, Utomo B, Islam M, Fauveau V, et al. The village-based midwife programme in Indonesia. Lancet. 2008;371(9620):1226–9. https://doi.org/10.1016/S0140-6736(08)60538-3.
108. National Research Council, Indonesian Academy of Sciences. Reducing maternal and neonatal mortality in Indonesia: saving lives, saving the future. Washington, DC: National Academies Press; 2013. Chapter 5, The quality of care. Available from: https://www.ncbi.nlm.nih.gov/books/NBK201699/.
109. Adegoke AA, Atiyaye FB, Abubakar AS, Auta A, Aboda A. Job satisfaction and retention of midwives in rural Nigeria. Midwifery. 2015;31(10):946–56. https://doi.org/10.1016/j.midw.2015.06.010.
110. Sandall J, Soltani H, Gates S, Shennan A, Devane D. Midwife-led continuity models versus other models of care for childbearing women. Cochrane Database Syst Rev. 2016;4:CD004667. https://doi.org/10.1002/14651858.CD004667.pub5.
111. Thaddeus S, Maine D. Too far to walk: maternal mortality in context. Soc Sci Med. 1994;38(8):1091–110. https://doi.org/10.1016/0277-9536(94)90226-7.
112. World Health Organization. International Confederation of Midwives, International Federation of Obstetricians and Gynecologists. Making pregnancy safer: the critical role of the skilled attendant [Internet]. Geneva: WHO; 2004. [cited 2025 Aug 22]. Available from: http://apps.who.int/iris/bitstream/handle/10665/42955/9241591692.pdf?sequence=1.
113. Podder L, Bhardwaj G, Siddiqui A, Agrawal R, Halder A, Rani M. Utilizing midwifery-led care units for enhanced maternal and newborn health in India: an evidence-based review. Cureus. 2023;15(8):e43214. https://doi.org/10.7759/cureus.43214.
114. Government of India, Ministry of Health and Family Welfare. Labour room quality improvement initiative (LaQshya) [Internet]. New Delhi: NHM. [cited 2025 Aug 21]. Available from: https://nhm.gov.in/index1.php?lang=1&level=3&sublinkid=1307&lid=690.
115. International Confederation of Midwives. Global standards for midwifery education [Internet]. The Hague (Netherlands): ICM; 2021. [cited 2025 Aug 27]. Available from: https://internationalmidwives.org/resources/global-standards-for-midwifery-education/.
116. Mahadalkar PS. Independent midwifery practice in India. Int J Curr Res. 2016;8:33–41. Available from: https://www.journalcra.com/article/independent-midwifery-practice-india.
117. Rao M, Rao KD, Kumar AS, Chatterjee M, Sundararaman T. Human resources for health in India. Lancet. 2011;377(9765):587–98. https://doi.org/10.1016/S0140-6736(10)61888-0.
118. United Nations Population Fund (UNFPA). The state of the world's midwifery 2021 [Internet]. New York: UNFPA; 2021. [cited 2021 Oct 4]. Available from: https://www.unfpa.org/sowmy.
119. Bogren M, Erlandsson K, Ternström E, Sharma B, Wagle RR, Berg M. Contextual factors influencing the implementation of midwifery-led care units in India. Women Birth. 2023;36(1):e134–41. https://doi.org/10.1016/j.wombi.2021.12.004.

120. Chiu P, Thiessen NJ, Idrees S, Leslie K, Kung JY. Nursing regulation in Canada: insights from a scoping review. PLoS One. 2025;20(5):e0323716. https://doi.org/10.1371/journal.pone.0323716.
121. Keighley T, World Health Organization Regional Office for Europe. European Union standards for nursing and midwifery: information for accession countries—revised and updated [Internet]. Copenhagen: WHO; 2009. [cited 2025 Aug 25]. Available from: https://iris.who.int/bitstream/handle/10665/107957/WHO-EURO-2009-8547-48319-71739-eng.pdf.
122. Brigante L, Drandic D, Maimburg RD. Updating the European Union's midwifery directive: advancing women's sexual and reproductive health and reinforcing professional standards within the midwifery profession. Sex Reprod Healthc. 2025; https://doi.org/10.1016/j.srhc.2025.101138.
123. World Health Organization Regional Office for Africa. Creating a common approach to regulation, educational preparation and practice: future direction for nursing & midwifery development in the African Region [Internet]. Brazzaville: WHO; 2016. [cited 2025 Aug 25]. Available from: https://apps.who.int/iris/bitstream/handle/10665/331472/9789290232643-eng.pdf.
124. Thiessen K, Heaman M, Mignone J, Martens P, Robinson K. Barriers and facilitators related to implementation of regulated midwifery in Manitoba: a case study. BMC Health Serv Res. 2016;16:92. https://doi.org/10.1186/s12913-016-1334-5.
125. World Health Organization. Global strategy on human resources for health: workforce 2030. Geneva: WHO; 2016.
126. Torrens C, Campbell P, Hoskins G, et al. Barriers and facilitators to the implementation of the advanced nurse practitioner role in primary care settings: a scoping review. Int J Nurs Stud. 2020;104:103443. https://doi.org/10.1016/j.ijnurstu.2019.103443.
127. Mahmood MA, Mufidah I, Scroggs S, Siddiqui AR, Raheel H, Wibdarminto K, et al. Root-cause analysis of persistently high maternal mortality in a rural district of Indonesia: role of clinical care quality and health services organizational factors. Biomed Res Int. 2018;2018:3673265. https://doi.org/10.1155/2018/3673265.
128. Watkins V, Nagle C, Kent B, Hutchinson AM. Labouring together: collaborative alliances in maternity care in Victoria, Australia—protocol of a mixed-methods study. BMJ Open 2017;7(3):e014262. doi:https://doi.org/10.1136/bmjopen-2016-014262.
129. Pulcini J, Jelic M, Gul R, Loke AY. An international survey on advanced practice nursing education, practice, and regulation. J Nurs Scholarsh. 2010;42(1):31–9. https://doi.org/10.1111/j.1547-5069.2009.01322.x.
130. Kilpatrick K, Savard I, Audet LA, et al. A global perspective of advanced practice nursing research: a review of systematic reviews. PLoS One. 2024;19(7):e0305008. https://doi.org/10.1371/journal.pone.0305008.
131. Stolee P, Hillier LM, Esbaugh J, Griffiths N, Borrie MJ. Examining the nurse practitioner role in long-term care: evaluation of a pilot project in Canada. J Gerontol Nurs. 2006;32(10):28–36. https://doi.org/10.3928/00989134-20061001-05.
132. Hill B. Exploring the development and identity of advanced practice nursing in the UK. Nurs Manag (Harrow). 2017;24(5):36–40. https://doi.org/10.7748/nm.2017.e1607.
133. Lewis R. The evolution of advanced nursing practice: gender, identity, power and patriarchy. Nurs Inq. 2022;29(4):e12489. https://doi.org/10.1111/nin.12489.
134. Pincha Baduge MSS, Garth B, Boyd L, et al. Barriers to advancing women nurses in healthcare leadership: a systematic review and meta-synthesis. EClinicalMedicine. 2023;67:102354. https://doi.org/10.1016/j.eclinm.2023.102354.
135. Kaphle S, Vaughan G, Subedi M. Respectful maternity care in South Asia: what does the evidence say? Experiences of care and neglect, associated vulnerabilities and social complexities. Int J Women's Health. 2022;14:847–79. https://doi.org/10.2147/IJWH.S341907.
136. Byrskog U, Akther HA, Khatoon Z, Bogren M, Erlandsson K. Social, economic and professional barriers influencing midwives' realities in Bangladesh: a qualitative study of midwifery educators preparing midwifery students for clinical reality. Evid Based Midwifery. 2019;17(1):19–26.

137. International Council of Nurses. Guidelines on advanced practice nursing [Internet]. Geneva: ICN; 2020. [cited 2024 Nov 15]. Available from: https://www.icn.ch/system/files/documents/2020-04/ICN_ANP%20Report_EN_WEB.pdf.
138. Hennessy D, Hicks C, Koesno H. The training and development needs of midwives in Indonesia: paper 2 of 3. Hum Resour Health. 2006;4:9. https://doi.org/10.1186/1478-4491-4-9.
139. Lopes-Júnior LC. Advanced practice nursing and the expansion of the role of nurses in primary health care in the Americas. SAGE Open Nurs. 2021;7:23779608211019491. https://doi.org/10.1177/23779608211019491.
140. Obata S, Iriyama S. Development and validation of a professional autonomy scale for Japanese midwives. Nagoya J Med Sci. 2023;85(3):555–68. https://doi.org/10.18999/nagjms.85.3.555.
141. Chiba Y, Hayashi R, Kita Y, Takeshita M. Care provided by midwives and the unmet needs of pregnant and postpartum women: a qualitative study of Japanese mothers. Heliyon. 2023;9(8):e18747. https://doi.org/10.1016/j.heliyon.2023.e18747.
142. van Soeren M, Hurlock-Chorostecki C, Goodwin S, Baker E. The primary healthcare nurse practitioner in Ontario: a workforce study. Nurs Leadersh (Tor Ont). 2009;22(2):58–72. https://doi.org/10.12927/cjnl.2009.20798.
143. Wilson A, Pearson D, Hassey A. Barriers to developing the nurse practitioner role in primary care—the GP perspective. Fam Pract. 2002;19(6):641–6. https://doi.org/10.1093/fampra/19.6.641.
144. Officer TN, McBride-Henry K. Perceptions of underlying practice hierarchies: who is managing my care? BMC Health Serv Res. 2021;21(1):911. https://doi.org/10.1186/s12913-021-06931-1.
145. Christmals CD, Armstrong SJ. The essence, opportunities and threats to Advanced Practice Nursing in Sub-Saharan Africa: a scoping review. Heliyon. 2019;5(10):e02531. Published 2019 Oct 4. https://doi.org/10.1016/j.heliyon.2019.e02531.
146. Laurant MG, Hermens RP, Braspenning JC, Akkermans RP, Sibbald B, Grol RP. An overview of patients' preference for, and satisfaction with, care provided by general practitioners and nurse practitioners. J Clin Nurs. 2008;17(20):2690–8. https://doi.org/10.1111/j.1365-2702.2008.02288.x.
147. Mihret MS, Alemu K, Beshah DT, Gezie LD, Erlandsson K, Lindgren H. Looking into opportunities for maternity continuum of care improvement within the primary health care system in Northwest Ethiopia: primary health care-oriented research. BMC Health Serv Res. 2025;25(1):518. https://doi.org/10.1186/s12913-025-12688-8.
148. Gross JM, McCarthy CF, Verani AR, Iliffe J, Kelley MA, Hepburn KW, et al. Evaluation of the impact of the ARC program on national nursing and midwifery regulations, leadership, and organizational capacity in East, Central, and Southern Africa. BMC Health Serv Res. 2018;18(1):406. https://doi.org/10.1186/s12913-018-3233-4.
149. McCarthy CF, Voss J, Salmon ME, Gross JM, Kelley MA, Riley PL. Nursing and midwifery regulatory reform in East, Central, and Southern Africa: a survey of key stakeholders. Hum Resour Health. 2013;11:29. https://doi.org/10.1186/1478-4491-11-29.
150. Cavagnero E, Daelmans B, Gupta N, Scherpbier R, Shankar A. Assessment of the health system and policy environment as a critical complement to tracking intervention coverage for maternal, newborn, and child health. Lancet. 2008;371(9620):1284–93. https://doi.org/10.1016/S0140-6736(08)60563-2.
151. van Meersbergen D. Task-shifting in The Netherlands. World Med J. 2011;57:126–30.
152. Scanlon A, Cashin A, Bryce J, et al. The complexities of defining nurse practitioner scope of practice in the Australian context. Collegian. 2016;23(2):129–42. https://doi.org/10.1016/j.colegn.2015.03.001.
153. Nove A, Pairman S, Bohle LF, et al. The development of a global midwifery education accreditation programme. Glob Health Action. 2018;11(1):1489604. https://doi.org/10.1080/16549716.2018.1489604.

154. Malya RM, Mahande MJ, Urstad KH, Rogathi JJ, Bø B. Perception of simulation-based education among nursing and midwifery students in Tanzania: a qualitative study. Adv Simul (Lond). 2025;10(1):8. https://doi.org/10.1186/s41077-025-00339-1.
155. Shakhman LM, Al Omari O, Arulappan J, Wynaden D. Interprofessional education and collaboration: strategies for implementation. Oman Med J. 2020;35(4):e160. https://doi.org/10.5001/omj.2020.83.
156. Leonardsen AL. The impact of clinical experience in advanced practice nursing education—a cross-sectional study of Norwegian advanced practice nurses' perspectives. Nurs Rep. 2023;13(3):1304–17. https://doi.org/10.3390/nursrep13030110.
157. Leggat SG, Balding C, Schiftan D. Developing clinical leaders: the impact of an action learning mentoring programme for advanced practice nurses. J Clin Nurs. 2015;24(11–12):1576–84. https://doi.org/10.1111/jocn.12757.
158. Hunter M, Smythe E, Spence D. Confidence: fundamental to midwives providing labour care in freestanding midwifery-led units. Midwifery. 2018;66:176–81. https://doi.org/10.1016/j.midw.2018.08.016.
159. Lawson B, Dicks D, Macdonald L, Burge F. Using quality indicators to evaluate the effect of implementing an enhanced collaborative care model among a community, primary healthcare practice population. Nurs Leadersh (Tor Ont). 2012;25(3):28–42. https://doi.org/10.12927/cjnl.2013.23057.
160. Fosah R, Llahana S. Barriers and enablers to leadership in advanced practice nursing: a systematic review. Int Nurs Rev. 2025;72(2):e70034. https://doi.org/10.1111/inr.70034.
161. Barry R, Green E, Robson K, Nott M. Factors critical for the successful delivery of telehealth to rural populations: a descriptive qualitative study. BMC Health Serv Res. 2024;24(1):908. https://doi.org/10.1186/s12913-024-11233-3.
162. Prata N, Weidert K, Dushimeyesu E, et al. Innovation through telemedicine to improve medication abortion access in primary health centers: findings from a pilot study in Musanze District, Rwanda. BMC Public Health. 2025;25(1):1681.
163. Mohan S, S HS. Usability and quality evaluation of the "E-Midwife" mobile application for nurse-midwives in obstetric complications: a randomized controlled trial. Int J Community Based Nurs Midwifery. 2023;11(4):247–56. https://doi.org/10.30476/IJCBNM.2023.98777.2264.
164. Gajarawala SN, Pelkowski JN. Telehealth benefits and barriers. J Nurse Pract. 2021;17(2):218–21. https://doi.org/10.1016/j.nurpra.2020.09.013.
165. Ahern S, Honardoost MA, Kartik A, et al. Monitoring performance and improving outcomes: characteristics and outputs of Australian clinical registries. Health Inf Manag J. 2025;0(0) https://doi.org/10.1177/18333583251345039.
166. Parker KJ, Hickman LD, Ferguson C. The science of clinical quality registries. Eur J Cardiovasc Nurs. 2023;22(2):220–5. https://doi.org/10.1093/eurjcn/zvad008.
167. Drury A, Boland V, Dowling M. Patient-reported outcome and experience measures in advanced nursing practice: what are key considerations for implementation and optimized use? Semin Oncol Nurs. 2024;40(3):151632. https://doi.org/10.1016/j.soncn.2024.151632.
168. Malapati SH, Edelen MO, Nthumba PM, Ranganathan K, Pusic AL. Barriers to the use of patient-reported outcome measures in low- and middle-income countries. Plast Reconstr Surg Glob Open. 2024;12(2):e5576. https://doi.org/10.1097/GOX.0000000000005576.
169. Stover AM, Haverman L, van Oers HA, Greenhalgh J, Potter CM. ISOQOL PROMs/PREMs in Clinical Practice Implementation Science Work Group. Using an implementation science approach to implement and evaluate patient-reported outcome measures (PROM) initiatives in routine care settings. Qual Life Res. 2021;30(11):3015–33. https://doi.org/10.1007/s11136-020-02564-9.

Global Healthcare Outcomes Improved by APN Clinical Autonomy

Richard Henker, Manila Prak, and Rebecca Silvers

Introduction

Advanced Practice Nurses (APNs) represent a globally recognized role of highly educated nurses who integrate advanced clinical, theoretical, and evidence-based knowledge to provide comprehensive patient care. According to the *International Council of Nurses (ICN) Guidelines on Advanced Practice Nursing* [45], advanced practice nurses are registered nurses who have acquired "the expert knowledge base, complex decision-making skills and clinical competencies for expanded practice, the characteristics of which are shaped by the context and/or country in which they are credentialed to practice." Advanced nursing practice is defined as extending

R. Henker (✉)
Department of Nurse Anesthesia, University of Pittsburgh School of Nursing, Pittsburgh, PA, USA
e-mail: rhe001@pitt.edu

M. Prak
Joint Commission International, Phnom Penh, Cambodia

Ministry of Health, Kingdom of Cambodia, Phnom Penh, Cambodia

Cambodian Association of Nurses, Phnom Penh, Cambodia

R. Silvers
Center for Global Nursing, University of California San Francisco, Institute of Global Health Sciences, San Francisco, CA, USA

Pediatric Neurosurgery & Critical Care Nurse Practitioner, San Francisco, CA, USA

UCSF Benioff Children's Hospitals, Oakland and San Francisco, CA, USA

UCSF School of Nursing, San Francisco, CA, USA

UCSF WHO Collaborating Centre for Emergency, Critical & Operative Care, San Francisco, CA, USA
e-mail: rebecca.silvers@ucsf.edu

A. Kapu et al. (eds.), *A Global View on Clinical Autonomy for Advanced Practice Nurses*, Advanced Practice in Nursing,
https://doi.org/10.1007/978-3-032-21458-4_9

and expanding the boundaries of nursing's scope of practice, characterized by the integration of theoretical and evidence-based knowledge at the graduate level [45, 51]. APN roles, often recognized in the literature as Nurse Practitioners (NPs), Clinical Nurse Specialists (CNSs), Nurse Anesthetists (NAs), and Nurse Midwives (NMs), share a unifying focus on improving access, quality, and continuity of care. The evolution of these roles has demonstrated that when APNs are empowered to function autonomously, outcomes such as patient safety, satisfaction, and care efficiency improve measurably [51].

Clinical Autonomy

Clinical autonomy is a defining feature of advanced practice nursing and a key determinant of its impact on patient and system outcomes. It encompasses the authority and accountability to utilize critical thinking for direct clinical judgments, initiate and modify treatment plans, prescribe medications, and manage care within a defined scope of practice. Core elements of clinical decision-making, professional accountability, interdisciplinary collaboration, and policy and regulatory support collectively enable APNs to optimize patient-focused care delivery. A growing body of evidence links higher levels of professional autonomy to reduced hospital readmissions, improved chronic disease management, and greater patient satisfaction [33, 37].

The autonomy of APNs also aligns closely with global health policy priorities articulated by the World Health Organization (WHO). Both the *Global Strategic Directions for Nursing and Midwifery 2021–2025* [54] and the *State of the World's Nursing Report 2025* [54] identify advanced practice nursing as essential to achieving Universal Health Coverage (UHC) and Sustainable Development Goal 3 (Good Health and Well-being). The 2025 report further expands workforce indicators to include advanced practice roles as a measurable component of system capacity, underscoring that nurses functioning at higher levels of scope directly contribute to improved access, quality, and efficiency of care [54].

The purpose of this chapter is to examine clinical autonomy in advanced practice nursing (APN) with a primary focus on how autonomy influences measurable patient and system outcomes. Rather than framing autonomy solely as a professional characteristic, the discussion emphasizes how decision-making authority affects quality of care, safety, access, continuity, and cost-effectiveness across diverse clinical contexts. Drawing on international regulatory, organizational, and cultural examples, the chapter illustrates how enabling APNs to practice to the full extent of their education and competencies improves performance at both the patient and health system level. In doing so, clinical autonomy is positioned as not only central to APN identity and role evolution but also as a necessary policy lever for strengthening workforce capacity, advancing health equity, and improving global health outcomes.

Conceptual Framework

The Relationship Between Autonomy and Healthcare Outcomes

Clinical autonomy among APNs is consistently linked to improved health outcomes, system efficiency, and professional satisfaction [41]. When APNs are empowered to make clinical decisions such as diagnosing, prescribing, and managing care, the timeliness and continuity of care improve, particularly in primary, critical care, and perioperative settings [41] [23]. Studies demonstrate that autonomous APN practice achieves outcomes comparable to or better than those of physicians in chronic disease management, acute care, and anesthesia services [13, 18, 31]. Greater professional autonomy also correlates with higher job satisfaction and lower turnover, contributing to workforce stability and improved quality of care [18, 40]. Conversely, restrictive regulatory environments and limited decision-making authority can reduce efficiency and undermine the cost-effectiveness of advanced practice roles. Thus, autonomy serves as both a clinical and systemic mechanism for advancing the quality, accessibility, and sustainability of healthcare services.

Models of APN Autonomy

Autonomy in advanced practice nursing is commonly conceptualized as a multidimensional construct encompassing the scope of practice, decision-making authority, and prescriptive rights [11, 31]. These dimensions form the structural basis of APN role effectiveness and delineate the boundaries among dependent, collaborative, and independent models of care. The scope of practice defines the range of activities APNs are authorized to perform, including assessment, diagnosis, treatment, and evaluation of patient outcomes. Decision-making authority reflects the extent to which APNs can exercise clinical judgment without mandatory physician oversight, while prescribing rights determine the degree of pharmacologic management permissible under law or institutional policy [31].

The interaction among these elements is further influenced by organizational culture, interprofessional relationships, and the availability of enabling policies [11, 40, 45]. The International Council of Nurses emphasizes that autonomy is shaped by the local context of education, legislation, and health system design, underscoring that advanced practice cannot be separated from its regulatory and institutional environment [45]

Variations in Regulatory Frameworks Across Countries and Regions [40]

Clinical autonomy varies widely across global jurisdictions. In North America, many US states and Canadian provinces grant nurse practitioners authority to assess, diagnose, treat, order and interpret tests, and prescribe within their regulated scope of practice. In Canada, nurse practitioners are regulated at the provincial and territorial level and are recognized as autonomous healthcare professionals with a broad scope of practice, but regulatory frameworks and specific practice authorities vary across jurisdictions, and national licensure has not yet been fully implemented. In Europe, the United Kingdom and Ireland support extensive prescriptive authority, while several continental European countries maintain more limited, collaborative models [31, 32]. Within the Asia–Pacific region, nations such as Australia and New Zealand have advanced regulatory frameworks, whereas others, including Japan, South Korea, and Taiwan, are progressing toward expanded scopes under physician-delegated structures [31]. In low- and middle-income countries, emerging models of advanced practice, supported by the World Health Organization (WHO) and ICN, are being developed to address workforce shortages and extend access to essential surgical, anesthesia, obstetric, and primary care services [54]. These differences reflect varying levels of system maturity and political will, yet the global trend continues toward enhancing APN autonomy as a key strategy for strengthening universal health coverage.

Integrative Perspective

Taken together, these models suggest that APN autonomy functions as both a professional attribute and a healthcare system outcome. It arises from education, regulation, and interprofessional trust and, in turn, produces measurable improvements in clinical performance and patient well-being. Conceptually, autonomy can be visualized as a dynamic interaction between four reinforcing domains—clinical decision-making, professional accountability, interdisciplinary collaboration, and regulatory support, each is essential for optimizing the contribution of APNs to contributing to health care system outcomes.

APN Roles and Outcomes

Nurse Practitioners (NPs)

Nurse practitioners (NPs) are often on the front lines of primary care delivery, particularly in settings facing physician workforce shortages. In the United States, where many states grant full practice authority, NPs independently diagnose and manage acute and chronic conditions, prescribe medications, and initiate referrals. A substantial body of evidence demonstrates that NP-led care in these settings is associated with outcomes comparable to those of physicians, including effective chronic disease management, high patient satisfaction, and similar or reduced emergency department utilization [27, 37, 49].

In other high-income countries, including Australia and the United Kingdom, NP roles are well established but generally function within more collaborative or delegated regulatory frameworks, with greater variability in prescriptive authority and independent decision-making when compared with the U.S. model [27, 31, 32]. Despite these differences, studies from these settings demonstrate that nurse-led care is safe and effective when supported by appropriate regulation and team-based models [27].

In resource-constrained settings, advanced practice nursing roles—often adapted to local regulatory environments—have been shown to address critical workforce gaps by expanding access to primary and chronic disease care in rural and underserved communities [44]. Evidence from sub-Saharan Africa demonstrates that nurse-led models of care safely manage large caseloads of patients with noncommunicable diseases, maternal health conditions, and infectious diseases, including HIV, with outcomes comparable to physician-led care and improvements in access and continuity of care [4, 24]. These findings align with global workforce priorities outlined in the *State of the World's Nursing* report, which emphasizes advanced nursing roles as essential to achieving universal health coverage and health equity [57].

Global Expansion of Nurse Practitioner Roles

The growing reliance on NPs to enhance primary care capacity in the United States parallels long-standing task-sharing models in many low- and middle-income countries (LMICs). Although educational pathways and regulatory frameworks differ across settings, evidence from LMICs demonstrates that nurse-led models of care can safely and effectively address workforce shortages, particularly in rural and underserved areas. Systematic reviews from sub-Saharan Africa show that nurses managing HIV, chronic disease, and maternal health services achieve clinical outcomes comparable to physician-led care, while improving access, continuity, and service availability [4, 24]. These findings support the role of advanced nursing practice as a pragmatic and evidence-based strategy for expanding primary care capacity in settings with limited physician supply.

Comparative International Evidence

A growing body of international research parallels the findings of Barnes et al. [2] on increased NP utilization. Htay and Whitehead [20] synthesized outcomes from multiple countries and concluded that NPs provide primary care that is comparable in safety, quality, and patient satisfaction to physician-delivered care, though consultation times tend to be longer. Similarly, Maier et al. [32] conducted a scoping review in an analysis across six nations and found that between 67% and 93% of routine primary-care services could be safely managed by NPs, supporting their substitution potential and contribution to system efficiency.

Evidence from Acute and Critical Care Settings

Comparable outcome patterns extend beyond primary care and into acute and critical care environments. Early work by Hoffman and colleagues helped establish the evidence base demonstrating the effectiveness of nurse practitioners in intensive care settings. Their studies showed that patient outcomes for those managed by acute-care nurse practitioners were equivalent to those managed by pulmonary or critical care fellows, including mortality, weaning success, and ventilator days [18]. A complementary time motion analysis by the same research team demonstrated that nurse practitioners and physician trainees distributed their time similarly across direct patient care, procedures, and documentation, reinforcing comparable role complexity and clinical workload. Although nurse practitioners spent more time with patients, families, and collaborating with other health care team providers [17].

Kleinpell et al. [23] expanded this evidence through multicenter observational research and systematic reviews evaluating advanced practice providers in high-acuity environments. Their work concluded that nurse practitioners and clinical nurse specialists contribute to improved care coordination, reduced complications, enhanced communication, and in many cases shorter length of stay—without compromising safety, mortality outcomes, or quality indicators [23].

Subsequent research has consistently confirmed and extended these findings. Landsperger et al. [26] reported no difference in 90-day survival between patients managed by nurse practitioners and those managed by resident teams in an academic medical ICU. Liao et al. [30] reinforced these findings in non-surgical ICU populations, demonstrating comparable mortality, length of stay, and readmission rates between NP-staffed and resident-staffed settings. Most recently, a 2024 study by Zhang et al. [58] found no significant differences in cardiac ICU or hospital mortality between patients managed by advanced practice providers and those managed by house staff teams.

Finally, meta-analytic evidence continues to support these outcome trends. Kreeftenberg et al. [25] concluded that across adult ICUs, advanced practice providers achieve equivalent patient outcomes—including mortality, ICU length of stay, and readmission—compared to physician trainees, while offering additional advantages such as care continuity and cost-effectiveness.

These studies provide evidence that the lack of outcome differences observed in primary care extends into high-acuity settings. Whether managing patients with chronic diseases in the community or critically ill patients in intensive care, nurse practitioners consistently demonstrate clinical competence, efficiency, and quality outcomes comparable to those of their physician counterparts (Table 1).

Case Example: LMIC Implementation

A recent case study from Uganda provides a practical example of NP integration into rural and peri-urban health systems. Nashwan [35] report that nurse-led HIV and maternal-health programs delivered clinical outcomes equivalent to physician-led models while extending service reach and improving efficiency in resource-limited districts. These findings echo the US experience described by Barnes et al. [2], where practices in rural areas increasingly relied on NPs to meet population health needs. Together, they demonstrate that advanced practice nurses can serve as adaptable components of interdisciplinary primary-care teams across diverse income settings.

Table 1 Evidence on nurse practitioner (NP) autonomy, outcomes, and system impact

Study	Design/setting	Sample/ population	Key findings	Outcome measures
Hoffman et al. [17]	Time–motion analysis, ICU	ACNPs vs physician trainees	Similar workload distribution; NPs spent more time with patients/families	Time allocation
Hoffman et al. [18]	Prospective cohort, medical ICU	ACNP-led vs fellow-led care	Equivalent mortality, ventilator days, and weaning success	Mortality, ventilator days
Kleinpell et al. [23]	Multicenter observational review	APPs in high-acuity settings	Improved coordination; similar mortality & LOS	Mortality, LOS, complications
Kreeftenberg et al. [25]	Meta-analysis, adult ICUs	APPs vs physician trainees	Equivalent ICU outcomes; continuity benefits	Mortality, LOS, readmissions
Landsperger et al. [26]	Prospective cohort, medical ICU	NP-led vs resident-led teams	No difference in 90-day survival	Survival, LOS
Maier et al. [32]	Scoping review across six countries	Primary care NPs	NPs can safely manage 67–93% of primary-care services	Quality, efficiency
Barnes et al. [2]	US workforce analysis	Primary care practices	NP utilization ↑ access in rural areas	Access indicators
Htay and Whitehead [20]	Systematic review	International primary care NPs	NP care comparable to physicians; high satisfaction	Safety, satisfaction
Liao et al. [30]	Retrospective cohort, non-surgical ICU	NP vs resident teams	Comparable mortality, LOS, readmissions	Mortality, LOS
Scanlon et al. [44]	LMIC implementation review	NP/APN roles in LMICs	Roles improve service availability, continuity	Access, continuity
Zhang et al. [58]	Multicenter cardiac ICU cohort	NP/APP vs housestaff	No difference in hospital/CICU mortality	CICU mortality
Nashwan et al. [35]	LMIC case study (Uganda)	NP-led HIV/ maternal programs	Outcomes equivalent to physicians; expanded reach	Maternal outcomes, access

Policy and Workforce Implications

Lessons from LMIC contexts reinforce the importance of supportive policy environments similar to full scope-of-practice laws in the United States for maximizing NP contributions. Regulatory clarity, standardized postgraduate training, and sustainable financing mechanisms remain essential for ensuring quality and integration. As value-based and team-based models expand globally, policymakers may look to both the United States and LMIC experiences for evidence that enabling advanced nursing practice can mitigate workforce shortages, particularly in rural areas where traditional physician supply remains limited.

Nurse Anesthetists

Nurse anesthetists play a vital role in addressing the global shortage of anesthesia professionals and expanding access to essential surgical and obstetric services. Recognized by the World Health Organization (WHO) as essential members of the surgical workforce, nurse anesthetists (NAs) are often the primary anesthesia providers in rural and underserved areas [10]. Their clinical autonomy directly influences patient safety, surgical capacity, and system resilience. The International Council of Nurses defines NAs as registered nurses with advanced preparation in anesthesia who provide care autonomously and collaboratively within interprofessional teams [21].

Evidence on Nurse Anesthetist Outcomes

Multiple studies have demonstrated that anesthesia care delivered by nurse anesthetists is safe, effective, and cost-efficient. Dulisse and Cromwell [13] analyzed over 481,000 Medicare surgical cases and found *no difference in mortality or anesthesia-related complications* between anesthesia care delivered by Certified Registered Nurse Anesthetists (CRNAs) and physician anesthesiologists. Hogan et al. [19] found that clinical practice patterns between CRNAs and anesthesiologists were comparable, while CRNAs delivered care at a lower overall cost [19]. Lewis et al. [29] conducted a systematic review published in the *Cochrane Database of Systematic Reviews*. More recent national analyses confirm these findings: Tarazi et al. [50] examined state-level variation in scope-of-practice laws and found that reducing restrictions on CRNA practice did not negatively impact patient safety, with no increase in anesthesia-related complications or adverse events. Taken together, this evidence demonstrates that CRNAs provide high-quality anesthesia care across a wide range of clinical settings (Table 2).

Regional Impact: Cambodia and Laos

At the Angkor Hospital for Children (AHC) in Cambodia and the Lao Friends Hospital for Children (LFHC) in Laos, locally trained nurse anesthetists supported through Health Volunteers Overseas (HVO) have transformed pediatric anesthesia services. Since 2015, nurse anesthetists at these institutions have implemented ultrasound-guided regional anesthesia programs, infection prevention protocols, and perioperative safety checklists that have measurably improved patient outcomes and reduced complication rates. Their growing autonomy has enabled consistent delivery of pediatric anesthesia in settings where physician anesthetists are scarce, contributing directly to surgical capacity, patient safety, and workforce sustainability. These models demonstrate how local investment in nurse anesthesia education and mentoring builds a sustainable model for increasing patient care while maintaining international standards of care (Table 3).

Table 2 Summary of key studies comparing outcomes by anesthesia provider type

Study	Design/setting	Sample/ population	Key findings	Outcome measures
Tarazi et al. [50]	National observational study using state-level regulatory variation	Multi-state sample of CRNA practice environments	States that reduced restrictions on CRNA scope of practice showed no negative impact on patient safety; loosening regulations did not increase adverse events	Patient safety indicators, anesthesia-related complications, and adverse event rates
Silber et al. [46]	Retrospective cohort, 194 hospitals	194,430 Medicare surgical cases	No significant difference in mortality or failure-to-rescue between anesthesiologist-directed and CRNA-delivered care	Mortality, failure-to-rescue
Pine et al. [39]	Retrospective analysis, 404 hospitals (USA)	481,440 Medicare surgical cases	Surgical mortality did not differ by anesthesia provider type	30-day mortality
Needleman and Minnick [36]	Retrospective cohort, 1086 hospitals (USA)	1.5 million maternal deliveries	No significant differences in maternal outcomes between anesthesia care models	Maternal complications, mortality
Simonson et al. [47]	Retrospective analysis, obstetric population (USA)	134,806 cesarean deliveries	No increase in anesthetic complications when CRNAs provided anesthesia independently	Anesthetic complications
Dulisse and Cromwell [13]	Retrospective analysis, Medicare claims (USA)	481,440 cases (opt-out vs non–opt-out states)	No harm or increase in mortality when CRNAs practiced without physician supervision	Mortality, postoperative complications
Rosseel et al. [43]	Longitudinal observational study (Haiti)	15,000 surgeries over 10 years	Non-physician anesthesia providers trained through NGO programs delivered safe anesthesia with low mortality	Anesthesia-related mortality and complications
Umutesi et al. [52]	Mixed-methods assessment, Western Kenya government hospitals	A multiple-level hospital system served by nurse anesthetists	Implementation of nurse anesthetists improved anesthesia safety indicators and expanded surgical access without an increase in adverse outcomes	Perioperative mortality, complication rates, and access to anesthesia services

Using the WHO Operative Encounter Registry to Drive Quality Improvement and Policy Reform

The development and implementation of the WHO Operative Encounter Registry (OER) represents an important advancement in measuring anesthesia care quality and demonstrating the value of clinical autonomy of nurse anesthetists, particularly

Table 3 Comparison of surgical volume and anesthesia workforce: Cambodia, Lao PDR, and United States

Indicator	Cambodia	Lao PDR	United States	Source/Notes
Population (approx.)	17 million	7.5 million	333 million	World Bank (55)
Surgical procedures per 100,000 population	419–1356	~620	9500–11,000	World Bank [53]
Total estimated surgical procedures (annual)	228,000–230,000	46,500	31–36 million	Calculated from rates × population
Physician anesthesia providers (per 100,000)	1.69	1.23	20.8	Law et al. [28]
Non-physician (nurse) anesthesia providers (per 100,000)	2.10	0.53	20.9	Law et al. [28]
Total anesthesia providers (per 100,000)	3.79	1.76	41.7	Computed from above
Estimated provider counts	290 physician; 361 non-physician	92 physician; 40 non-physician	69,000 anesthesiologists; 60,000 CRNAs	Derived from workforce registries

in low- and middle-income countries (LMICs). Established through collaboration between the World Health Organization and the Global Alliance for Surgical, Obstetric, Trauma, and Anesthesia Care (G4 Alliance), the OER provides a standardized framework for collecting operative and anesthesia indicators using the DHIS-2 platform. The tool was formally introduced during the 77th World Health Assembly in 2024, signaling its potential role in strengthening national surgical and anesthesia information systems. Early feasibility work in Lao PDR, Kenya, and Pakistan demonstrated that the OER can effectively capture case mix, safety metrics, complications, and clinical recovery measures, creating a mechanism to track performance and generate evidence where none previously existed. This is especially relevant in settings where nurse anesthetists provide the majority of perioperative care. Research already suggests that scaling the anesthesia workforce in LMICs, particularly through well-trained nurse anesthetists, improves access to surgical services [52]. The OER adds the critical next step: the ability to measure outcomes and demonstrate impact.

The OER can strengthen clinical autonomy by equipping nurse anesthetists with meaningful performance data, enabling them to engage in evidence-informed decision-making, advocate for resources, and participate in national quality improvement and policy discussions. As additional sites join and the dataset grows, the OER has the potential to provide the first multi-country dataset describing anesthesia care delivered by nurse anesthetists in LMICs, moving beyond narrative justification to measurable outcomes. In doing so, it reinforces a central premise of advanced practice nursing: autonomy paired with accountability strengthens care quality, expands access, and advances health care system equity.

Clinical Nurse Specialists (CNSs)

Clinical Nurse Specialists (CNSs) are advanced practice nurses who combine expert clinical judgment with systems-level leadership to strengthen care delivery and improve patient outcomes. Their practice spans direct patient care, consultation, staff and patient education, research translation, and leadership in program development. CNSs are frequently positioned at the interface of clinical operations and organizational strategy, ensuring that policies, protocols, and evidence-based standards are both feasible and effectively implemented at the point of care. Their expertise is most visible in high-acuity or complex environments such as critical care, oncology, perioperative services, and infection prevention, where care coordination, risk mitigation, and rapid decision-making are central to patient safety.

Impact on Patient Outcomes

Substantial evidence from high-income health systems demonstrates that CNS involvement contributes to measurable improvement in both clinical and operational outcomes. In a meta-analysis, Newhouse et al. [37] reported that CNS-led models reduced length of stay, improved patient satisfaction, and decreased care delivery costs compared with traditional models. Similarly, Donald et al. [12] found that CNS-directed chronic disease management programs improved clinical stability and reduced hospital readmissions. These effects are attributed not only to advanced clinical assessment and consultation skills but also to CNS leadership in applying evidence-based frameworks, optimizing workflows, and enhancing continuity across care transitions.

Quality Improvement and Patient Safety Leadership

CNSs are instrumental in translating quality improvement (QI) science into practice. Their work frequently begins with identifying variation or gaps in care using tools such as chart audits, safety event reviews, process mapping, or gap analysis to determine where improvements are needed. Based on these findings, CNSs lead or co-lead initiatives grounded in recognized QI methods, including Plan–Do–Study–Act (PDSA) cycles, root-cause analysis, and implementation science frameworks. Such approaches support iterative testing, rapid feedback, team engagement, and sustained practice change.

Through these structured methods, CNSs help close the gap between current and optimal performance, increasing adherence to clinical guidelines, reducing preventable harm, and improving safety culture. Their ongoing monitoring and evaluation ensure that improvements are durable, scalable, and aligned with system goals such as accreditation standards, national quality metrics, or benchmarking initiatives.

Infection Prevention and Critical Care

CNS leadership is strongly associated with improved outcomes in infection prevention and critical care. Studies such as Harlan et al. [16], Richardson and Tjoelker [42] have demonstrated reductions in central line–associated bloodstream infections (CLABSI) following CNS-led implementation of surveillance programs, staff coaching, standardization of procedures, and use of quality improvement methodologies. In addition, a Clinical Nurse Specialist–led CAUTI prevention initiative showed that rates of catheter-associated urinary tract infection dropped from 16.67 to 0 cases per 1000 catheter days following the implementation of a best-practice bundle that included education, competency assessment, and adherence audits, with sustained reductions in catheter utilization and improvements in documentation practices [38]. These results reinforce the alignment among CNS practice, regulatory standards, and value-based care outcomes.

Evidence from diverse settings supports similar trends. In Japan, CNS leadership in an open intensive care unit was associated with reductions in ICU mortality and fewer patients requiring mechanical ventilation [15], offering early international evidence of CNS impact outside North American contexts. Collectively, these findings underscore that CNS expertise in systems leadership, change management, and QI science can meaningfully improve outcomes across specialties.

Global and LMIC Perspectives

Although CNS roles are primarily formalized in high-income settings, their core functions—mentorship, quality improvement, and coordination of complex care—are increasingly recognized as critical to health system strengthening in low- and middle-income countries (LMICs). Emerging evidence from resource-constrained hospitals shows that nurse-led and interprofessional training programs in surgical site infection prevention can improve clinicians' knowledge, self-reported adherence to evidence-based practices, and perioperative infection-control behaviors, even where supplies and infrastructure are limited [22]. These models, alongside studies demonstrating that targeted nursing interventions can reduce surgical site infection rates and improve wound healing in high-risk surgical populations, suggest that CNS-type leadership roles may represent a scalable strategy for driving quality improvement in low-resource hospitals (Table 4).

Nurse Midwives

Nurse Midwives practicing autonomously are integral to improving maternal and newborn outcomes worldwide. The WHO emphasizes midwife-led care as a critical strategy to reduce maternal and neonatal mortality [54]. Autonomous nurse midwifery practice includes conducting antenatal visits, managing labor and delivery, and providing postpartum and newborn care [54].

Table 4 Summary of key studies evaluating clinical nurse specialist outcomes

Study	Design/setting	Population/ specialty	Key findings	Outcome measures
Fukuda et al. [15]	Observational before–after cohort	Adult ICU, Japan	Introduction of a CNS as head nurse was associated with significantly lower ICU mortality and fewer patients requiring mechanical ventilation	ICU mortality; mechanical ventilation prevalence
Cheung et al. [9]	Narrative review and role evaluation	Cancer services coordination	CNS participation supported earlier triage, efficient care coordination, and improved patient education and service navigation	Care coordination efficiency; education quality; referral timeliness
Smith and Greenwood [48]	Observational evaluation of CNS-led specialty care	Renal specialty services	CNS involvement improved care continuity, resource utilization, and patient monitoring in long-term renal disease management	Continuity of care; resource use metrics; clinical monitoring indicators

Evidence Linking Midwifery Autonomy to Improved Maternal and Newborn Outcomes in LMICs

Growing evidence demonstrates that when midwives are enabled to practice autonomously through the support of regulation, appropriate training, and a clearly defined scope of practice, maternal and newborn outcomes improve without compromising safety. Studies from low- and middle-income countries (LMICs) indicate that midwife-led models of care are associated with higher rates of vaginal birth, reduced reliance on unnecessary cesarean sections and episiotomy, and improved continuity of care. The strongest outcomes are seen in settings where midwives are integrated into primary health care systems and empowered to lead antenatal, intrapartum, and postpartum care. Evidence also highlights that clinical autonomy alone is insufficient; supportive health system conditions such as clinical mentorship, adequate staffing, equitable deployment, and regulatory oversight are necessary to translate professional authority into improved clinical outcomes. The table below summarizes key peer-reviewed studies contributing to this evidence base (Table 5).

Summary Interpretation

Across LMIC contexts, research consistently demonstrates that when midwives are permitted to practice autonomously—within supportive regulatory, organizational, and educational environments—maternal and newborn outcomes improve, quality of care strengthens, and reliance on unnecessary interventions decreases. These findings reinforce the importance of autonomy not merely as a professional

Table 5 Evidence on outcomes of autonomous or nurse midwife-led care in LMICs

Study	Setting	Design	Key findings related to outcomes
Fikre et al. [14]	Multiple LMICs	Systematic review and meta-analysis	Midwife-led care is associated with higher spontaneous vaginal birth, lower emergency cesarean rate, and reduced episiotomy use without compromising safety.
Callander et al., [5]	Bangladesh, Pakistan, sub-Saharan Africa	Multi-country case study	Midwife-led birthing centers improved access to care, reduced unnecessary intervention, and supported continuity of care
Michel-Schuldt et al., [34]	Multiple LMICs	Integrative review	Midwife-led models showed improved continuity, respectful maternity care, and patient experience; authors also noted variation in standards of practice, regulation of midwifery roles, and supportive infrastructure
Adnani et al. [1]	LMIC global analysis	Evidence review	Highlights that autonomy, when paired with supportive health systems and regulation, correlates with improved maternal–newborn outcomes
WHO Evidence Brief, 2024 [56]	Global LMIC context	Policy synthesis	Identifies midwife-led continuity models as a cost-effective approach to reducing maternal and neonatal morbidity in resource-constrained settings

privilege, but as a health system strategy with direct implications for safety, access, equity, and performance.

Case Study: Cambodia—The Impact of Midwives on Maternal and Newborn Health Outcomes

Background

Cambodia has experienced one of the most rapid improvements in maternal and newborn health in Southeast Asia. Midwives have been central to this progress, particularly in rural and decentralized settings where physicians remain scarce. Their expanding scope, leadership roles, and growing contribution to primary care have positioned midwives as essential providers in achieving national health priorities and advancing Universal Health Coverage (UHC).

Role of Midwives in the Health System

Midwives serve as the backbone of Cambodia's primary healthcare (PHC) network. In many health centers, particularly outside major cities, midwives are the primary clinicians responsible for antenatal care, intrapartum management, postnatal follow-up, health education, and family planning. As physician density remains low (especially in rural areas), midwives frequently hold formal leadership roles such as Health Center Chief, where they oversee:

- Clinical decision-making and triage.

- Staff supervision and mentorship.
- Supply chain and budgeting.
- Implementation of Ministry of Health standards.

Their autonomy reflects practical task-sharing based on need, and is foundational to continuity of maternal and newborn care.

Strengthening Care Through Collaboration and System Integration

Midwives work closely with Village Health Support Groups (VHSGs), referral hospitals, and national partners to ensure seamless care pathways. This interprofessional coordination supports early risk identification, timely referral, and postpartum follow-up. These relationships also link community-level practice with national maternal and newborn health strategies, ensuring local implementation aligns with policy goals.

Documented Impact on Patient Outcomes

Cambodia's health indicators demonstrate dramatic progress aligned with midwifery expansion, improved training standards, and strengthened regulatory oversight:

Indicator	2000	2014	2022	National Target
Maternal mortality ratio (deaths per 100,000 live births)	437	170	154	<70 by 2034
Neonatal mortality rate (per 1000 live births)	–	18	8	<6 by 2034
Skilled birth attendance	–	89%	>90%	Sustained
Facility-based delivery	–	–	88.2%	96% by 2034
≥4 antenatal care visits	–	–	74.9%	95% by 2034

Notably, the reduction in neonatal mortality (51% decline between 2014 and 2022) demonstrates effective transition from access to quality—an achievement realized 8 years ahead of national targets [6, 8].

Current Workforce Status and Persistent Challenges

Despite progress, the midwifery workforce remains below required levels to meet future population needs:

- Midwife density: 6.8 per 10,000 population [3, 7].
- Licensure gap: Only 62.5% of registered midwives hold a valid practice license [8].
- Urban–rural distribution inequities remain pronounced [7].
- Attrition and dual employment signal system-level retention barriers [7].

Without targeted investment, Cambodia risks regression in maternal and newborn outcomes as childbirth volumes rise and case complexity increases.

Strategic Investment Priorities (2025–2034)

To sustain momentum, national and partner strategies are prioritizing:

- Competency-based education and standardized clinical preceptorship.
- Mandatory continuing professional development (CPD).
- Equitable deployment and rural retention incentives.
- Strengthened regulatory oversight and midwifery governance.
- Safe, dignified work environments and professional recognition.

These investments aim not only to expand the workforce but to ensure quality, accountability, and consistency of care delivery.

Conclusion

Cambodia's rapid improvement in maternal and newborn outcomes illustrates the transformative role of midwives when supported through education, regulation, and system integration. Continued investment in the midwifery workforce remains one of Cambodia's most cost-effective paths toward UHC and the Sustainable Development Goals. Strengthening midwives' leadership, practice autonomy, and professional infrastructure will be essential to ensure no woman or newborn is left behind.

Barriers to APN Autonomy

Although advanced practice nurses (APNs) have demonstrated positive effects on access, quality, and efficiency of care, their ability to practice autonomously remains limited in many health systems. Persistent legal, regulatory, and institutional barriers constrain APNs from applying their full range of competencies. Inconsistent legislation, fragmented credentialing, and restrictive supervision requirements continue to narrow clinical authority even in countries that recognize advanced practice roles [21, 32].

Beyond policy constraints, a critical gap in systematically measured outcomes continues to hinder progress. While studies demonstrate comparable or superior outcomes in settings where APNs have high decision-making authority, the evidence base remains uneven across regions and practice domains [40, 49]. In many low- and middle-income countries, the absence of rigorous data linking APN autonomy to patient and system outcomes weakens arguments for reform and limits political traction.

The *State of the World's Nursing 2025* report calls for greater investment in research and data systems to document the contribution of advanced practice roles to national health goals [57]. Without outcome-driven evidence, efforts to expand the scope of practice, standardize regulation, and integrate APNs into workforce planning remain vulnerable to resistance from traditional professional hierarchies. Strengthening the empirical foundation linking autonomy to measurable outcomes is therefore a strategic priority for advancing policy recognition and sustainable role integration globally.

Strategies to Promote APN Autonomy Globally

Promoting Advanced Practice Nurse (APN) autonomy is a strategic pathway to improving health outcomes, particularly in systems facing workforce shortages and growing demands for high-quality, cost-effective care. The *State of the World's Nursing 2025* report highlights that countries with supportive policy environments enabling advanced practice roles demonstrate greater progress toward Universal Health Coverage (UHC) and more equitable service delivery [57].

Strengthening regulatory frameworks and scope-of-practice laws ensures that APNs can apply their full clinical expertise, which has been linked to improved chronic disease management, reduced wait times, and higher patient satisfaction [49]. Evidence-based policy reform—grounded in measurable outcomes—provides the foundation for sustainable role integration.

Integration of APNs into national health policy and workforce planning enables data-driven deployment of advanced nursing roles in underserved areas. Embedding APNs in strategic planning aligns their contributions with population health targets and facilitates the collection of national outcome data to guide policy refinement.

Investment in APN education and leadership development correlates with higher quality and safety metrics across health systems. Graduate-level preparation and mentorship cultivate leadership capacity to drive evidence-informed practice and innovation, amplifying the role of APNs as catalysts for system improvement.

Finally, interprofessional collaboration and physician partnership remain essential for achieving outcome-oriented autonomy. Support from physicians and administrative champions helps integrate APN-led models of care, strengthening continuity, efficiency, and teamwork—all measurable determinants of better patient outcomes.

Collectively, these strategies advance not only professional autonomy but also the evidence base linking APN practice to tangible improvements in health system performance and population health.

Conclusion

Clinical autonomy lies at the center of Advanced Practice Nursing's contribution to modern healthcare systems. Evidence consistently demonstrates that when APNs are empowered to practice to the full extent of their education and scope, patient outcomes improve—manifested in greater access to care, higher satisfaction, reduced hospitalizations, and more efficient use of resources. Yet autonomy remains unevenly supported by regulation, education, and institutional culture. Strengthening the evidence base that links APN clinical autonomy to measurable system outcomes is essential for shaping policy and investment decisions. As highlighted in the *State of the World's Nursing 2025* report, advancing autonomy is not solely a professional aspiration but a strategic imperative for achieving Universal Health Coverage (UHC) and sustainable global health equity. The future of nursing's impact will depend on translating autonomy into action—and outcomes—across every level of practice and policy.

References

1. Adnani QES, Nurfitriyani E, Merida Y, Khuzaiyah S, Okinarum GY, Susanti AI, Adepoju VA, Hashim SH. Ninety-one years of midwifery continuity of care in low and middle-income countries: a scoping review. BMC Health Serv Res. 2025;25(1):463. https://doi.org/10.1186/s12913-025-12612-0.
2. Barnes H, Richards MR, McHugh MD, Martsolf G. Rural and nonrural primary care physician practices increasingly rely on nurse practitioners. Health Aff (Millwood). 2018;37(6):908–14. https://doi.org/10.1377/hlthaff.2017.1158.
3. C. M. Council. Midwife registration and licensing records. C. M. Council; 2024.
4. Callaghan M, Ford N, Schneider H. A systematic review of task- shifting for HIV treatment and care in Africa. Hum Resour Health. 2010;8:8. https://doi.org/10.1186/1478-4491-8-8.
5. Callander EJ, Scarf V, Nove A, Homer C, Carrandi A, Abdullah AS, Clow S, Halim A, Mbalinda SN, Nabirye RC, Rahman AKMF, Rasheed SI, Turk AM, Bazirete O, Turkmani S, Forrester M, Mandke S, Pairman S, Boyce M. Midwife-led birthing centres in Bangladesh, Pakistan and Uganda: an economic evaluation of case study sites. BMJ Glob Health. 2024;9(3):e013643. https://doi.org/10.1136/bmjgh-2023-013643.
6. Cambodia MoH. Cambodia demographic and health survey 2021–22. N. I. o. Statistics; 2023. https://www.dhsprogram.com/pubs/pdf/FR377/FR377.pdf?utm_source=chatgpt.com.
7. Cambodia MoH (2024). National health workforce development plan 2024–2033.
8. Cambodia MoH. Health strategic plan 2025–2034. M. o. H. (Cambodia); 2025. https://his-mohcambodia.org/public/fileupload/HEALTH%20STRATEGIC%20PLAN%202025-2034_Eng%20Final.pdf.
9. Cheung V, Brown J, Julius A, Mitchell L, Moura S, Jin R. Guiding the clinical nurse specialist role in oncology within Princess Margaret cancer Centre. Can Oncol Nurs J. 2022;32(3):357–65. https://doi.org/10.5737/23688076323357.
10. Cohen C, Baird M, Koirola N, Kandrack R, Martsolf G. The surgical and anesthesia workforce and provision of surgical services in rural communities: a mixed-methods examination. J Rural Health. 2021;37(1):45–54. https://doi.org/10.1111/jrh.12417.
11. Delamaire M-L, Lafortune G. Nurses in advanced roles: a description and evaluation of experiences in 12 developed countries, OECD Health Working Papers; 2010. https://doi.org/10.1787/5kmbrcfms5g7-en.
12. Donald F, Kilpatrick K, Reid K, Carter N, Martin-Misener R, Bryant-Lukosius D, Harbman P, Kaasalainen S, Marshall DA, Charbonneau-Smith R, Donald EE, Lloyd M, Wickson-Griffiths A, Yost J, Baxter P, Sangster-Gormley E, Hubley P, Laflamme C, Campbell-Yeo M, Price S, Boyko J, DiCenso A. A systematic review of the cost-effectiveness of nurse practitioners and clinical nurse specialists: what is the quality of the evidence? Nurs Res Pract. 2014;2014:896587. https://doi.org/10.1155/2014/896587.
13. Dulisse B, Cromwell J. No harm found when nurse anesthetists work without supervision by physicians. Health Aff (Millwood). 2010;29(8):1469–75. https://doi.org/10.1377/hlthaff.2008.0966.
14. Fikre R, Gubbels J, Teklesilasie W, Gerards S. Effectiveness of midwifery-led care on pregnancy outcomes in low- and middle-income countries: a systematic review and meta-analysis. BMC Pregnancy Childbirth. 2023;23(1):386. https://doi.org/10.1186/s12884-023-05664-9.
15. Fukuda T, Sakurai H, Kashiwagi M. Impact of having a certified nurse specialist in critical care nursing as head nurse on ICU patient outcomes. PLoS One. 2020;15(2):e0228458. https://doi.org/10.1371/journal.pone.0228458.

16. Harlan MD, Kennell JS, Lucas W, Ren D, Tuite PK. A clinical nurse specialist–led quality improvement initiative to identify barriers to adherence to a bundle for central line maintenance. Clin Nurse Spec. 2022;36(2):99–108. https://doi.org/10.1097/nur.0000000000000657.
17. Hoffman LA, Tasota FJ, Scharfenberg C, Zullo TG, Donahoe MP. Management of patients in the intensive care unit: comparison via work sampling analysis of an acute care nurse practitioner and physicians in training. Am J Crit Care. 2003;12(5):436–43.
18. Hoffman LA, Tasota FJ, Zullo TG, Scharfenberg C, Donahoe MP. Outcomes of care managed by an acute care nurse practitioner/attending physician team in a subacute medical intensive care unit. Am J Crit Care. 2005;14(2):121–30. quiz 131-122
19. Hogan PF, Seifert RF, Moore CS, Simonson BE. Cost effectiveness analysis of anesthesia providers. Nurs Econ. 2010;28(3):159–69.
20. Htay M, Whitehead D. The effectiveness of the role of advanced nurse practitioners compared to physician-led or usual care: a systematic review. Int J Nurs Stud Adv. 2021;3:100034. https://doi.org/10.1016/j.ijnsa.2021.100034.
21. International Council of Nurses. (2021). Guidelines on advanced practice nursing: nurse anesthetists.. https://www.icn.ch/system/files/documents/2021-05/ICN_Nurse-Anaesthetist-Report_EN_WEB.pdf.
22. Khan MNA, Verstegen DML, Shahid A, Dolmans DHJM, van Mook WNA. The impact of interprofessional task-based training on the prevention of surgical site infection in a low-income country. BMC Med Educ. 2021;21(1):607. https://doi.org/10.1186/s12909-021-03046-3.
23. Kleinpell RM, Grabenkort WR, Kapu AN, Constantine R, Sicoutris C. Nurse practitioners and physician assistants in acute and critical care: a concise review of the literature and data 2008–2018. Crit Care Med. 2019;47(10):1442–9. https://doi.org/10.1097/ccm.0000000000003925.
24. Kredo T, Adeniyi FB, Bateganya M, Pienaar ED. Task shifting from doctors to non-doctors for initiation and maintenance of antiretroviral therapy. Cochrane Database Syst Rev. 2014;7(7):CD007331. https://doi.org/10.1002/14651858.CD007331.pub3.
25. Kreeftenberg HG, Pouwels S, Bindels A, de Bie A, van der Voort PHJ. Impact of the advanced practice provider in adult critical care: a systematic review and meta-analysis. Crit Care Med. 2019;47(5):722–30. https://doi.org/10.1097/ccm.0000000000003667.
26. Landsperger JS, Semler MW, Wang L, Byrne DW, Wheeler AP. Outcomes of nurse practitioner-delivered critical care: a prospective cohort study. Chest. 2016;149(5):1146–54. https://doi.org/10.1016/j.chest.2015.12.015.
27. Laurant M, van der Biezen M, Wijers N, Watananirun K, Kontopantelis E, van Vught A. Nurses as substitutes for doctors in primary care. Cochrane Database Syst Rev. 2018;7(7):CD001271. https://doi.org/10.1002/14651858.CD001271.pub3.
28. Law TJ, Lipnick MS, Morriss W, Gelb AW, Mellin-Olsen J, Filipescu D, Rowles J, Rod P, Khan F, Yazbeck P, Zoumenou E, Ibarra P, Ranatunga K, Bulamba F. The global anesthesia workforce survey: updates and trends in the anesthesia workforce. Anesth Analg. 2024;139(1):15–24. https://doi.org/10.1213/ane.0000000000006836.
29. Lewis SR, Nicholson A, Smith AF, Alderson P. Physician anaesthetists versus non-physician providers of anaesthesia for surgical patients. Cochrane Database Syst Rev. 2014;(7) https://doi.org/10.1002/14651858.CD010357.pub2.
30. Liao MT, Chang HC, Chen CK, Cheng LY, Lin TT, Keng LT. Outcomes of daytime nurse practitioner-staffed versus resident-staffed nonsurgical intensive care units: a retrospective observational study. Aust Crit Care. 2022;35(6):630–5. https://doi.org/10.1016/j.aucc.2021.10.004.
31. Maier CB, Aiken LH. Task shifting from physicians to nurses in primary care in 39 countries: a cross-country comparative study. Eur J Pub Health. 2016;26(6):927–34. https://doi.org/10.1093/eurpub/ckw098.
32. Maier CB, Barnes H, Aiken LH, Busse R. Descriptive, cross-country analysis of the nurse practitioner workforce in six countries: size, growth, physician substitution potential. BMJ Open. 2016;6(9):e011901. https://doi.org/10.1136/bmjopen-2016-011901.

33. McMenamin A, Turi E, Schlak A, Poghosyan L. A systematic review of outcomes related to nurse practitioner-delivered primary care for multiple chronic conditions. Med Care Res Rev. 2023;80(6):563–81. https://doi.org/10.1177/10775587231186720.
34. Michel-Schuldt M, McFadden A, Renfrew M, Homer C. The provision of midwife-led care in low-and middle-income countries: an integrative review. Midwifery. 2020;84:102659. https://doi.org/10.1016/j.midw.2020.102659.
35. Nashwan AJ. Transforming primary care in LMICs through advanced practice nursing. Lancet Prim Care. 2025;1(3) https://doi.org/10.1016/j.lanprc.2025.100033.
36. Needleman J, Minnick AF. Anesthesia provider model, hospital resources, and maternal outcomes. Health Serv Res. 2009;44(2 Pt 1):464–82. https://doi.org/10.1111/j.1475-6773.2008.00919.x.
37. Newhouse RP, Stanik-Hutt J, White KM, Johantgen M, Bass EB, Zangaro G, Wilson RF, Fountain L, Steinwachs DM, Heindel L, Weiner JP. Advanced practice nurse outcomes 1990-2008: a systematic review. Nurs Econ. 2011;29(5):230–50. quiz 251
38. Pajerski DM, Harlan MD, Ren D, Tuite PK. A clinical nurse specialist-led initiative to reduce catheter-associated urinary tract infection rates using a best practice guideline. Clin Nurse Spec. 2022;36(1):20–8. https://doi.org/10.1097/nur.0000000000000643.
39. Pine M, Holt KD, Lou YB. Surgical mortality and type of anesthesia provider. AANA J. 2003;71(2):109–16.
40. Poghosyan L, Boyd DR, Clarke SP. Optimizing full scope of practice for nurse practitioners in primary care: a proposed conceptual model. Nurs Outlook. 2016;64(2):146–55. https://doi.org/10.1016/j.outlook.2015.11.015.
41. Poghosyan L, Kueakomoldej S, Liu J, Martsolf G. Advanced practice nurse work environments and job satisfaction and intent to leave: six-state cross sectional and observational study. J Adv Nurs. 2022;78(8):2460–71. https://doi.org/10.1111/jan.15176.
42. Richardson J, Tjoelker R. Beyond the central line–associated bloodstream infection bundle: the value of the clinical nurse specialist in continuing evidence-based practice changes. Clin Nurse Spec. 2012;26(4):205–11. https://doi.org/10.1097/NUR.0b013e31825aebab.
43. Rosseel P, Trelles M, Guilavogui S, Ford N, Chu K. Ten years of experience training non-physician anesthesia providers in Haiti. World J Surg. 2010;34(3):453–8. https://doi.org/10.1007/s00268-009-0192-2.
44. Scanlon A, Murphy M, Smolowitz J, Lewis V. Advanced nursing practice and advanced practice nursing roles within low and lower-middle-income countries. J Nurs Scholarsh. 2023;55(2):484–93. https://doi.org/10.1111/jnu.12838.
45. Schober, M., Lehwaldt, D., Rogers, M., Steinke, M., Turale, S., Pulcini, J., Roussel, J., & Stewart, D. (2020). Guidelines on advanced practice nursing. https://www.icn.ch/system/files/documents/2020-04/ICN_APN%20Report_EN_WEB.pdf
46. Silber JH, Kennedy SK, Even-Shoshan O, Chen W, Koziol LF, Showan AM, Longnecker DE. Anesthesiologist direction and patient outcomes. Anesthesiology. 2000;93(1):152–63. https://doi.org/10.1097/00000542-200007000-00026.
47. Simonson DC, Ahern MM, Hendryx MS. Anesthesia staffing and anesthetic complications during cesarean delivery: a retrospective analysis. Nurs Res. 2007;56(1):9–17. https://doi.org/10.1097/00006199-200701000-00002.
48. Smith S, Greenwood M. The value of renal clinical nurse specialists: future potential and current challenges in the United Kingdom. Semin Oncol Nurs. 2024;40(6):151750. https://doi.org/10.1016/j.soncn.2024.151750.
49. Stanik-Hutt J, Newhouse RP, White KM, Johantgen M, Bass EB, Zangaro G, Wilson R, Fountain L, Steinwachs DM, Heindel L, Weiner JP. The quality and effectiveness of care provided by nurse practitioners. J Nurse Pract. 2013;9(8):492–500.e413. https://doi.org/10.1016/j.nurpra.2013.07.004.
50. Tarazi WW, Ghosh P, Ferrara EE, Ume N, Hogan PF, Parker ED. Impact of reduced restrictions in scope of practice of nurse anesthetists on patient safety across states. J Nurs Regul. 2025; https://doi.org/10.1016/j.jnr.2025.10.003.

51. Tracy MF, O'Grady ET, Phillips SJ. Hamric & Hanson's advanced practice nursing : an integrative approach. 7th ed. Elsevier; 2023.
52. Umutesi G, McEvoy MD, Starnes JR, Sileshi B, Atieli HE, Onyango K, Newton MW. Safe anesthesia care in Western Kenya: a preliminary assessment of the impact of nurse anesthetists at multiple levels of government hospitals. Anesth Analg. 2019;129(5):1387–93. https://doi.org/10.1213/ane.0000000000004266.
53. World Bank. Number of surgical procedures (per 100,000 population). World Bank; 2025. https://data360.worldbank.org/en/indicator/WB_WDI_SH_SGR_PROC_P5.
54. World Health Organization (2021). Global Strategic Directions for Nursing and Midwifery 2021–2025. https://apps.who.int/iris/handle/10665/344562.
55. World Bank. World Development Indicators. Population, total for 2023. Available at: World Bank DataBank. Accessed May 25, 2026. https://databank.worldbank.org/.
56. World Health Organization (2024). WHO urges expansion of lifesaving midwifery care for women and babies. https://www.who.int/news/item/16-10-2024-who-urges-expansion-of-lifesaving-midwifery-care-for-women-and-babies.
57. World Health Organization (2025). State of the world's nursing 2025: investing in education, jobs, leadership and service delivery. ISBN 978-92-4-011023-6. https://www.who.int/publications/i/item/9789240110236.
58. Zhang RS, Zhang P, Bailey E, Ho A, Rhee A, Xia Y, Schimmer H, Bernard S, Castillo P, Grossman K, Dai M, Singh A, Padilla-Lopez M, Nunemacher K, Hall SF, Rosenzweig B, Katz JN, Link N, Keller N, Bangalore S, Alviar CL. Comparing outcomes between advanced practice providers and Housestaff teams in the cardiac intensive care unit. JACC Adv. 2024;3(11):101312. https://doi.org/10.1016/j.jacadv.2024.101312.

Leaders Empower Full APN Clinical Practice Authority

Janet A. Dewan, Cecelia Chuchu Kpangbala-Flomo, Annie Camacho-Trusso, Peachy Quitugua, and Assumpta Yamuragiye

...Achieving full practice authority is mainly due to ... trailblazer APRN leaders...they unlocked the doors for us, but it took local nurses to open the door and walk through [1].

Abbreviations

APN	Advanced Practice Nurse
APRN	Advanced Practice Registered Nurse
BON	Board of Nursing
BS	Bachelor Degree
CNMI	Commonwealth of the Northern Mariana Islands
CNM	Certified Nurse Midwife

J. A. Dewan (✉)
Bouvé College of Health Science Nurse Anesthesia Program, Northeastern University, Boston, MA, USA
e-mail: J.dewan@northeastern.edu

C. C. Kpangbala-Flomo
Liberian Board of Nursing and Midwifery, Monrovia, Republic of Liberia

A. Camacho-Trusso · P. Quitugua
Commonwealth Healthcare Corporation, Garapan, MP, USA

A. Yamuragiye
College of Medicine and Health Sciences, School of Health Sciences, Department of Anestheisa, University of Rwanda, Kigali, Rwanda

A. Kapu et al. (eds.), *A Global View on Clinical Autonomy for Advanced Practice Nurses*, Advanced Practice in Nursing,
https://doi.org/10.1007/978-3-032-21458-4_10

CRNA	Certified Registered Nurse Anesthetist
CNO	Chief Nursing Officer
CPD	Continuing Professional Development
FPA	Full Practice Authority
IFNA	International Federation of Nurse Anesthetists
ICN	International Council of Nurses
KHI	Kigali Health Institute
LANA	Liberian Association of Nurse Anesthetists
LBNM	Liberian Board of Nursing and Midwifery
LMA	Liberian Midwife Association
LNA	Liberian Nurses Association
MOH	Ministry of Health
MS/MA	Master Degree
NCNM	Rwanda National Council of Nursing and Midwifery
NGO	NON Governmental Organization
NPA	Nurse Practice Act
NSPM	Non-Surgical Pain Management
NP	Nurse Practitioner
PhD	Doctoral Degree
Phebe	Phebe Ester Bacon College of Nursing and Midwifery
UR	University of Rwanda
US	United States
WHO	World Health Organization

This chapter will highlight three central leadership roles and illustrate them with distinct but overlapping illustrations of dynamic leadership: the education leader, the policy maker/regulator leader, and the clinical leader. Examples of real-world champions for FPA in each domain illustrate the diversity of leadership focus and authority. Although the manifestation of APN roles may vary with specialty, developing and authorizing FPA falls under a variety of intermingled nurse leadership spheres and can be actualized in different contexts and at varying rates. Vision, consistency, resilience, flexibility, and collaboration are core leadership attributes. Leaders envision a future where APNs practicing to their full scope at the top of their licenses can flourish without impediments. Leaders understand and use their positions, specialty knowledge, and influence to facilitate autonomous APN practice, leading to increased access to high-quality, timely patient-centered care. They build on advances gradually while courageously seizing opportunities for rapid progress. Most effectively when those in leadership domains collaborate and assemble a coherent, progressively realized full scope practice structure for APNs, they create, then protect the milieu for APN practice that best meets health system and patient needs.

For APNs, the prospect of achieving FPA starts in their education programs. It's there that nurses develop advanced critical thinking and independent decision making as core FPA competencies in disciplines that require integrating complex intellectual, technical, and social skills. Once educated to form autonomous decisions to guide evidence-based patient care, the graduate or practicing APN needs authorization, employment opportunities, license protection, and practice support shaped by policy makers/regulators who oversee nursing license recognition, and nurse-led regulation. This is most often accomplished through a legally authorized Board of Nursing (BON) or Nursing Council, though it may sometimes include other credentialing/certification bodies or Ministries of Health (MOH). Formal authorization distinguishes FPA from autonomous practice that evolves simply because of circumstances, such as skilled health worker resource limitation. The fact that nursing at all levels is regulated, virtually everywhere in the world, assures that people can expect an adequately scrutinized quality of care that is in their best interest from nurses who hold a nursing license. Besides supporting FPA, policymakers can remove legal and special interest barriers to nurse autonomy. And finally, practicing to full license and education scope and demonstrating the value of APN patient-centered care rests on the clinical leaders who model and actualize FPA. They take their authorized opportunity to walk through the open door, continuously advance their practice, and improve patient outcomes by using and improving their skills and knowledge to deliver care that reflects the top capacity of their licenses and training.

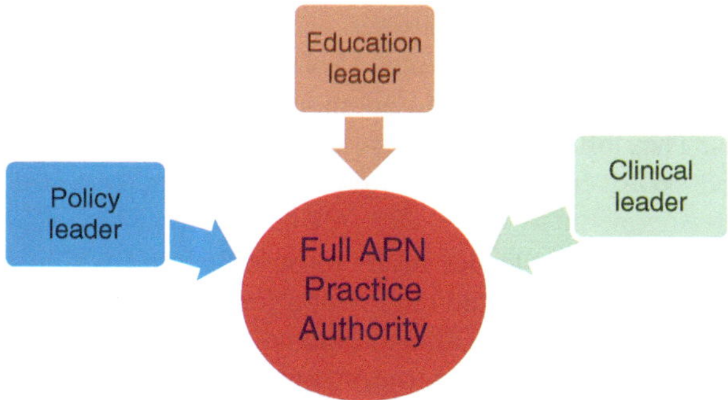

Leadership and FPA

The Educator Leader

The template that prepares nurses for FPA lies in APN education. The International Council for Nurses (ICN) suggests that a graduate degree, Master's (MS) or higher, should be entry level for APN practice [2]. In some under-resourced or remote areas, earning an MS in nursing may be aspirational or currently impossible to attain, but the visionary educator sets progressively realizing the MS degree for APNs as a goal. Having international standards for APN practice helps educators envision the goal of specialist credentialed nurse education. Additionally, as a scaffold for meeting global standards, validated, published guides authoritatively convince administration authorities, outside of the nursing department, and government policy makers to support advancing programs toward delivering the recognized global standard. The International Council of Nurses (ICN) has published APN practice guides and some specialty guides, including those specific to nurse anesthesia, that can inform knowledge and experiential aspects of education to develop FPA competencies [2, 3].

Beyond specialty knowledge and skill acquisition and supervised practice opportunities, APN educators design curricula that develop the critical thinking that is crucial for graduate APN autonomous clinical decisions. Student APNs use critical assessment and intervention design competency with preceptor backup while in training, learning to practice to the fullest extent of their education and licenses after graduation. Educator leaders bear the responsibility for developing clinicians prepared to realize specialty practice autonomy both in advanced skill and professional competency. The education leader must stay current as APN specialty roles continuously evolve to meet student and health system needs. They incorporate state-of-the-art techniques and training for emerging subspecialty knowledge and advanced skill, such as independent prescription authorization, chronic pain management, neonatal and pediatric care, psychiatric interventions, emergency and critical care, and autonomous obstetric care.

Educators are student-focused. Besides assuring formal curricula and teaching techniques that develop critical thinking, APN preparation methods aim to produce graduates who are ready to also lead autonomous clinical practice and evolving role definitions. They often also facilitate ongoing professional development that assures updated skills, credentials, and continued competency for those already practicing.

The APN nurse educator leader needs to be influential within their academic institutions to secure resources and recognition for students at an affordable price. For areas where MS degrees remain aspirational, the visionary educator develops and promulgates realistic planning toward that goal, supported by global ICN and specialty guidelines [2, 3]. The International Federation of Nurse Anesthetists (IFNA) has published a context-adapted model for MS nurse anesthesia education and supports a global accreditation process for nurse anesthesia programs that incorporates CANMED competencies. This could serve as an example of a competency validated transnational graduate degree guide for other specialties [4]. The education leader develops and mentors faculty and engages in scholarship and advocacy that raise the nursing academic division to the level expected by degree-granting institutions. Nurse educator leaders are responsible for shaping graduates to be ready for FPA.

Education Leaders Prepare APN Graduates to Walk Through the FPA Door

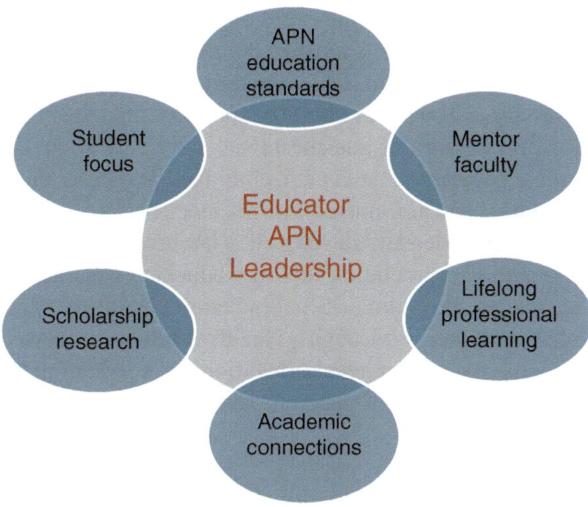

Components of educator leadership

Rwanda: From Apprenticeship to Diploma to Graduate Degree: The Evolution of APN Anesthesia Specialist Education in a Resource-Limited Setting

The 1994 genocide, which followed years of civil war, left Rwanda with a decimated health sector and a dire need for skilled health professionals to meet basic health needs. There was no formal anesthesia specialty training for nurses, technicians, or physicians. Nurses who were working as anesthetists had learned in an apprenticeship model, usually under visiting foreign anesthetists. Skills and knowledge competency were inconsistent and unregulated.

The first nurse anesthesia formal training became part of the accelerated health system infrastructure rebuilding after the 1994 genocide. A Ugandan-trained Rwandan anesthetist, the visionary leader Charles Rangira MMed RA, returned to Kigali and resolved that he would do something to assure safe anesthesia for the citizens of Rwanda. He established and led the formal diploma in anesthesia program, which started in 1996 at the Kigali Health Institute (KHI). Students were experienced nurses or those with science backgrounds and completed a 3-year anesthesia diploma program. Graduate anesthetists, frequently working alone, were expected to make autonomous decisions and interventions at the level for which they were prepared and equipped. Their practice rights were authorized by the Rwandan Allied Health Professions Council. The KHI diploma program laid the foundation for steady progress toward full scope advanced practice for graduate anesthetists that continues today. By 2010, the KHI program had graduated almost 200 anesthetists, greatly expanding the cadre of formally trained anesthesia providers in the public hospitals that serve most of the population [5, 6].

In 2013, the anesthetist program transitioned to a bachelor's (BS) degree in anesthesia at the University of Rwanda (UR). This program includes two years of basic nursing education and 2 years of anesthesia specialty education, divided between didactics and clinical experience and is currently the entry-level anesthetist credential. Graduates are nurses and non-nurses with a science background. Simultaneously, nurse anesthesia education leaders developed a BS bridge program at UR to raise the academic credentials of practicing diploma-educated anesthetists to the degree level of the university program's BS graduates. Certified Registered Nurse Anesthetist (CRNA) volunteers, through a Health Volunteers Overseas (HVO) affiliation, expand faculty for degree-level education by conducting one-month core modules assigned by the Rwandan program administrators to reflect their curriculum sequence [7].

As the education level for entry anesthetists advanced at UR, developing faculty became a crucial step to advancing to global APN standards. The Rwandan MOH strategic plan calls for health worker development intended to increase the quality and quantity of skilled health workers and educators [8]. Support from the Rwandan MOH and NGOs funded MS and PhD options for nurse anesthesia educators through the country's 4x4 scholarship program [9]. Currently, there are three PhD-prepared nurse anesthetist education leaders, as well as others who have earned MS degrees, on the UR faculty.

With appropriately credentialled faculty and recognizing the advantage of meeting the global APN MS degree standard for nurse anesthetists, the anesthesia faculty leadership worked tirelessly with the nursing and health science departments at UR, where other APN disciplines already offer MS degrees, and the Rwandan Nursing Council, to develop a post-BS Nurse Anesthesia MS program. Multilevel government health and education ministries granted approval of a post-graduate MS in Nurse Anesthesia and Critical Care in early 2025. The first cohort of 25 students entered the 2–3 year program in September 2025. The value of nurse anesthetists and critical care specialty nurses during the 2024 Marburg Virus Disease outbreak, their contributions and sacrifices, highlighted the importance of assuring readiness and empowering FPA specialty skilled and knowledgeable clinicians who are prepared to lead in critical response before unexpected health emergencies occur [10, 11].

The education trajectory for nurse anesthesia in Rwanda highlights anesthetist education leadership from the creation of training at KHI, inspired by Rangira, through university bachelors credential, transition to master's post-graduate specialty nursing credentials that meet ICN APN criteria. At each phase, the education program's success reflects the leadership of former and current UR program administrators and faculty. The transition, the vision, knowledge dissemination, resilience, negotiation, and tireless advocacy of a succession of education leaders have been the key to the progressive and non-dependent success. Though the depth of education has evolved, anesthesia education in Rwanda has always prepared graduates for professionally autonomous practice because many anesthetists work in solo practices. Their authority to practice as anesthetists and their practice scope is established by the Rwanda Allied Health Professions Council. Launching an MS in nursing degree program represents progress toward recognizing nurse anesthesia through the APN lens with NCNM credentials and practice regulation. Unsurprisingly, with training more physician anesthetists, who work almost exclusively in urban medical centers, anesthetists cite decreased role autonomy in teaching hospitals compared with rural practice. Graduates of the MS in Anesthesia and Critical Care Nursing Program will be prepared to fill an APN niche. It remains for health sector authorities to create positions where they can use their skills to the full extent of their license and education preparation. New APNs will be mentored in their role in clinical leadership and will be MS-prepared nurses regulated as APNs by the Rwandan National Nursing and Midwifery Council (NCNM), rather than only the current anesthetist authorization for technical and nurse anesthetists issued by the health professions council [6].

Rwanda's nurse anesthesia training example shows that a succession of strong education leaders can evolve specialty practice programs from non-degree, but formal context appropriate training, to progressive academic degree credentials that optimize student and health system needs while preserving the FPA professional heritage embedded in Rwandan anesthesia education.

The Nurse Regulator and Policy Leader

Graduates of APN programs who have acquired the skills and knowledge for FPA also need a legal right to practice to the full extent of their training if they are to experience authorized clinical autonomy and title protection. Although the use of terms may overlap, formal authorization distinguishes FPA from autonomous practice based solely on circumstances without formal authorization, such as that seen when skilled health worker resources are scarce. The APN license and other credentials to practice should reflect their advanced nursing practice privilege. To optimize their contributions to the health sector, APNs need employment options that utilize their full scope of skills and knowledge and recognize the value of their roles. In the public sector, it is often the MOH or other government authority that assigns public sector job ranks and salary structure based on the level of training credentials. Nursing regulators, policy makers and local health system administration leaders develop strategies through formal and informal routes to assure nurses educated for FPA can actualize it without impediments. The value of APNs practicing at the top of their license permissions and policy makers advancing permissions when needed is well documented, but impediments exist in both the global South and North. These often reflect outdated hierarchical regulatory structures, lack of employment opportunities, and poorly developed role definitions and can potentially affect health equity [12–14].

Nurse policy and regulatory leaders promulgate the rules under which APNs practice. They are public servants. Their influence will vary with government and professional structure, but they are the gatekeepers who lead in interpreting compliance with role delineations. Surveyed European APNs cite lack of nursing practice and education regulation as one significant barrier to successfully establishing their roles [15].

Nurse policy and regulation leaders codify the FPA scope for all recognized categories of APNs. For example, in the United States it is a program accreditation requirement that APNs are educated to practice autonomously. However, since in the US federalist governance system, nursing statutes, usually nurse practice laws (NPA), are passed by individual state legislatures with input from BONs and others, there can be some variation in APN practice scope among states. Autonomous BONs then write the regulations to reflect but not exceed the practice act statutory language. Nursing and other professional boards' written regulations carry the force of law and define role parameters for APRNs practicing in a particular state. Ongoing efforts have secured specialty-specific prescriptive practice for the majority of APRNs in most US states and FPA without physician supervision or collaboration requirements in many. Still, the right to FPA is not assured for all APNs everywhere in the US system and may still be further restricted at the facility or local level.

In the Rwandan example, the authority to practice as anesthetists is granted by the Allied Health Professions Council, although the Rwandan NCNM awards other APN nursing licenses. Graduates of the new MS in Anesthesia and Critical Care Nursing Program will be licensed under the NCNM. In the contrasting example, below, we highlight the role of nurse policy makers and regulators in the Liberian Board of Nursing and Midwifery (LBNM) and MOH, authorizing APN credentialing and an education program for nurse anesthetists who were already independently practicing for decades without a nursing board APN designation [16, 17]. In the practice leader example on Saipan, visionary nurse regulatory leaders preempted the potential right to FPA for APNs by including all specialties in the nurse practice act, then amending it to specifically incorporate autonomous practice language, before there were even specialists in some named disciplines prepared for FPA on the islands [18, 19].

Global resources, legal practice scope, and context vary with supply and need. When APN nursing practice is recognized as an advanced role and authorized by autonomous nurse regulatory and policy leaders, who are appointed or elected to represent the public interest, it systematically reassures the public of the quality of care they can expect. The policy leader mandate blends public interest with safe APN practice autonomy that maximizes benefits for citizens and health systems.

Policy Leaders with Vision Unlock the Door to FPA for APNs

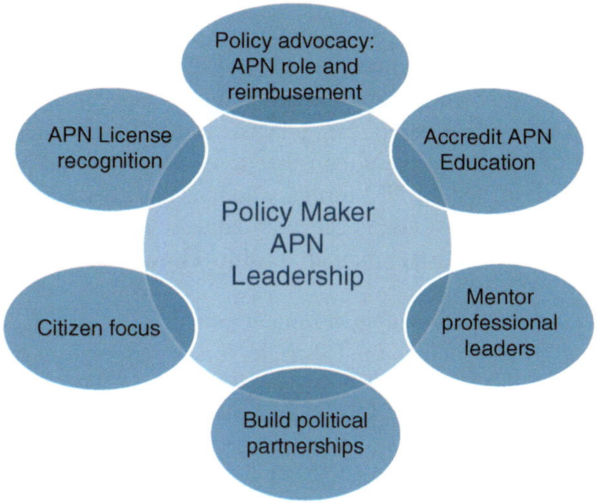

Policy advocacy: APN role and reimbusement
APN License recognition
Accredit APN Education
Policy Maker APN Leadership
Citizen focus
Mentor professional leaders
Build political partnerships

Components of policy leadership

Liberia: Advancing APNs Toward FPA in Liberia Through Nurse-Led Regulation

The Liberian Board for Nursing and Midwifery (LBNM) was recognized in 1949, making it one of the country's longest-serving regulatory bodies. Its scope is highlighted in the 1976 Liberian Public Health Law. A 2016 amendment to the statute formally recognized the LBNM board as the autonomous sole regulator of nursing, advanced practice nursing, and midwifery. The scope of LBNM autonomy means it is the only licensing authority for nurses, advanced practice nurses, and midwives. It also owns the responsibility to accredit its education and training programs in Liberia [16].

Although Liberia, a West African democracy, is classified as a low-income country, nursing education is well developed. Nurses represent the largest sector of the health workforce in Liberia, which makes the nursing regulatory body, LBNM, a powerful force in the health system. The LBNM Mission is to serve the public interest by overseeing nursing education and practice. Its Vision describes the scope of their oversight of the profession.

> MISSION: "To protect the public's health and safety by ensuring that all nurses and midwives are competent, ethical practitioners with the knowledge and skills required to provide high quality and safe health services to the people of Liberia." [17]

VISION: "To serve as the ultimate authority in regulating the nursing and midwifery professions in Liberia and ensure professional excellence in nursing and midwifery education and practices." [17]

Success in governance demands collaboration with other agencies, especially the MOH. The Chief Nursing and Midwifery Officer (CNMO) at the Liberian MOH is currently a licensed APN who grasps the significance of specialty advanced practice to the health system when APNs can practice at the top of their licenses. Her appointment shows a recognition of the value of nurses and the APN role within the Liberian health system. The LBNM formally defines the advanced practice nurse as nurses with at least a year of added specialty education in the categories of nurse midwives, nurse anesthetists, mental health clinicians, and other clinical specialists.

The LBNM works closely with government ministries, especially the MOH, and also professional groups such as the Liberian Nurses Association (LNA), Liberian Association of Nurse Anesthetists (LANA), and Liberian Midwives Association (LMA). As a component of initial nurse and APN specialty licensure, in addition to verifying graduation from approved programs, the LBNM also collaborates with educators, content experts, and professional associations such as LNA, LANA, or LMA to design and assess performance on the required entry to practice exams. In a new initiative, formal Continuing Professional Development (CPD) credits are collated by the Liberian nurse-led organization, Nursing Online Liberia, repository. In 2023, the LBNM enacted a plan to require designated CPD credits for license renewal. Nurse anesthetists led by LANA and Liberian educators, along with LBNM and US partners, have designed a CPD program where practicing anesthetists can obtain specialty-relevant CPD credits [20].

The LBNM also accredits nursing program curricula. Their formal approval has influence beyond the single program. As an example, in 2016–2017, anesthesia faculty, with consultants, under the leadership of Phebe-Ester Bacon Anesthesia Program (Phebe) Director, Wilmot Fassah, completely revised the nurse anesthesia curriculum. The revision was based on IFNA global competency standards adapted to the Liberian context and was in line with LBNM education standards [21]. In 2018, after Phebe was internationally reviewed and was awarded the IFNA program Recognition, the LBNM declared the revised nurse anesthesia curriculum to be the Liberian national curriculum for nurse anesthetist education. It is housed at LBNM. This means that any other nurse anesthetist education program opened in Liberia would have to follow the official LBNM curriculum that adheres to LBNM education and context-appropriate global standards to gain approval.

Nurse policy leaders, such as the esteemed Registrar of the LBNM and the CNMO at the MOH, collaborate with the government and private entities to ensure that the scope of APN education and title recognition is understood and that it reflects society's needs for safe, basic, and advanced practice nursing care.

They are the trusted link between the citizens of Liberia and nurse practitioners.

The Clinical Leader

Even when there are opportunities for nurses to graduate from advanced practice specialty programs that prepare them for full scope practice and then gain regulatory approval with license recognition and employment in positions where they can practice at the top of their licenses, it takes clinical leaders to fully realize and advance the APN role to FPA for the benefit of patients and health systems. The Future of Nursing Report (2020–2030) calls on clinical nurses to act as leaders in achieving health equity. APNs who complete advanced education and hold added role responsibilities are assumed to be clinical leaders. As they guide while designing and implementing care, they are the models for the added value of their additional education, skills, and independent decision making when they are able to function with FPA in their professional roles [22, 23].

Clinical nurse leaders focus on using their education, authorization, and advanced skills to improve the quality of and access to the best patient care. They innovate and expand their practice scope, learning new skills and new ways of using their expertise. They identify gaps in the evidence-based care available to patients and work to eliminate them. This may include scholarship, often implementing research into practice using quality improvement methods or adding additional education or certification to their specialty credential, as best practice advances with new knowledge. The formality and recognition of advanced roles vary among countries, with some awarding the graduation title (nurse practitioner (NP), nurse anesthetist, nurse midwife, clinical specialist) without APN licensing privileges that would elevate their authorized practice scope above the basic nursing credential. At times, this leads to APNs working below their level of training because FPA employment has not been developed or protected. At other times, APNs may leave the public sector for private clinics, potentially impeding health equity. Some countries have tiered programs for the NP scope of practice. In Finland, for example, nurses graduate with a BS degree for basic clinical practice, then have options for extra training to secure limited prescriptive authority or advanced practice specialties in MS programs of varying lengths and clinical focus. Doctoral education is also available along with specialty non-degree programs [24].

The Saipan exemplar of clinical leadership highlights the challenges and opportunities for two APNs, a nurse midwife, and a nurse anesthetist, practicing in the Commonwealth of the Northern Mariana Islands (CNMI) who became leaders because they had guaranteed FPA. Despite being a US territory, APNs face significant challenges accessing required education for specialties from their remote location, but forward-thinking nurse policy leaders included FPA from the onset in revised statutory language. They unlocked the door to FPA so that, when ready, the APNs were able to walk through without hesitation or impediment, to improve care [18, 19].

Clinical Leaders, Prepared by Educator Leaders, Pass Through the Door to FPA, Which Policy Makers Unlock

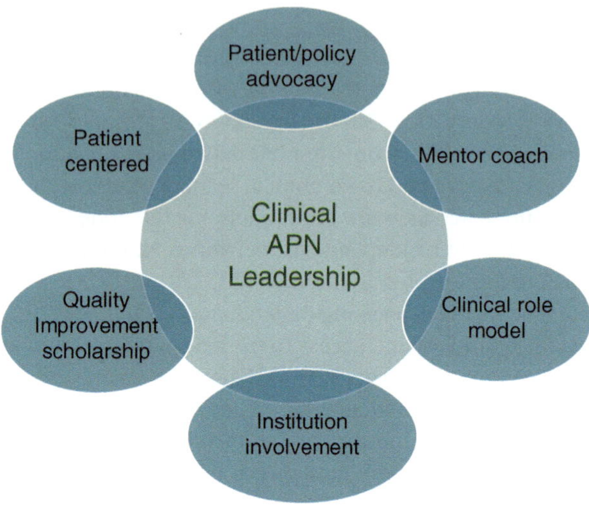

Components of clinical APN leadership

Saipan: Clinical Full Scope Practice Expands Maternity, Surgical, and Pain Services

On the Island of Saipan, capital of the CNMI, an unincorporated US territory in the Western Pacific, there are no APN education programs. Education is the limiting step to developing advanced practice nurse roles. Nurses face many barriers to enrolling in off-island programs, making attaining the credentials for APN practice difficult for native islanders. Basic nursing education is at the associate degree level on Saipan. Any nurse aiming for APN status must first complete a BS degree in nursing, often online, then find an APN program that accepts clinical rotations on the island or relocate off island for required clinical experiences. With no local APN education program, nurses would need to enroll in US mainland or off-island programs for nurse anesthesia, midwifery, clinical specialist, or nurse practitioner specialties. In fact, even to take specialty board exams, nurses need to travel many hours off-island to approved testing sites. Authorization for practice follows US regulations. This means graduation from an approved program is necessary for the certification required by the boards of nursing for advanced practice licensure, similar to mainland US requirements.

Statutory groundwork authorizes FPA for clinical APN leaders on Saipan. A forward-thinking nurse regulatory leader participated in drafting the CNMI Nurse Practice Act (NPA) in 2003, establishing an autonomous nurse-led board that incorporated all APRN specialties, even those with no nurses yet practicing in the roles, for licensure. In 2009, the visionary nurse policy leader helped guide an amendment to the NPA that includes the stipulation for practice autonomy for all APNs. Once educated, this unlocked the door to FPA for all practicing APNs [18, 19].

Prior to the statutory amendment for APN autonomy, nurse midwives practiced only in labor and delivery supervised by physicians. Current licensure with FPA elevates nurse midwife practice scope to the top of their licenses and training. Certified Nurse Midwives (CNM) now function independently and have expanded their roles to include family planning, women's health, and complex deliveries, such as shoulder dystocia, obstetric hemorrhage, or vaginal birth after Caesarean section. They act as surgical first assistants and have admitting privileges. They can own and operate clinics and serve in leadership roles on the BON and in the institution hierarchy, including acting as head of OBGYN services. As clinical leaders, they precept student nurses, run hospital-based emergency training, operate clinics, and run community outreach health teaching. Without the FPA assured in the NPA amendment by policy leaders, their potential contributions would never have materialized [19].

There are barriers to optimizing specialty APN contributions in the CNMI, where there is no on-island access to APN education. As an example, accredited nurse anesthesiology education involves rigorous academic and clinical requirements of over 650 cases in specific categories and over 2000 clinical hours before graduation, and to gain permission to sit for the National Certifying Exam. Even if a mainland program affiliated with the hospital on Saipan for clinical experiences, the case distribution required for certification would not be available on the island [25]. Relocating to attend an accredited program is the only option for native nurses who want to be CRNAs. Consequently, Saipan relies on the addition of visiting short-term contract CRNAs to fill anesthesia needs. In 2019, one DNAP-prepared CRNA returned to her native Saipan after nurse anesthesiology education in Washington DC. Her robust anesthesia training was evident as CRNAs independently delivered expert care for patients across the lifespan. Since then, the CRNA role at the only hospital in the CNMI has expanded with CRNAs independently managing complex caseloads.

The returned native CRNA assumed a leadership position in the anesthesia department and sought opportunities to fill gaps that expanded anesthesia services for patients. She started a labor epidural service in 2021 and increased the number and variety of peripheral nerve blocks for surgical analgesia. In 2022, the gap in chronic pain management necessitated the transfer of Saipan's patients to other Pacific Islands for care. After being supported to obtain formal non-surgical pain management certification (NSPM), she opened and now runs the first nurse-led clinic on the island, treating chronic pain with steroid injections and other modalities. Still, the expanding CRNA practice on Saipan counts on recruiting CRNAs from the US mainland because of the difficulty with education access on the island. Besides clinical leadership, the Saipan CRNAs now precept nursing students with an OR rotation to expose learners to the CRNA role.

The open door to FPA has created the landscape for a full license scope of practice for APNs on Saipan. Clinical leadership extends beyond clinical care for individual patients to department management, independent nurse-led clinics, institution leadership, and mentoring the next generation of clinicians. With FPA embedded in the APN title, the island now has a psychiatric care clinic run by an NP, prenatal clinics managed by CNMs, and a CRNA-run chronic pain clinic. Statutory FPA license validity opened opportunities for not only clinical practice leadership but for APN leadership in the health sector that expands and improves access to equitable, patient-centered care.

Conclusion

Nurse leaders have a profound impact when they support and enable full scope independent practice for APNs. How nurse leadership contributes to FPA is nuanced by resources, history, and social context, but without a doubt, when autonomous clinical practice for APNs is realized, it reflects the vision, actions, and coordinated influence of nurse leaders. From a global perspective, the names or categories of APN specialties and their national level recognitions and associated titles vary. But in every situation, fostering APN full scope practice at the top of a nurse's license authorization and training has been shown to be in the best interest of patients and health systems [26–28].

The influences of the three leadership domains are intermingled and overlapping, but all three are essential to realizing the APN's potential for FPA and its impact on patients, health equity, and society. The education leader is student-focused, developing APNs ready to practice with the advanced skills, knowledge, and decision-making needed for FPA. The policy/regulator leader serves to represent the public and oversees nursing's safe contributions to the health of citizens, while considering individuals and society. For clinical leaders, FPA allows them to use their full array of clinical and professional skills to deliver evidence-based, compassionate patient-centered care and to model and expand their roles.

Education opportunities for nurses develop their advanced specialty skills, preparing them to independently use critical decision-making to deliver care. Education leaders guide the programs that bring students to the door of autonomous practice. Specialty education can have an established progressive path to accreditation, as in the United States, or a unique trajectory shaped by external events, as in Rwanda and Liberia, or may be unavailable to nurses without additional resources, as on Saipan.

Education access does not guarantee FPA. It falls on policymakers at nursing regulatory boards and MOHs, as well as health system administrators, to authorize and approve APN advanced practice programs that safely meet their health system needs. Globally, nurse regulation is developed almost everywhere but varies in authority and autonomous decision scope. State laws in the United States, where licensure for APNs is not nationally authorized but regulated by states, can limit or expand APN practice in regulation, sometimes by specialty or academic credential. In Liberia and Saipan, practice authorization is led by autonomous nursing regulatory boards. In Rwanda, the Nursing Council does not exercise oversight for nurse anesthetist's scope of practice, which is delineated by an allied health professions board. In some examples, nursing boards and other policy and professional leaders license nurses but may still be developing important expanded criteria to distinguish the specialty title of the APN licensee, or may themselves be impeded in autonomous decisions by competing interests. Visionary health system administrators, regulators, and other government entities ensure license privileges are formally authorized and create positions within health systems where APNs can flourish as specialized autonomous clinicians who promote health equity. Understanding the value of the top of the APN license scope for FPA roles is crucial and requires documentation, professional advocacy, and modeling that illustrate the added value to health systems when unencumbered advanced nurse specialty practice is formally authorized, guaranteed, and protected.

Clinical leaders emerge when they practice to the full scope of their licenses. They lead by prioritizing equitable patient-centered care. They integrate new knowledge and skills to fill gaps in access to care. On Saipan, APN clinical nurse leaders expanded their practice to include services that had previously been denied to the island's citizens. They show the value of a legally recognized FPA for APNs in diverse specialties. Leaders collaborate, pass on their knowledge, and mentor others to optimize health equity by providing and expanding access to APN FPA care for all. The clinical leader realizes that no matter how well-intentioned, with expert skill and deep knowledge, their ability to flourish in their practice rests on education and policy leader contributions. Clinical leaders enter through the FPA door and lead their colleagues to endorse independent patient-centered care assessments and interventions when they are enabled to practice at the top of their licenses.

Visionary leaders shape the education, authorization, and practice landscape essential for Full Practice Authority. In any specialty or location, when APNs approach and pass through the open door to the autonomous full scope practice, patients and health systems benefit.

References

1. Trusso, AC; "clinical full scope". personal communication. 2025.
2. International Council of Nurses. Guidelines for advanced practice nursing. Geneva: ICN; 2020. ISBN: 978-92-95099-71-5.
3. International Council of Nurses. Guidelines for the advanced practice of nurse anesthesia. Geneva: ICN; 2021. ISBN: 978-92-95099-85-2.
4. International Federation of Nurse Anesthetists; Masters Model Curriculum. IFNA education committee. 2016. https://ifna.site/download/masters-model-curriculum. Accessed July 2025.
5. Martin RF. Rangira C. d'Arc Uwambazimana J. Desai SP. The history and evolution of anesthetic care in Rwanda. J Anesth Hist 2017 ;3(1):5–11. doi:https://doi.org/10.1016/j.janh.2016.12.004. Epub 2016 Dec 27.
6. Rwandan Allied Health Professions Council. Scope of practice for non-physician anesthetists. 2017. https://rahpc.org.rw/storage/documents/January2018/Cr6UXIIDnHz5jkdApoRH.pdf. Accessed Aug 2025.
7. Health Volunteers Overseas. Specialty Programs Anesthesia. https://hvousa.org/specialty-areas/anesthesia/. Accessed Aug 2025.
8. Rwanda Ministry of Health. 4×4 Reform: a path to quality health care in Rwanda. 2025. https://www.moh.gov.rw/index.php?eID=dumpFile&t=f&f=95973&token=991cc48dad7e712c7d5645533c2e06ed7fb39708. Accessed Aug 2025.

9. Rwanda Ministry of Health. Health Sector Strategic Plan V; June 2024–July 2029. https://www.moh.gov.rw/index.php?eID=dumpFile&t=f&f=118060&token=fe26ea0d43c122279f8009690afa707ae65f5853.
10. Yamuragiwe A, Ufashingabire C, Gallant K, Dewan J. Marburg virus disease: the lived experience of nurse anesthetists at three Kigali referral hospitals. AANA congress oral presentation, AANA Foundation. Aug 2025. Nashville TN.
11. Nutt CP. Marberg virus disease in Rwanda—centering both evidence and equity. NEJM. 2025; https://doi.org/10.1056/NEJMp2415557.
12. Schorn MN. Myers C. Barosso J. et.al. Results of a national survey: ongoing barriers to APRN practice in the United States. Policy Polit Nurs Pract 2022;23(2):118–129. Doi:https://doi.org/10.1177/15271544221076524.
13. Kleinpell R, Myers CR, Schorn MN. Addressing barriers to APRN practice: policy and regulatory implications during Covid-19. J Nurs Regul. 2023;14(1):13–20. https://doi.org/10.1016/s2155-8256(23)00064-9.
14. Torrens C.Campbell P. Hoskins G. et.al. Barriers and facilitators to the implementation of the advanced nurse practitioner role in primary care settings : a scoping review. Int J Nurs Stud 2020;104(103443). doi:https://doi.org/10.1016/j.inurstu.2019.103443.
15. Unsworth J, Greene K, Ali P, et al. Advanced practice nurse roles in Europe: implementation challenges, progress and lessons learned. Int Nurs Rev. 2022;71(2) https://doi.org/10.1111/inr.12800.
16. Liberian Board of Nursing and Midwifery. Admmendment to grant autonomy to LBNM. 2016. http://13.201.94.201/wp-content/uploads/2024/01/lbnm_act.pdf.
17. Liberian Board of Nursing and Midwifery. https://home.lbnm.gov.lr/. Accessed Aug 2025.
18. Northern Mariana Islands Commonwealth Legislature. Nurse Practice Act CNMI PL 14-62. https://nmibon.info/wp-content/uploads/2019/06/pl14-62.pdf.
19. Northern Mariana Islands Commonwealth Legislature. Ammendment to Nurse Practice Act. PL 16-34. https://www.cnmilaw.org/pdf/public_laws/16/pl16-34.pdf.
20. Nursing online Liberia. CPD for nurses. https://www.nursingonlineliberia.org. Accessed Aug 2025.
21. IFNA. Nurse Anesthesia licensure and education in Liberia. 2022. https://ifna.site/app/uploads/2019/01/Liberia-2019.pdf. Accessed Aug 2025.
22. Pulcini J, Street N, Purcell S. The nurse practitioner as leader. In: Thomas S, Rowles J, editors. Nurse practitioners and nurse anesthetists: The evolution of global roles. Springer; 2023. p. 95–101.
23. National Academies of Sciences, Engineering, and Medicine; National Academy of Medicine; Committee on the Future of Nursing 2020–2030; Flaubert JL, Le Menestrel S, Williams DR, et al., editors. The future of nursing 2020–2030: charting a path to achieve health equity. Washington (DC): National Academies Press (US); 2021 May 11. Summary. Available from: https://www.ncbi.nlm.nih.gov/books/NBK573919/. Accessed Aug 2025.
24. Suutarla A, Sulosaari V, Heikkila J. The NP role and practice in Finland. In: Thomas S, Rowles J, editors. Nurse practitioners and nurse anesthetists: the evolution of the global roles. Springer; 2023. p. 181–95.
25. Council on Accreditation of Nurse Anesthesiology Programs. Accreditation Standards. https://www.coacrna.org/wp-content/uploads/2024/03/Standards-for-Accreditation-of-Nurse-Anesthesia-Programs-Practice-Doctorate-editorial-rev-February-2024-1.pdf.
26. Poghosyan L, Maier CB. Advanced practice nurses globally: responding to health challenges, improving outcomes. Int J Nurs Stud. 2022;132:104262. https://doi.org/10.1016/j.ijnurstu.2022.104262. Epub 2022 Apr 26. PMID: 35633596; PMCID: PMC9040455
27. Kleinpell R, Kapu A, Woo B, Wentao Z. Nurse practitioner outcomes evaluation. In: Thomas S, Rowles J, editors. Nurse practitioners and nurse anesthetists: the evolution of the global roles. Springer; 2023. p. 119–27.
28. BJ MM. The impact of nurse practitioner laws on preventable hospitalizations. J Health Econ. 2025;103:103044. ISSN.0167–6296. https://doi.org/10.1016/j.jhealeco.2025.103044.

Clinical Autonomy as a Driver of Innovation: A Global Perspective

Brett Morgan

Innovation in healthcare is the deliberate design, testing, and scaling of new or significantly improved products, services, processes, and policies that measurably enhance patient outcomes, equity, safety, experience, workforce wellbeing, and value [22, 23]. It couples human-centered insight with clinical evidence, data, and enabling technologies such as telehealth, AI, and remote monitoring, and is implemented within regulatory, ethical, and financial constraints [6, 22, 23]. Innovation spans care models, payment and delivery methods, diagnostics and therapeutic approaches, and public health, requiring multidisciplinary collaboration, iterative experimentation, rigorous evaluation, and accountable adoption, so that the benefits are consistently affordable and accessible for diverse populations across settings and the continuum of care [6, 22, 23].

Advanced Practice Nurses (APRNs) are prepared at the graduate level to evaluate patients, diagnose, order and interpret tests, and initiate and manage treatments across settings such as primary care, acute care, specialty services, and maternity care [1, 2]. Their preparation and role in healthcare delivery positioned them to be impactful drivers for innovation. The Future of Nursing 2020–2030 consensus study argues that nurses need supportive work environments and autonomy to achieve health equity and modernize care delivery, highlighting the removal of scope-of-practice barriers as critical [22, 23]. Together, these sources position autonomy not as a privilege but as an operational requirement for innovation—the ability to design, deploy, and continuously improve new models of care [1, 2, 22, 23].

Evidence consistently shows that APRNs deliver high-quality care that has been shown to be comparable to that of physicians. This legitimizes nurse-led redesigns of care pathways and provides a strong empirical base for value-based designs that scale APRN-led approaches to delivering healthcare. This chapter will explore the

B. Morgan (✉)
College of Health and Human Sciences, Western Carolina University, Cullowhee, NC, USA
e-mail: morganb@wcu.edu

A. Kapu et al. (eds.), *A Global View on Clinical Autonomy for Advanced Practice Nurses*, Advanced Practice in Nursing,
https://doi.org/10.1007/978-3-032-21458-4_11

importance of clinical autonomy in supporting APRN innovation and will provide real examples of APRNs who have led in changing the way that care has been delivered. We will identify key characteristics of innovative APRNs and link those to the important role autonomy plays in supporting successful APRN-driven change.

APRN Autonomy Improving the Development and Adoption of New Technology

APRNs, including nurse practitioners (NPs), certified nurse-midwives (CNMs), clinical nurse specialists (CNSs), and certified registered nurse anesthetists (CRNAs, sit at the intersection of direct patient care, clinical decision-making, and systems leadership. This frontline vantage point makes APRNs uniquely positioned to shape the development and adoption of new healthcare technologies. APRNs contribute across the technology lifecycle: co-design, pilot, evaluation, and spread. As embedded clinicians, they notice friction points that designers cannot see. APRN innovators frequently contribute to technology development by participating in pilot studies, quality-improvement projects, and interdisciplinary design teams. Their clinical expertise helps refine technologies such as telehealth platforms, electronic health record workflows, remote patient monitoring systems, and AI-supported decision tools. By providing feedback on usability, workflow integration, and patient impact, APRNs help developers create solutions that fit naturally into care delivery rather than disrupting it. Their feedback improves usability, safety, and workflow integration, and this tight alignment of design with clinical practice is a key reason APRN-led efforts produce technologies that clinicians actually use.

Evidence and existing national policy demonstrate that APRN autonomy accelerates design, testing, implementation, and scale of technologies such as telehealth, remote patient monitoring (RPM), and AI-supported decision tools, while improving access, quality, equity, and value [22, 23, 32]. When empowered to practice to the full extent of their training, APRNs lead co-design with developers, pilot technology in real clinical workflows, and drive change management, all with measurable gains in patient engagement, clinician usability, and organizational readiness [6, 9].

Autonomy gives APRNs the decision rights to move from idea to action by enabling them to select appropriate digital tools, adapt care pathways, and create important clinical connections without waiting for external sign-off. The Future of Nursing 2020–2030 explicitly links removal of scope-of-practice barriers to innovation and equity, arguing that nurses need authority to deploy technology-enabled solutions across settings [22, 23]. In practice, autonomy strengthens APRNs' role in interdisciplinary collaboration. As independent decision-makers, APRNs can engage confidently with technology developers, informaticists, and organizational leaders, contributing clinical insight that improves usability, safety, and patient-centered design. This leadership role is especially important when adopting emerging technologies such as artificial intelligence, where clinical judgment and ethical

Table 1 APRN technology innovators

Name and credentials	Role/specialty	Technology/ innovation	Impact/notable achievements
Roxanne McMurray, DNP, APRN, CRNA	Certified Registered Nurse Anesthetist	McMurray Enhanced Airway (MEA), a first-of-its-kind distal pharyngeal airway device	Improves ventilation and patient safety during sedation and anesthesia; demonstrates CRNA-led medical device innovation
Elleanor Griffiths, RM, MSc	Senior Lead Informatics Midwife (UK)	Digital health systems for maternity care	Leads digital transformation efforts; integrates clinical midwifery expertise into system development and interoperability
Mirini Kim, DNP, RN, CPNP-PC	Head of Nursing, PocketRN	Virtual care model using video, AI, and remote patient monitoring	Expands access to care; augments clinical workflows; refines virtual care protocols; scales telehealth services
Jane Hartman, MSN, APRN, PNP-BC	Clinical Nurse Specialist & Pediatric Nurse Practitioner, Cleveland Clinic	High-line™ IV tubing device	Improves safety, reduces line entanglements, adapts to pediatric care needs; developed via prototyping, engineering collaboration, and end-user feedback

oversight are critical. Furthermore, APRN autonomy supports innovation in underserved and rural settings, where access to physicians may be limited. Autonomous APRNs can leverage technology to expand care access, reduce disparities, and improve outcomes without waiting for external authorization. Ultimately, autonomy empowers APRNs to transform clinical insight into action, accelerating the development and adoption of healthcare technologies that improve efficiency, equity, and quality of care.

The following table (Table 1) highlights the notable contributions of APRNs who have led the development and implementation of innovative healthcare technologies. It showcases a range of specialties, emphasizing how each APRN role has leveraged their expertise to advance patient care, enhance clinical workflows, and integrate emerging digital and medical technologies [10–12, 14, 17, 18, 20, 21, 28–31].

Autonomy Supports Innovations that Increase Access to Care

Autonomy is fundamental to enabling APRNs to develop and implement innovations that increase access to care. [22, 23] APRNs often practice on the frontlines of healthcare delivery, particularly in underserved, rural, or medically underserved areas. In these settings, the ability to make independent clinical decisions allows APRNs to respond quickly to patient needs and implement interventions that improve care access. For example, in rural primary care clinics where physicians may be scarce, autonomous nurse practitioners can develop telehealth programs or mobile health initiatives that extend specialty services to remote patients. [9, 34] By having the authority to assess, diagnose, and manage care without needing constant physician oversight, APRNs can pilot digital platforms, remote monitoring systems, or community-based interventions that directly increase patient reach [9, 32]. Without autonomy, such initiatives may be delayed or stifled by bureaucratic requirements, limiting their potential impact.

Autonomy also enables APRNs to drive innovation grounded in clinical insight [22, 23]. Because they spend significant time with patients and understand workflow challenges, APRNs are ideally positioned to identify problems that could be addressed through technology or process redesign [6]. For instance, a clinical nurse specialist in a hospital may notice delays in patient triage due to inefficient data entry. With autonomy, they can design and implement a digital triage tool or mobile application that streamlines patient assessment and prioritization. Similarly, nurse midwives can implement electronic maternity records or patient-facing apps that enhance prenatal care access [12, 31], particularly for populations facing transportation, socioeconomic, or geographical barriers. Autonomy ensures that APRNs can make decisions about which innovations to pursue, how to adapt them to their clinical context, and how to implement them safely and effectively.

Autonomous APRNs also play a critical role in expanding equitable access to care [22, 23]. Many underserved populations face barriers such as long travel distances, a lack of specialty providers, or limited health literacy. APRNs with the freedom to act independently can tailor technology-driven interventions to meet these needs [9, 32]. For instance, nurse practitioners and nurse midwives can implement mobile health platforms that deliver culturally relevant education and symptom monitoring directly to patients' phones. [9] Autonomous practice allows them to adapt these tools to the specific needs of diverse communities, ensuring that technology does not simply replicate existing disparities but actively reduces them. Furthermore, autonomy empowers APRNs to advocate for systemic changes, such as policy modifications or reimbursement structures, that facilitate broader access to technology-enabled care [22, 23, 34].

Autonomy allows APRNs to leverage their clinical insight, lead technology development, implement solutions efficiently, and adapt interventions to the needs of diverse populations [22, 23]. By removing barriers to independent practice, healthcare systems enable APRNs to function as innovators, problem-solvers, and advocates, translating frontline knowledge into practical, scalable, and equitable solutions. As healthcare continues to evolve, supporting APRN autonomy will be essential to ensuring that technological advancements and process innovations reach all patients, especially those in underserved communities [1, 7], [27], ultimately improving outcomes and access for the populations who need care most.

This table (Table 2) highlights a selection of advanced practice nurses (APRNs) and nurse leaders who have made significant contributions to healthcare innovation, clinical autonomy, and access to care. It showcases nurse midwives, clinical nurse specialists, advanced practice nurses, and nurse practitioners from diverse

Table 2 Nursing innovators who increased access to care

Name	Role/credential	Innovation/contribution	Impact on access or autonomy
Margaret Hewitt	Nurse Midwife, USA	Created the first hospital-based nurse midwife practice in Minnesota (1971); established patient-centered birth planning and one of the earliest single-room birthing units	Advanced clinical autonomy by embedding midwives in hospital settings, allowing independent management of births, prenatal/postpartum care, and midwife-led interventions; expanded scope and legitimacy of nurse midwives
Dorothy Brooten, JoAnne M. Youngblut, Linda Brown	Clinical Nurse Specialists (CNS). USA	Developed CNS-led prenatal home-visit model for high-risk pregnant women; provided half of prenatal care at home, including teaching, counseling, and follow-ups	Increased access to care by reducing barriers like transportation and childcare; improved outcomes, including fewer preterm births and hospitalizations; exemplifies how CNS-led service models expand equity in care delivery
Cecilia Ndungu	Advanced Practice Nurse (APN), Kenya	Global nursing leader promoting digital health, policy, leadership, and health system strengthening; Afro Region Co-chair of Nursing Now Challenge	Expanded access to care through leadership, digital health integration, and innovative health service delivery models in underserved populations; promotes the NP/APN role in health policy and system reform
Sylvanus Kampo	Nurse Practitioner / Nurse Anesthesiologist, Ghana	Senior lecturer and head of anesthesia and intensive care at CKT-UTAS; research in anesthesia, perioperative care, pain management, and training programs	Increased access to anesthesia and critical care in Ghana, particularly in district and regional hospitals, contributes to workforce development and training of future anesthesia providers; bridges clinical practice, education, and research

international settings, each of whom has implemented novel care models, digital health initiatives, or education and training programs that address gaps in healthcare delivery. By illustrating their key innovations, contributions, and impacts, the table demonstrates how APRNs leverage advanced clinical expertise, leadership, and creativity to expand access, improve patient outcomes, and redefine the scope and influence of nursing practice [5, 15, 16, 19, 25, 26, 36].

Autonomy Strengths Entrepreneurship and Local Business Development

APRNs are uniquely positioned to drive innovation that not only improves healthcare delivery but also stimulates community business development [4, 22–24]. Their advanced clinical expertise, combined with an understanding of population health and community needs, enables APRNs to identify gaps in care and develop entrepreneurial solutions that generate economic and social value [1, 2, 7]. By creating nurse-led clinics, mobile health units, telehealth platforms, and specialty service centers, APRNs establish healthcare enterprises that serve as both healthcare access points and economic engines within their communities [9, 32, 34]. These ventures often create employment opportunities for healthcare staff, administrative personnel, and allied health professionals, thereby contributing directly to local economies [22, 23, 36].

APRNs often leverage community-responsive service models to foster business growth. For example, nurse practitioners may establish primary care practices in underserved areas, opening clinics that integrate pharmacy services, wellness programs, nutrition counseling, and chronic disease management [1, 2, 22, 23]. Such practices not only meet critical healthcare needs but also attract ancillary businesses, including medical supply vendors, diagnostic laboratories, and health education providers [6, 36]. Similarly, nurse midwives who develop birth centers or maternity-focused wellness programs often partner with local businesses such as lactation consultants, postpartum care services, and complementary therapy providers, creating a local ecosystem of health-related commerce [15, 16, 31]. These initiatives demonstrate that APRN-led innovation can catalyze broader economic activity while addressing pressing health needs [22, 23].

Telehealth and digital health innovations spearheaded by APRNs are another mechanism through which community business development is supported. APRNs designing virtual care platforms, remote patient monitoring programs, or AI-enabled triage services often contract with technology companies, software developers, and IT support teams [9, 32, 34]. These partnerships provide local employment opportunities and stimulate investment in regional tech infrastructure, creating a multiplier effect that extends beyond the clinic walls [12, 28, 29]. In addition, APRN-led health education and prevention programs can spur demand for wellness products, fitness centers, and home health technologies, further contributing to the growth of local enterprises [26, 37].

APRNs also play a critical role in public health entrepreneurship, translating clinical insight into business models that serve vulnerable populations. For instance, a CNS or NP may identify barriers to chronic disease management in low-income neighborhoods and develop mobile clinics or community health hubs that operate as sustainable business entities [22, 23, 36]. By billing for services, offering preventive care packages, and providing subscription-based health programs, APRNs create self-sustaining models that improve health outcomes while circulating revenue within the community [5]. This approach not only enhances access to care but also fosters local job creation, professional development opportunities, and economic resilience [19, 22, 23].

Furthermore, APRN innovation often encourages local investment and collaboration. As APRNs pilot new care delivery methods or health technology solutions, they frequently attract partnerships with hospitals, universities, public health agencies, and private investors [4, 24]. These collaborations can lead to incubator programs, funding for community health initiatives, and the establishment of ancillary service providers, all of which strengthen the community's business ecosystem [10, 21, 30]. In this way, APRN-led ventures not only address unmet healthcare needs but also cultivate a culture of entrepreneurship and economic development within the community [22, 23].

By translating clinical expertise into sustainable enterprises that generate employment, APRN innovation fosters partnerships and stimulates local economic growth [22, 23, 36]. Whether through nurse-led clinics, birth centers, telehealth platforms, or community health initiatives, APRNs demonstrate that improving health and strengthening the local economy are mutually reinforcing goals [1, 2]. By bridging clinical innovation and entrepreneurship, APRNs serve as both healthcare leaders and catalysts for community-level economic resilience, illustrating the broader societal impact of advanced nursing practice [4, 24].

This table (Table 3) highlights a selection of APRNs who have combined clinical expertise with entrepreneurial vision to create innovative healthcare and wellness businesses. Each of these APRNs has leveraged their advanced training to address unmet healthcare needs in their communities, improve patient outcomes, and expand access to specialized care. Beyond clinical impact, their ventures have generated meaningful local economic benefits, including employment opportunities, partnerships with allied health professionals, and the stimulation of ancillary business activity. By illustrating the intersection of nursing innovation, patient-centered care, and business leadership, this table demonstrates the critical role APRNs play not only in advancing healthcare delivery but also in supporting local communities and economies [3, 4, 8, 13, 17, 18, 24, 33, 35, 37].

Table 3 APRN entrepreneurs

APRN	Title/ credentials	Innovation/ business	Clinical/community impact	Economic/local business contribution
Marqueta Abraham	DNP, APRN, PMHNP-BC	Founder and owner of **CLR mind psychiatry, LLC**	Provides comprehensive mental health services (children, adolescents, adults, veterans); focuses on evidence-based, personalized care for underserved populations, especially the African American community	Expands local mental health workforce, creates jobs for clinicians and administrative staff, increases access to psychiatric care in Memphis, and reduces health disparities
Nicolle Gonzales	BSN, RN, MSN, CNM	Founder and executive director of **changing woman initiative (CWI)**	Provides culturally grounded maternal health care for indigenous families; offers prenatal care, home services, doula support, nutrition programs, and wellness resources; working to establish the first native American-focused birthing center	Creates healthcare jobs for midwives, doulas, and support staff; supports local indigenous communities economically through health-focused programs; stimulates local supply chains for birthing and wellness services
Ladan Eshkevari	PhD, CRNA, L.ac., FAAN	Co-CEO and founder of **Avesta Ketamine and wellness**	Developed ketamine-assisted therapy for treatment-resistant mental health and chronic pain; integrates anesthetic expertise with innovative, patient-centered treatment models	Generates local economic activity by employing clinical, administrative, and support staff; fosters partnerships with pharmacies, labs, and allied health professionals; attracts regional patients, boosting ancillary local services
Melanie Speed	APRN, NP-C, CANS	Founder of **flawless MedSpa and the Beverly Hills MedSpa**	Provides advanced aesthetic medicine services (injectables, plasma treatments, thread lifts, hair restoration); trains other clinicians in advanced techniques	Drives local economic growth through clinic employment, education of clinicians, and service-based revenue; attracts clients regionally, increasing business for local suppliers and allied services

Final Thoughts

Innovation in healthcare depends not only on new technologies or delivery models but on the authority and expertise of the clinicians positioned to implement them effectively. This chapter has demonstrated that clinical autonomy is a foundational enabler of innovation for APRNs. When APRNs are empowered to practice to the full extent of their education and training, they serve as catalysts for meaningful change—bridging frontline clinical insight with system-level transformation. Autonomy is therefore not merely a professional issue, but a strategic imperative for advancing access, quality, equity, and value across the healthcare continuum.

Throughout this chapter, evidence and real-world examples have shown that APRNs are uniquely positioned to lead innovation because of their proximity to patients, deep understanding of care workflows, and interdisciplinary roles. Autonomous APRNs drive the development, testing, and adoption of healthcare technologies by identifying unmet needs, co-designing solutions with developers, and ensuring that innovations align with real clinical practice. Whether advancing telehealth, remote patient monitoring, digital maternity records, or novel medical devices, APRNs translate clinical challenges into scalable, patient-centered solutions that improve outcomes and usability. Autonomy accelerates this process by allowing APRNs to move efficiently from idea to implementation without unnecessary regulatory or organizational delays.

The chapter also highlighted how APRN autonomy expands access to care, particularly for underserved, rural, and marginalized populations. Autonomous practice enables APRNs to deploy technology-enabled care models, home-based services, mobile clinics, and culturally responsive interventions that overcome geographic, socioeconomic, and structural barriers. Importantly, APRN-led innovations do not simply increase access; they advance equity by tailoring solutions to the specific needs of diverse communities and advocating for systemic change. In this way, autonomy supports innovation that is not only efficient but also just and inclusive.

Beyond clinical innovation, APRN autonomy strengthens entrepreneurship and local economic development. Nurse-led clinics, telehealth enterprises, birth centers, and specialty practices demonstrate how APRNs convert clinical expertise into sustainable business models that generate employment, stimulate local economies, and reinvest resources into community health. These ventures illustrate that healthcare innovation and economic resilience are mutually reinforcing outcomes when APRNs are empowered to lead. By integrating care delivery with business development, APRNs extend their impact beyond individual patients to entire communities.

In summary, this chapter affirms that APRN autonomy is essential to the future of healthcare innovation. Removing scope-of-practice barriers unlocks the full potential of APRNs as innovators, leaders, and entrepreneurs who can respond rapidly to evolving healthcare needs. As healthcare systems confront rising costs, workforce shortages, and persistent inequities, supporting APRN autonomy offers a high-value strategy for sustainable transformation. Investing in autonomous APRN practice is ultimately an investment in a more accessible, equitable, and innovative healthcare system—one that is better equipped to meet the needs of patients and communities now and in the future.

References

1. AANP. Literature on quality of nurse practitioner practice. 2025. Available at: https://www.aanp.org/advocacy/advocacy-resource/position-statements/quality-of-nurse-practitioner-practice. Accessed 23 Dec 2025.
2. AANP Literature on nurse practitioner cost effectiveness. 2025. Available at: https://www.aanp.org/advocacy/advocacy-resource/position-statements/nurse-practitioner-cost-effectiveness. Accessed 23 Dec 2025.
3. Abraham M. CLR Mind Psychiatry, LLC: about us. 2023. Available at: https://www.clrmind-psychiatry.com. Accessed 23 Dec 2025.
4. American Nurses Association. ANA Innovation Awards—Winners. 2023. Available at: https://www.nursingworld.org/practice-policy/innovation/events/awards2/winners/. Accessed 23 Dec 2025.
5. Brooten D, Youngblut JM, Brown LP. The impact of a nurse specialist home care intervention on high-risk prenatal patients. J Obstet Gynecol Neonatal Nurs. 2001;30(2):181–9. https://doi.org/10.1111/j.1552-6909.2001.tb01535.x.
6. Brown T, Wyatt J. Design thinking for social innovation. In: Stanford Social Innovation Review, Winter; 2010. p. 31–5. Available at: https://ssir.org/articles/entry/design_thinking_for_social_innovation. Accessed 23 Dec 2025.
7. Buerhaus P, Perloff J, Clarke S, O'Reilly-Jacob M, Zolotusky G, DesRoches CM. quality of primary care provided to Medicare beneficiaries by nurse practitioners and physicians. Med Care. 2018;56(6):484–90. https://doi.org/10.1097/MLR.0000000000000908. Available at: https://europepmc.org/article/MED/29613873. Accessed 23 Dec 2025.
8. Changing Woman Initiative. Our work and mission. 2024. Available at: https://changingwomaninitiative.com. Accessed 23 Dec 2025.
9. Charalambous J, Hollingdrake O, Currie J. Nurse practitioner-led telehealth services: a scoping review. J Clin Nurs. 2023;33(3):839–58. https://doi.org/10.1111/jocn.16898. Available at: https://onlinelibrary.wiley.com/doi/epdf/10.1111/jocn.16898. Accessed 23 Dec 2025.
10. Cleveland Clinic ConsultQD. Nursing innovation provides solution for COVID-19 challenges and beyond. 2020. Available at: https://consultqd.clevelandclinic.org/nursing-innovation-provides-solution-for-covid-19-challenges-and-beyond. Accessed 23 Dec 2025.
11. Cleveland Clinic Magazine. Jane Hartman, MSN, APRN, CPNP-PC (Profile). 2022. Available at: https://magazine.clevelandclinic.org/2022-fall/jane-hartman. Accessed 23 Dec 2025.
12. Digital Health. Maternity app and electronic health record to be rolled out in Wales. 2025. Available at: https://www.digitalhealth.net/2025/01/maternity-app-and-electronic-health-record-to-be-rolled-out-in-wales/. Accessed 23 Dec 2025.
13. Eshkevari L., Avesta Ketamine & Wellness. Ketamine-assisted therapy and integrative mental health care. 2023. Available at: https://avestaketaminewellness.com. Accessed 23 Dec 2025.
14. FreePatentsOnline. IV tubing carriage system — Patent application US 20230293808. 2023. Available at: https://www.freepatentsonline.com/y2023/0293808.html. Accessed 23 Dec 2025.

15. Hewitt M. The development of hospital-based nurse-midwifery practice. J Nurse Midwifery. 1973;18(4):1–7.
16. International Confederation of Midwives. Midwifery autonomy and scope of practice. The Hague: ICM; 2014. Available at: https://www.internationalmidwives.org. Accessed 23 Dec 2025.
17. Johns Hopkins School of Nursing. Ladan Eshkevari: innovating mental health and pain management. Johns Hopkins Nursing Magazine; 2022. Available at: https://nursing.jhu.edu. Accessed 23 Dec 2025.
18. Johns Hopkins School of Nursing. Breaking the mold: Alumni talk with Mirini Kim. 2022. Available at: https://nursing.jhu.edu/magazine/articles/2022/03/breaking-the-mold-alumni-talk-with-mirini-kim/. Accessed 23 Dec 2025.
19. Kampo S, Asare A, Ofori-Kwakye K. Expanding access to anesthesia services in Ghana: the role of nurse anesthetists. Anesth Analg. 2019;129(1):234–40. https://doi.org/10.1213/ANE.0000000000003921.
20. McMurray Medical. MEA — distal pharyngeal airway (product information). 2025. Available at: https://www.mcmurraymed.com/. Accessed 23 Dec 2025.
21. Medical Alley. McMurray Medical receives national innovation award for airway device. 2023. Available at: https://medicalalley.org/mcmurray-medical-receives-national-innovation-award-for-airway-device/. Accessed 23 Dec 2025.
22. National Academies of Sciences, Engineering, and Medicine. The future of nursing 2020–2030: charting a path to achieve Health equity. Washington, DC: The National Academies Press; 2021. Available at: https://www.nmnec.org/wp-content/uploads/2021/05/Future-of-Nursing-2020-2030.pdf. Accessed 23 Dec 2025.
23. National Academies of Sciences, Engineering, and Medicine. Highlights: the future of nursing 2020–2030. 2021. Available at: https://nap.nationalacademies.org/resource/25982/Highlights_Future%20of%20Nursing_4.30.21_final.pdf. Accessed 23 Dec 2025.
24. National Academy of Medicine. Emerging nurse leaders and innovators. Washington, DC: NAM; 2022. Available at: https://nam.edu. Accessed 23 Dec 2025.
25. Ndungu C. Advancing digital health and nursing leadership for universal health coverage in Africa. Afr J Nurs Midwifery. 2021;23(2):1–10.
26. Nursing Now. Nursing now challenge: leaders profiles. 2022. Available at: https://www.nursingnow.org. Accessed 23 Dec 2025.
27. Perloff J, DesRoches CM, Buerhaus P. Comparing the Cost of Care Provided to Medicare Beneficiaries Assigned to Primary Care Nurse Practitioners and Physicians. Health Serv Res. 2016;51(4):1407–23. https://doi.org/10.1111/1475-6773.12425.
28. PocketRN. PocketRN publishes clinical study highlighting efficacy of novel virtual nursing care model. 2023. Available at: https://www.pocketrn.com/blog/pocketrn-publishes-clinical-study-highlighting-efficacy-of-novel-virtual-nursing-care-model. Accessed 23 Dec 2025.
29. PR.com. New study from PocketRN and Stanford Health Care reveals efficacy of nurse-led care via telehealth. 2023. Available at: https://www.pr.com/press-release/897383. Accessed 23 Dec 2025.
30. Protolabs. Cleveland Clinic device saves PPE, increases patient freedom. 2020. Available at: https://www.protolabs.com/resources/blog/cleveland-clinic-device-saves-ppe-increases-patient-freedom/. Accessed 23 Dec 2025.
31. Royal College of Midwives. Elleanor Griffiths — Digital Midwife (profile). 2024. Available at: https://rcm.org.uk/team/elleanor-griffiths/. Accessed 23 Dec 2025.
32. Schultz MA. Telehealth and remote patient monitoring innovations in nursing practice: state of the science. Online J Issues Nurs. 2023;28(2) Available at: https://ojin.nursingworld.org/globalassets/ojin/tableofcontents/vol-28-2023/no2-may-2023/telehealth-and-remote-patient-monitoring-innovations-in-nursing-practice_state-of-the-science_ojin.pdf. Accessed 23 Dec 2025.
33. Speed M. Flawless MedSpa: about. 2024. Available at: https://www.flawlessmedspabh.com. Accessed 23 Dec 2025.

34. Telehealth.HHS.gov. Telehealth policy updates. 2025. Available at: https://telehealth.hhs.gov/providers/telehealth-policy/telehealth-policy-updates. Accessed 23 Dec 2025.
35. The Beverly Hills MedSpa. Clinical services and professional training. 2024. Available at: https://www.thebeverlyhillsmedspa.com. Accessed 23 Dec 2025.
36. World Health Organization. State of the world's nursing 2020: investing in education, jobs and leadership. Geneva: WHO; 2020. Available at: https://www.who.int/publications/i/item/9789240003279. Accessed: 23 Dec 2025.
37. World Health Organization. Mental health and community-based care. Geneva: WHO; 2022. Available at: https://www.who.int. Accessed 23 Dec 2025

Regional Variations and Reflections on Autonomous APN Practice

Eileen M. Stuart-Shor, Rebecca Silvers, Kanata Akter,
Maura M. Brain, Bonisile Nsibandze, and Ama Taplah

Introduction

This chapter tells the story of how a midwife, nurse anesthetist, pediatric acute-care nurse practitioner, primary care nurse practitioner, and family nurse practitioner describe their day-to- day advanced practice nursing (APN) work in Bangladesh, Liberia, Eswatini, and the United States. The variations in role and region are intentional to provide a global snapshot of clinical autonomy for APNs. Their stories are embedded in a framework that explores the levels of autonomy of advanced practice nurses and examines the factors that facilitate or restrain their ability to practice independently [1].

The advanced practice nurse role, for this chapter, uses the International Council of Nurses (ICN) definition as a "registered nurse who acquired the expert knowledge

E. M. Stuart-Shor (✉)
Department of Anesthesia, Critical Care and Pain Medicine, Beth Israel Deaconess Medical Center, Boston, MA, USA

University of Massachusetts Boston, Manning College of Nursing and Health Sciences, Boston, MA, USA

Boston-Africa Anesthesia and Critical Care Collaborative, Boston, MA, USA
e-mail: Eileen.Stuart-Shor@umb.edu

R. Silvers
Center for Global Nursing, University of California San Francisco, Institute of Global Health Sciences, San Francisco, CA, USA

Pediatric Neurosurgery & Critical Care Nurse Practitioner, San Francisco, CA, USA

UCSF Benioff Children's Hospitals, Oakland and San Francisco, CA, USA

UCSF School of Nursing, San Francisco, CA, USA

UCSF WHO Collaborating Centre for Emergency, Critical & Operative Care, San Francisco, CA, USA
e-mail: rebecca.silvers@ucsf.edu

A. Kapu et al. (eds.), *A Global View on Clinical Autonomy for Advanced Practice Nurses*, Advanced Practice in Nursing,
https://doi.org/10.1007/978-3-032-21458-4_12

base, complex decision-making skills and clinical competencies for expanded practice, the characteristics of which are shaped by the context and country in which they are credentialed to practice" [2]. This definition assures that education that prepares the APN with an expert knowledge base, complex decision-making skills, and clinical competencies for expanded practice is the base for autonomous APN practice. Further, acknowledging that the characteristics of APN practice are shaped and bounded by country context and need is important to understanding regional differences in practice. APNs provide care to communities as well as patients and families across the lifespan with acute, chronic, and/or complex conditions. Their clinical autonomy is associated with varying amounts of independence, empowerment, and valuation for autonomous practice [1]. The boundaries of independent/autonomous practice are delineated by the scope of practice (what services an APN is legally permitted to provide) within the confines of practice authority (restricted, full), which states whether the APN can evaluate, diagnose, treat, and prescribe medications independently, without physician supervision or mandatory collaboration.

Development and global emergence of the APN role arose in response to global health demands, changing and more complex patient needs, health systems challenges, including inequitable access and a critical health worker shortage. In the United States, the genesis of the APN role (1965) was in response to healthcare shortages, particularly in primary care and rural health. The role has since evolved across the care continuum (disease prevention, health promotion, acute and chronic illness management, and palliative care) to improve the health and well-being of all Americans with a specific focus on eliminating health disparities. Uptake of the APN role in Africa was accelerated in response to the HIV crisis, which stressed an already overwhelmed and fragile healthcare system with crippling healthcare worker shortages. In 2008, the World Health Organization (WHO), fueled by a sense of urgency to contain the HIV epidemic in Africa, disseminated its report on Task Shifting [3]. This report recommended that non-physician clinicians (APNs are specifically included in this category) can safely and effectively undertake most clinical tasks. They noted that the use of APNs is associated with good outcomes, shows minimal differences compared to medical doctors, and increases access to care [3]. Based on

K. Akter
Hope Foundation for Women and Children of Bangladesh, Cox's Bazar, Bangladesh

International Council of Midwives, ICM Fellow Executive Sponsorship Leadership Programme, Cox's Bazar, Bangladesh

M. M. Brain
Massachusetts General Hospital, Bullfinch Medical Group, Boston, MA, USA

B. Nsibandze
Department of General Nursing Science, Faculty of Health Sciences, University of Eswatini, Mbabane, Eswatini

A. Taplah
John F. Kennedy Memorial Medical Center, Monrovia, Liberia

Program Coordinator, TNIMA/JFK Anesthesia Program, Monrovia, Liberia these recommendations, Ministries of Health in Africa began to shift care to non-physician clinicians (including APNs) using protocols. Gradually, the concept transitioned to task sharing, which acknowledged the advanced educational preparation and complex clinical decision making provided by APNs, and formalization of the role within countries [4]. Other resource-constrained countries with fragile healthcare systems and healthcare worker shortages applied the lessons learned from HIV to meet the need to reduce unacceptably high maternal and child mortality rates and to improve access to lifesaving surgical and anesthetic care. Recent large studies have supported the APN role globally in responding to health challenges and improving outcomes, finding care was equal to or superior to the comparator (e.g. physicians) when compared across several categories and a wide range of clinical settings, patient populations, and acuity level [5]. Of significance, these outcomes were reported in both developed and developing countries. Despite these positive outcomes, studies note that APNs continue to struggle with titling, title protection, regulation development, credentialing, and barriers to practice [6].

While there is evidence of the variability in the integration of advanced practice nursing roles globally, research related to clinical autonomy of the APN in different world regions is limited [7]. Lockwood and colleagues proposed a framework to understand the factors associated with autonomous practice, identifying four themes: ANP stepping up, ANP living it, ANP bounce-back ability, and ANP setting in motion (Fig. 1) [1]. *Stepping up* is demonstrated by the nurse transitioning from their current role to the APN role and taking on advanced clinical responsibilities and scope of practice. APNs master more advanced clinical tasks (such as complex clinical decision making, diagnosis, and treatment plans) and can complete a visit or episode of care without physician oversight. *Living it* involves a sense of enabling clinical autonomy within their day-to-day practice (the working environment), contributing to professional support and a sense of achievement. Enabling environments were described as having collaborative working relationships as opposed to a

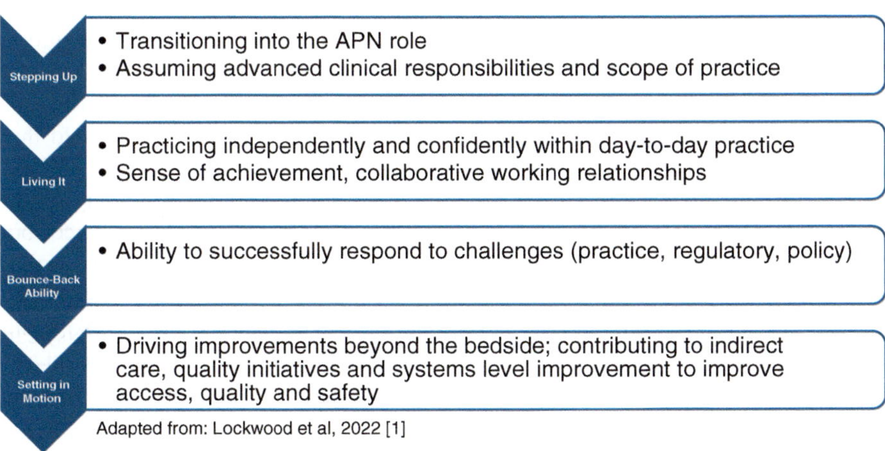

Fig. 12.1 Factors Associated with Autonomous APN Practice

hierarchical structure. Nurses in APN roles need *bounce-back ability*, the ability to regain control and balance when faced with challenges that threaten their ability to practice autonomously. Sociocultural and service-level challenges, regulatory/policy restraints on practice, and interprofessional conflicts were all areas where APNs needed the ability to bounce back in order to succeed in autonomous practice. *ANP setting in motion* acknowledges the responsibility of APNs to contribute to indirect care activities, quality initiatives and systems-level improvements in order to improve access, quality, and safety of care [1, 8].

In order to practice autonomously, APNs need to step up to the advanced care skills and responsibilities inherent in the role, live the role fully integrated into an enabling environment, bounce back from threats to autonomy, and set in motion enhancements in the care they deliver to promote high-quality, safe, accessible care and autonomous practice. In a recently reported large study that examined 117 systematic reviews, Kilpatrick and colleagues reported that there was highly consistent evidence that APNs provided similar or superior care compared to physician or usual care across a wide range of clinical settings, patient populations, and acuity levels [7]. They also reported that autonomous or full scope of practice enhanced patient, provider, and health systems level outcomes. In an editorial that introduced a volume of *The International Journal of Nursing Studies* dedicated entirely to reporting clinical outcomes of APN practice globally, Poghosyan and colleagues noted that APNs provided clinically- and cost-effective care but need enabling environments to practice efficiently [5]. These observations, made in both developed and developing countries, call for innovative ways of thinking about clinical autonomy to more fully understand clinical autonomy and regional variance (and its impact), and to extend the conversation beyond the pillars of education, practice, and policy.

Vignettes: Stories from the Field

To better understand the current practice environment for Advanced Practice Nurses (APNs) and its implications for practicing autonomously, we elected to describe the experience of practicing APNs in several countries across different WHO Regions in a series of vignettes. Essentially, these vignettes are stories from the field that describe the lived experience of the APN, embedded in the country context. These stories are not intended to be construed as research, a systematic review, or an exhaustive description of the role and how providers perceive their practice, but rather as individual examples that can provide insights and questions for further consideration. Utilizing the framework proposed by Lockwood and colleagues to unpack the practice characteristics influencing autonomy [1, 8], APNs from Bangladesh, Liberia, Eswatini, and the United States share their country context and their clinical journey towards full-scope, autonomous practice.

A Midwife in Bangladesh

Background and Country Context

The story of modern midwifery in Bangladesh is one of vision, commitment, and transformation. Only a decade and a half ago, the country faced alarmingly high rates of maternal and newborn deaths. Many women lost their lives each year due to preventable complications in pregnancy and childbirth, often because skilled birth attendants were unavailable in rural and remote areas. Against this backdrop, in 2010, the Prime Minister made an impotant announcement: Bangladesh would train and deploy 3000 professional midwives to strengthen safe motherhood. This political commitment set in motion a nationwide movement that has since redefined maternal and newborn health in the country and acknowledged the global evidence that midwives save lives.

Education: Initially, as a measure to fill a critical gap, a 6-month post-basic training programme was introduced for registered nurses, producing the first generation of midwives trained to international standards. By 2012, the government launched a three-year Diploma in Midwifery, formally recognizing midwifery as an independent profession. Since then, the journey of midwifery education has been marked by steady expansion and innovation. Different educational models emerged, including direct-entry three-year diploma programmes, a two-year post-basic and a BSc in Midwifery, providing midwives with advanced qualifications and leadership opportunities. The commitment to high-quality education has also been reinforced through international collaboration. More than 150 Bangladeshi faculty members earned Master's degrees in Sexual and Reproductive Health from Dalarna University in Sweden, while others pursued PhDs abroad. Locally, a Master's curriculum in Midwifery is being developed, ensuring the sustainability of faculty expertise. Accreditation, skill-lab training, peer mentorship, and clinical internships have further strengthened the academic environment, laying the foundation for a competent and confident midwifery workforce.

Regulation, Credentialing, and Professionalization: The Bangladesh Nursing and Midwifery Council (BNMC) has played a critical role in regulating the profession. It oversees accreditation of institutions, licensing of midwives, and continuing professional development. Re-licensing every 5 years, tied to evidence of ongoing training, has ensured that midwives remain updated with international standards. Alongside regulatory growth, the profession has also organized itself. The Bangladesh Midwifery Society (BMS), formed in 2010, has emerged as a strong advocate for midwives. With young leaders championing advocacy, policy dialogue, and professional visibility at national and global levels, with the help and guidance of the ICM.

Practice Climate and Impact: Graduates of the diploma and post-basic training programmes began deployment at sub-district and union-level health facilities from 2016 onward, and now posts have been created in District-level hospitals with plans to create posts in Medical College Hospitals. Currently, over 2000 Midwives have been deployed through the government, and their presence has translated into measurable improvements: women reported more respectful maternity care, facility births increased, and complications were better managed at the community level. The midwifery workforce has not only shaped health outcomes in stable settings but also played a vital role in humanitarian response. Around 500 midwives are currently serving Rohingya refugees and host communities, providing lifesaving maternal and newborn health services in some of the most challenging conditions. For midwives to practice effectively, enabling environments are essential. The Directorate General of Nursing and Midwifery (DGNM), in collaboration with UNFPA and other partners, has introduced clinical mentorship, supportive supervision, and Centers of Excellence. These centers not only support newly deployed midwives but also demonstrate the effectiveness of midwife-led maternity care units, influencing health managers and policymakers to embrace the model nationwide.

Despite meaningful gains in the education, regulation, and deployment of midwives in Bangladesh, there are challenges that remain to be addressed. Many communities and even some health professionals are not fully aware of the distinct role of midwives, often confusing them with staff nurses. Midwives are sometimes underutilized in facilities and assigned tasks outside their scope, and there is a lack of clear role definition and supportive supervision in some settings. Shortages of experienced midwifery educators and mentors and an inconsistent quality of midwifery training institutions across the country are a challenge to producing and scaling up qualified, well-trained midwives. Limited access to continuing professional development and higher studies (e.g., Bachelor's/Master's in Midwifery) challenges practicing midwives to remain current and able to function as leaders in maternal and child health. In the area of infrastructure and resources, many health facilities lack adequate equipment, supplies, drugs, and space for midwife-led care. Midwives are primarily concentrated in urban or semi-urban areas, while rural areas often face shortages despite high maternal and newborn needs. Retention is difficult in remote postings due to safety, workload, and lack of incentives. Policy and systems challenges, including incomplete integration of midwives into the national health system hierarchy, limited leadership positions in policy and pay scales, and benefits that do not reflect the workload and responsibility midwives carry. There are also challenges related to workload and burnout due to high caseloads and constrained resources, as well as the unique gender-based challenges midwives face as a female-dominated profession. To fully realize the potential of midwives to improve maternal and newborn health outcomes in Bangladesh, there will need to be coordinated efforts by the government, Bangladesh Nursing and Midwifery Council, international partners, and the midwives themselves to develop and deploy locally relevant solutions to the challenges.

Today, midwives in Bangladesh are gaining recognition as central to achieving universal access to sexual, reproductive, maternal, newborn, and adolescent health (SRMNAH) services. Their scope extends beyond childbirth to include antenatal and postnatal care, newborn resuscitation, family planning, cervical cancer screening, and gender-based violence prevention. They have become trusted frontline providers who provide dignified, respectful care. Bangladesh's vision is ambitious: to deploy more than 20,000 midwives by 2030, ensuring that every woman, regardless of geography or socioeconomic status, can give birth safely under the care of a skilled professional. Investment in midwifery education and practice is not only a moral and health imperative but also an economic one. Global evidence suggests that every dollar invested in midwives yields up to a 16-fold return in lives saved and unnecessary interventions averted.

Personal Reflections on My Midwifery Practice

I have been a midwife for 7 years now. My experience of *Stepping Up* and moving into midwifery practice was a good experience, which I attribute to having had strong support and a supportive environment as a new midwife. I attended a three-year diploma in midwifery training that was excellent. During my training, I heard stories of the plight of the Rohingya refugees, particularly women and children, which fueled my desire to serve as a midwife in the region when I finished my training. After passing the final exam at the conclusion of the training program, I had a 6-month internship at an NGO supported field hospital that provided care within the Rohingya refugee community. Despite the challenging conditions in the refugee community, it was a beautiful training environment for me, supported by experienced midwives, doctors, pediatricians, and gynecologists. In this hospital setting, I saw many complicated cases and got to see how the experienced midwives, pediatricians, and gynecologists managed the patients. The NGO field hospital created a friendly environment for midwives to learn in the clinical setting. After completing my internship, I served as a provisional midwife at the same hospital system, providing care during the prenatal, birth, and post-natal continuum. Now my job is supported by a private/public (national/international) partnership where I serve as a midwife mentor/coordinator. I practice in both the primary health care center (PHC), where there are no doctors present, and at the field hospital, where I have strong support for learning to manage complicationed patients.

Reflecting on my experience practicing as a midwife (*ANP-living it*), I would say that I practice independently but refer to my physician colleagues whenever the situation requires more complex care than we can provide in our environment. In the Primary Health Care Center (PHC), there are no physicians. Midwives provide comprehensive maternal and newborn health care, including promoting universal access to sexual, reproductive, maternal, newborn, and adolescent health (SRMNAH). I manage most patient care visits independently and have my midwife colleagues and the nurses in the PHC to consult with if I have a question. But if the situation requires escalation of care, I refer to the hospital. In my practice at the PHC, I am confident providing a full scope of service care for women during an uncomplicated birth, as well as many complicated births. For example, if a woman experiences post-partum hemorrhage (PPH), I can usually manage the patient in the PHC community setting, but if she requires a transfusion, I refer her to the hospital. Of course, my patients were also important mentors for me as a midwife. Because I work in the refugee community, I had a lot to learn about the needs and culture of my patients. Gaining trust in the community was critical to their willingness to come to the PHC facility and allow me to care for them. Having them trust me required that I learn about and trust their culture and desires for the birth experience.

Midwifery is a new profession in Bangladesh, which is a challenge for us. Although we have strong Bangladeshi midwives, we are few and the profession is new. I have been very grateful for the international midwives who work with the NGO and provide hands-on mentoring for us. By watching them practice respectful maternity care and being exposed to the full scope of midwifery practice, I have learned so many things. There are many challenges to practicing independently in Bangladesh, but the environment in which I work is supportive of midwives. Initially, physicians were not used to the role, and that was a challenge, but over time, that issue has lessened. Perhaps the biggest challenge is working with individuals from a different culture (Rohingya) and coping with the shortages that can be expected in a refugee community. I would say the international midwife mentors have been the biggest support in my learning to meet challenges and develop as a midwife (*ANP bounce-back ability*). I also sought opportunities to advance my training outside my work environment. I attended and became a master trainer for Helping Mothers Survive, a program that provides health workers with skills in prevention, detection, and management of the leading causes of maternal deaths, including bleeding after birth, pre-eclampsia and eclampsia. This, and other educational programs, increased my confidence in my midwifery skills and were important in my journey as a clinician.

Since I became a midwife 7 years ago, there have been several opportunities for me to be involved in indirect care and to contribute to service level improvements (*ANP-Setting in Motion*). As part of my job responsibilities, I mentor midwives in training and new midwives, to ensure that they deliver high-quality, safe midwifery care that meets our SOP (standard operating procedures). I enjoy this part of my role as I can give back to the new midwives what was given to me and can contribute to the safe, high-quality, respectful care our mothers and newborns deserve. Interacting with and learning from the refugee community is also important to me. We go into the community to teach about safe mother and baby care throughout the perinatal time and encourage pregnant women to give birth in a health facility. We also learn from the community how to deliver culturally sensitive, respectful maternity care, which is important to building trust. Spending time in the community and learning about the women's needs and strengths created opportunities for me to advocate for them within the NGO and in a variety of media outlets.

The story of midwifery in Bangladesh is a testament to political will, global partnership, and local determination. From the Prime Minister's 2010 commitment, to the vibrant profession it is today, midwifery has today emerged as an essential cornerstone of the country's health system. The journey is not without challenges, but the progress made to date demonstrates that midwives are not only birth attendants, but they are also agents of change, advocates of dignity, and guardians of life.

Kanata Akter, Diploma in Midwifery, BSc in Midwifery(Post Basic)—Ongoing, is a Midwife in Bangladesh (WHO South Asia Region)

A Nurse Anesthetist in Liberia

Background and Country Context

The story of nurse anesthesia in Liberia is one of courage, resilience, and rebuilding because Liberian Nurse Anesthetists believe that every Liberian has a right to safe anesthesia and surgery. Surgery is recognized as a core component of primary care and universal health coverage (UHC), integral to the realization of the right to health. In Liberia (a small West African country designated as a low-income country by the World Bank) however, there is a dire shortage of anesthesia providers, and this shortage limits the ability of everyday Liberians to receive essential, life-saving anesthesia care. Shortages of healthcare workers were exacerbated by the 14-year civil war and the Ebola epidemic. These two devastating incidents led to a complete setback to the government of Liberia and its healthcare system. In 2015, while the government was making efforts to put the broken pieces back together after the civil war and rebuild the country, the deadly Ebola virus outbreak occurred. Over 4800 Liberians and foreign nationals died. Over 160 Liberian health workers' lives were taken away by the Ebola virus, bringing a sharp decrease in the number of health workers and access to health care facilities [9]. In 2025, no county in Liberia meets the Lancet Commission Recommendation on Global Surgery 2030 recommended number of anesthesia providers (10 per 100,000 individuals) [10]. Against this backdrop, Liberian nurse anesthetists, with the support of government and international funding and technical partners, have been striving to strengthen the number and quality of nurse anesthesia providers and attain universal access to safe anesthesia in Liberia. They are doing this by building a highly skilled, resilient, sustainable network of nurse anesthesia educators and providers.

Education: Educating nurse anesthetists within Liberia is deeply embedded in the country's history. The first programs were deployed in 1976. Initially, nurse anesthetists were educated primarily by visiting foreign faculty and non-governmental organizations (NGOs). Beginning in 2016 with the country's effort to rebuild the healthcare system and worker cadres after the devastation of Ebola, the training for nurse anesthetists transitioned from a foreign-faculty dependent system to a Liberian-led system. At this point they developed a locally tailored, competency-based curriculum for training Nurse Anesthetists that is aligned with the education standards set by the International Federation of Nurse Anesthetists and International Council of Nurses [11, 12]. The curriculum was approved and adopted by the Liberian Board for Nursing and Midwifery (LBNM) in 2017 as the national training curriculum to be used by any accredited training school. To gain entry to a nurse anesthetist program, applicants must be Registered Nurses licensed by the Liberian Board for Nursing and Midwifery and preferably with 2 years of acute care experience. In 2022 training was upgraded from a post-basic nursing Diploma in Nurse Anesthesia to a post basic nursing Bachelor's Degree in Nurse Anesthesia.

Regulation, Credentialing and Professionalization: The Liberian Board for Nursing and Midwifery (LBNM), established by law in 1949, is the autonomous sole regulator for nursing, advanced practice nursing and midwifery in Liberia. They are also the sole accreditor for nursing, advanced practice nursing and midwifery training programs in Liberia. They recognize Nurse Anesthetists as one cadre of Advanced Practice Nurses. After successful completion of an accredited nurse anesthetist program, graduates apply to the LBNM to sit for the national entry-to-practice nurse anesthetist examination, and then if successful, for recognition as a Nurse Anesthetist in the Advanced Practice Nurse role. Nurse anesthetists work in both the public sector (government facilities) and the private sector (private hospitals and health centers). The Liberian Ministry of Health assigns public sector job ranks and sets the salary structure for level of training credentials. Of note, the current Chief Nursing and Midwifery Officer at the MOH is an experienced nurse anesthetist. While her role is to represent all of nursing and midwifery, her experience as a nurse anesthetist, positions her well to advocate for safe, high-quality anesthetic and surgical care. The Liberian Association of Nurse Anesthetists (LANA) has been an important professional organization in the country advocating for high quality, safe anesthesia care in the country as well as the scaling up of practicing nurse anesthetists and improvements in quality-of-life issues (pay, working conditions etc.) inherent in the role. They collaborate closely with individual nurse anesthetists, nurse anesthesia education programs, the LBNM and the MOH to assure that their membership has the education, resources, infrastructure and support necessary to practice to their full capability. LANA has played a vital role in professionalizing the field and in shaping national policy and global collaborations.

Practice Climate and Impact Nurse anesthetists (NAs) are the primary providers of anesthesia in Liberia and practice independently [13]. In the urban setting they typically have nurse anesthetist colleagues, and more recently physician anesthesiologist colleagues, to consult with, but in the rural setting, they are often the sole anesthesia provider in the facility. Despite the challenges inherent in resource constrained settings, workforce shortages and a fragile health system, NAs in Liberia have demonstrated their ability to deliver high quality, safe anesthesia care in both urban and rural areas. They provide full-service anesthesia across the peri-operative care continuum (pre-operative, procedure, post-operative and critical care), tailored to the resources available in the setting (rural and urban). Recent attention to scaling up the production of practice-ready nurse anesthetists has resulted in the government re-opening a second nurse anesthesia education program at the national hospital which had been closed since 2012. International partnerships continue to support and strengthen anesthesia care in Liberia, but the focus has shifted to these partnerships being Liberian led. For the past 5 years, Liberian nurse anesthetists have joined with NA colleagues in Boston to discuss difficult cases. These transnational Anesthesia Grand Rounds are virtual. The Liberian NAs identify and present a case that has local relevance and the Boston CRNA provides a review of best practices from the literature. The rounds have wide visibility with most providers in the country joining as they can. The scaling up of continuing professional development education (CPD), in collaboration with the educational programs, LANA and international partners provides ongoing support for evidence-based, high quality, safe and dignified anesthesia care.

Personal Reflections on my Nurse Anesthetist Practice

My journey as a nurse anesthetist (NA) in Liberia mirrors the journey (progress and challenges) of the country. In 2008, the MOH, with support from the World Bank, re-established its nurse anesthesia program at the national hospital. This was done in response to the urgent demand for anesthetic providers and was designed to fill immediate gaps in surgical and obstetric care. I felt privileged to be part of the cohort of nurses who were asked to step up to meet this challenge. Despite concerns about how I would manage to balance school, work, and raising my young children, I accepted the challenge and enrolled in this nurse anesthetist training program. As a Bachelor's-prepared nurse, I had a strong foundation to begin this 18-month specialty training. Academically, I felt that the nurse anesthesia training program was strong, and I received excellent clinical mentoring, which was important as I began my first job as a NA. When I graduated in 2011, I made the decision to remain at the national hospital because the need was so great. And so, very soon after graduation, I started my first job as a nurse anesthetist at the hospital and was immediately assigned to cases on my own. At that time, conditions at the hospital were extremely difficult: there was only one outdated, closed-off anesthesia machine to serve four operating rooms. With no ventilators, nurse anesthetists performed manual bagging using Ambu bags for General Anesthesia. Monitoring relied on stethoscopes, direct observation with eyes on chest movement, and hand on pulse checks. In those early days, I depended on the few nurse anesthetists at the hospital to guide and mentor me in this early phase of my career. These experienced nurse anesthetists (trained outside the country, mostly in the global south) provided me with an example of high-quality, safe anesthetics and mentored me to develop my skills as a nurse anesthetist. They also taught me to be resilient, to practice under challenging conditions, and to advocate for the patient. There was one nurse anesthetist who stood out in my mind. She was excellent at pediatric anesthesia, and she inspired me to focus on meeting the needs of this critically underserved group, children. It took a year to begin to feel comfortable in the role, and I attribute my success to the support of these experienced, kind, wise nurse anesthetists (*ANP-Stepping Up*).

I have been a nurse anesthetist for 14 years now and feel that my professional journey is symbolic of both the progress and challenges of anesthesia in Liberia. I practice independently, meaning I take full responsibility for the full range of anesthesia care that I deliver (pre-operative, procedure, post-operative, and critical care), and have full authority to provide these services. As I gained experience, my confidence in my skills as a nurse anesthetist increased. However, the changing needs of the country, with the increased volume and complexity of surgical cases performed, required me to expand my skills. After the civil war, and particularly after Ebola, visiting surgeons began to come to Liberia to perform more complex operations, and these procedures required more advanced anesthesia techniques. Many times, they brought anesthesiologists as part of the surgical team, and this became an opportunity to learn from these experienced clinicians. International partnerships and mentors have been important to my journey as a nurse anesthetist. When I decided to focus on improving the quality and safety of pediatric anesthesia, I looked for opportunities to obtain advanced qualifications that strengthened both my practice and my leadership role. I participated in a Smile Train training in Nigeria and received a Certificate in *Nursing Care Saves Lives,* a training that focuses on providing high-quality, safe nursing care for children before and after cleft surgery. I brought that knowledge back to our hospital to improve the anesthetic care of children in general, and to support the Smile Train surgical team when they came to my hospital to provide this lifesaving and life-enhancing surgery for Liberian Children. Through international partners, I have been able to improve my skills in Basic Life Support (BLS), enhance my ability to teach in the clinical setting (Certificate in Advanced Anesthesia Education; BIDMC/BAAC), update my knowledge of best practices (Anesthesia Update; Harvard Medical School), and serve on the leadership committee that hosts monthly BAAC Virtual Anesthesia Grand Rounds. I also sought out opportunities within Liberia to improve my ability to collect and use data to solve problems, graduating with a Master of Public Health in Epidemiology in 2019 (ANP—*Living it*).

Despite the advances made in anesthesia care since I began to practice in 2011, challenges remain. The primary challenges include issues around professional recognition and identity. NAs are often undervalued or mistaken for general nurses, and there is often an overlap of responsibilities between doctors and nurses. There are resource and infrastructure challenges, such as shortages of drugs and modern equipment. In the training environment, there are insufficient simulation labs and training equipment, and few opportunities for postgraduate education. There is weak integration of NAs into the national health hierarchy. Salary scales often do not reflect responsibilities or education, and there are few scholarships and career advancement pathways. Burnout is a real issue with shortages of providers, heavy caseloads, and long hours. These challenges are real and provide obstacles to high-quality safe care and autonomous practice, but day after day we respond to the challenges. Nurse anesthetists in Liberia have also practiced in crisis contexts. During the Ebola and Covid Pandemics and in remote areas where resources were scarce, NAs remained on the frontlines. My early experiences managing patients without ventilators or monitors reflect the adaptability of Liberia's anesthesia workforce in the most difficult settings, and from these experiences, I learned that leadership and advocacy were essential buffers to challenges. I apply these lessons not only to the patient care I deliver, but to my role as an educator and mentor (*ANP-Bounce back ability*). At my hospital, through concerted, persistent advocacy, infrastructure has improved from one broken machine to ten anesthesia machines (six brand new and four partially functional). Supplies of resuscitation drugs and basic monitoring tools have improved, though costly anesthetics remain limited, and the introduction of capnography (donated by international partners) marked a turning point in patient safety.

As my career advanced, I was able to focus on the non-clinical aspects of my work (ANP-B*eyond the basics*), including mentoring, education, and advocacy. It was my honor and privilege to be recently appointed as the coordinator of the nurse anesthesia education program that reopened at my hospital. This position allows me to advocate for modern resources such as simulation labs and strong clinical mentorship and to educate the next generation of NAs. International partnerships have been instrumental in my ability to grow in my profession. One area that I am particularly proud of is my work to improve the care of children needing anesthesia, with a focus not only on the safety of the anesthesia but also on providing age-appropriate and dignified care for the children. International partnerships have also supported my growth as a leader and advocate. Serving on the leadership committee for BAAC Virtual Anesthesia Grand Rounds has broadened my perspective and provided meaningful professional connections.

The story of nurse anesthesia in Liberia is a story of survival and transformation. Today, nurse anesthetists in Liberia are recognized as essential to achieving universal access to safe anesthesia and surgery, obstetric care, and emergency response. Their scope of practice extends from general and regional anesthesia to airway management, pain relief, critical care, and resuscitation. My journey has embodied this expanded role, serving not only as a provider but also as an educator, mentor, and advocate for the profession. Liberia's vision is ambitious to scale up the number of trained NAs to meet the needs of its 5.7 million people. I will end my reflection with a thought: *We are not where we want to be, but we are not where we were* — and we (NAs) are up to the challenge!

Ama A Taplah, BSc, RN, NA, MPH, is a practicing Nurse Anesthetist, OR Manager and Nurse Anesthetist Supervisor, John F Kennedy Medical Center, and Coordinator, TNIMA/JFK Anesthesia Program in Liberia (WHO Africa Region)

A Family Nurse Practitioner in Eswatini

Background and Context

Advanced practice nursing has been the goal of the health care system in Eswatini, informed by the country's health care landscape. The healthcare delivery framework of the country is primary health care, and the backbone of the healthcare delivery system is the nursing profession. A ground-breaking landscape assessment study was conducted in 2017 as part of a needs assessment for a nursing educational program [14]. Findings indicated that the family nurse practitioner role was needed as a matter of urgency. Thus, the need for APNs in eSwatini is both an urgent and a transformative one, given the country's health care challenges and aspirations for universal health coverage [15]. Several contextual drivers exist for the urgent need of the APN cadre. First and foremost, the country has a high disease burden. Eswatini faces significant morbidity and mortality rates from non-communicable diseases such as cancers, diabetes mellitus, hypertension, communicable diseases including HIV and AIDS, and pulmonary tuberculosis [16]. A majority of the population, around 70%, reside in the rural areas where there is limited access to physicians and under-resourced health care services [17]. Because of this, an urgent need for APN practice exists where the current nursing workforce is practicing at the top of their scope of RN practice. Additionally, there is a critical shortage of nurses at the primary health care level. The FNP program was launched as a strategic response to the overwhelming shortage of the healthcare workforce, disease burden, and geographical location of the population.

*Education***:** The strategic response by the education sector to the needs of the country was the launch (2017) of the first-ever graduate-level FNP programme at the University of Eswatini in partnership with international partners, with the aim of strengthening primary health care delivery. A competency-based curriculum tailored to meet local Eswatini population needs was developed using the PEPPA framework (Participatory, Evidence-based, Patient-focused Process for Advanced Practice Nursing) [18]. This framework guided curriculum design, policy integration, and scope of practice development. The programme goals include a focus on training nurses to provide expanded access to primary health care across the life span, which helps bridge access gaps in underserved areas of the country. The programme also fosters collaboration between educators, clinicians, and policy makers to strengthen the health care system. Admission criteria include a bachelor's degree from an accredited university or college and a second-class second division pass (2ii) or equivalent.

The FNP curriculum is a three-year, part-time, competency-based curriculum that runs over six semesters with foundational modules such as pathophysiology, advanced health assessment, pharmacology, research, thesis, and an FNP internship of 528 hours, including child and adolescent, adult and elderly, and mental health care. The curriculum is tailored to meet the health needs of the Eswatini population with an emphasis on clinical competence, independent practice, and responsiveness to community needs. Because this was a new role, there were no FNPs practicing in the country who could serve as preceptors. Despite initial challenges in clinical placements of the students and preceptorship in the clinical area, placements were successfully implemented, and medical officers, who are primarily family physicians, offered to assist students in the clinical space. This led to interdisciplinary collaboration. For educators to teach in the program, the University of Eswatini regulations require a master's degree in nursing with a specialization in FNP and a PhD in Nursing.

Regulation and Credentialing The regulation of FNPs in Eswatini is guided by the Eswatini Nursing Council (ENC), which operates under the Nurses and Midwives Act of 1965, as amended [19]. The ENC is responsible for defining scopes of practice, setting licensure standards, and ensuring public safety through professional oversight [20]. Recent developments have seen the approval of a formal Scope of Practice (SOP) for FNPs, which was completed in 2017 prior to program implementation. The SOP outlines their expanded clinical authority, including diagnosis, treatment, and some prescribing rights. This SOP was developed using the PEPPA framework to ensure alignment with local health needs and policy priorities. The Ministry of Health is mandated to update national guidelines, including the Standard Treatment Guidelines and Essential Medicines List (Ministry of Health, 2021), which is important to FNP practice to allow them expanded access to prescribing. However, that has not yet happened, which is a significant impediment to FNPs practicing autonomously and to the approved scope of practice.

In order to practice as an FNP in Eswatini, the FNP must have graduated from an accredited program and completed supervised clinical rotations in an approved health facility, have a current Eswatini RN license, be registered with the ENC as an FNP, agree to practice within the Scope of Practice, and engage in Continuing Professional Development. The ENC formally recognizes FNPs as a distinct cadre within advanced practice nursing. This recognition is embedded in regulatory documents such as the Scopes of Practice for all nursing cadres in Eswatini and supported by policy integration efforts led by the Ministry of Health. The ENC also provides a bar (an epaulette worn on the shoulder of the FNP uniform) that is a visible distinction of the FNP role. The FNP role is now acknowledged in strategic health planning, with emphasis on its contribution to universal health coverage, equity, and community-based care. Importantly, there is growing acceptance of the role among professional stakeholders and communities, who view FNPs as competent,

Policy engagement around the FNP role in Eswatini is in its infancy, yet active and still evolving. The Ministry of Health has endorsed the FNP role and is working to integrate it into national health strategies. However, full policy integration, including deployment, career progression, and salary scales, is still in progress. Deployment is a thorny issue in the sense that it is an activity that is handled by another Ministry, which is the Ministry of Labour that is responsible for recruitment and placement of civil servants. Of note, Policymaking has involved educators, regulators, clinicians, and international partners. This inclusive approach has fostered shared ownership but requires stronger coordination and accountability mechanisms. The FNP role is aligned with National Health Goals and supports Eswatini's commitment to Universal Health Coverage (UHC), the Sustainable Development Goals (SDGs), and the WHO Global Strategic Directions for Nursing and Midwifery. However, there is a need for clearer legislation that defines APN roles, protects their autonomy, and ensures equitable deployment across the health care system in settings where they are needed the most.

Practice Climate: The emergence of the Family Nurse Practitioner (FNP) role in Eswatini marked a pivotal shift in the country's health workforce strategy. As advanced practice nurses, FNPs are trained to deliver comprehensive, autonomous care across the lifespan, particularly in underserved and rural settings. However, the success of this role depends not only on education and clinical competence but also on the broader practice climate, which is shaped by policy, professional networks, and government support. Several conditions have supported the emergence and growth of the FNP role in Eswatini. First and foremost, strategic educational partnerships were key to the development of the FNP programme. These partnerships were instrumental because they provided technical expertise, landscape assessment, curriculum design support, and faculty development. Also, the use of the PEPPA Framework (The Participatory, Evidence-based, Patient-focused Process for Advanced Practice Nursing) (PEPPA) framework [18] guided the development of the FNP role, ensuring alignment with Eswatini's health care sector priorities and stakeholder needs.

Furthermore, the Ministry of Health, through the Eswatini Nursing Council, has shown commitment by approving the FNP scope of practice and proposing updates to national guidelines such as the Standard Treatment Guidelines and Essential Medicines List. Although this is still pending, there is hope that the FNPs will be considered when revision of this document commences in the future. There is growing support and acceptance of the family nurse practitioner role amongst stakeholders and communities. This emphasizes the value of improving health care access and health outcomes. Gradually, communities and health professionals have come to recognize the value of FNPs in improving access, continuity, and quality of care, especially in rural clinics where physician coverage is limited. Faculty at the University of Eswatini have played a key role in mentoring students, conducting research, and advocating for the integration of APNs into the health system.

Hindering Factors and Practice Challenges Despite the progress made in the education and practice pillars, several barriers continue to constrain the full integration of the FNP role in Eswatini. Regulatory ambiguity remains the main hindering factor. While the Eswatini Nursing Council has approved a scope of practice for FNPs, broader regulatory mechanisms such as prescribing authority, deployment protocols, and remuneration structures remain underdeveloped in the country, making it difficult to fully integrate the role. This also leads to fragmented policy implementation. Although policy-level support exists, implementation across regions and facilities is uneven. Some health managers remain unclear about how to deploy and support FNPs effectively in clinical practice. Resource constraints such as financial limitations, staff shortages, and a lack of equipment in rural facilities hinder the optimal utilization of FNPs. Access to continuing Professional Development (CPD) opportunities is limited, especially in remote areas. Without structured CPD pathways, FNPs risk stagnation in clinical competence and leadership development. Limited clinical infrastructure speaks to the practice of FNP students before graduating from the program. FNP students initially faced challenges securing appropriate clinical placements due to the novelty of the role and lack of awareness among supervising clinicians; however, this has improved over time with the support of physicians, particularly in Family Medicine.

Personal Reflections on my FNP Educator Experiences

I was educated in the FNP role in Botswana at the university, completing a 1-year didactic training and over 600 h of clinical affiliation in primary healthcare settings. As a student, I observed and was mentored by experienced FNPs who practiced autonomously and with a full scope of practice. I also benefited from my interactions with Botswanan and Cuban Family Medicine doctors, both of whom were supportive of the FNP role and were generous in sharing their time and expertise. The Cuban doctors were particularly strong in family medicine. In Cuba, the pride of their healthcare system is a strong primary care model, and the Cuban physicians were very skilled at community immersion and delivering locally-tailored care. After graduation, I returned to Eswatini, where I did not have the opportunity to practice clinically since the regulatory mechanisms to practice had not yet been put in place. But I did have the privilege of helping to shape FNP education in Eswatini and to be part of developing and implementing the FNP program at our university, and participating in the policy process for role credentialing.

Teaching in the FNP program is my primary role within the University. My personal experience with the FNP program has been both challenging and rewarding. *Stepping up* as an educator in advanced practice nursing required me to transition from an undergraduate educator role and guide students in both theoretical and practical settings. Drawing from my educator experiences and my clinical training as an FNP, I learned to design learning experiences, mentor students in clinical placements, and assess their competencies effectively, contributing to their development as competent family nurse practitioners. This experience strengthened my skills in adult learning principles, communication skills, and ability to explain concepts clearly, fostering critical thinking and promoting attainment of the FNP clinical competencies among students. Throughout this process, I had support from international partners who were experienced FNP clinicians and educators with extensive practice experience. I also had support from our LiSwati nurses and family medicine doctors who supported the FNP role and its contribution to primary care.

Living the FNP program first hand allowed me to understand the demands and rigor of advanced practice nursing education. I witnessed the integration of theory and practice and appreciated the challenges that students face in balancing clinical duties and academic requirements as well as the smooth transition from the general nursing role to the advanced practice role.

The journey, as it continues, has not been without challenges. Managing time between clinical responsibilities, teaching duties, and program expectations requires careful planning (*ANP-Bounce back ability*). Resource limitations such as occasional shortage of teaching materials and clinical supervision tested my problem-solving skills. Additionally, the diverse preparedness of students necessitates adapting teaching methods to meet varied learning needs. Also, the geographical location of students must be taken into consideration when planning online classes. Navigating program logistics such as organizing and coordinating clinical rotations, logging clinical hours, and determining student support needed to complete internship added another layer of complexity.

Despite these challenges, the FNP program has been transformative for my professional development (*ANP Setting in Motion).* I have experienced mentorship and support from international partner faculty who were providing technical expertise when the program started in 2017. I have also strengthened my leadership and mentoring skills, learned to adapt teaching strategies, and reinforced the importance of resilience and lifelong learning as an educator. I am currently working as both an educator and the program coordinator for this program. In my capacity as the coordinator, I am also responsible for securing internship placements for our students.

This is usually not an easy task because most medical officers in the country are not familiar with the FNP cadre thus for some there is a lot of hesitation with regards to accepting the responsibility to mentor the students in the clinical area. My practice has been solely confined in the education space of the FNP role. As the FNP role advances in the country, the FNP program has also fostered the growth of capable educators. I have experienced seeing one of our own former students joining the faculty as an educator. It is a rewarding experience as well when feedback from employers of our graduates commend them on their clinical skills. To me these successes point towards a positive direction with regards to acceptance of the cadre in clinical practice. As an educator, I am not directly required to have direct patient care. I do have direct patient care during clinical placements when I supervise students.

The practice climate for Family Nurse Practitioners in Eswatini is marked by both promise and complexity. Strategic partnerships, policy engagement, and professional advocacy have laid a strong foundation for APN role development. Yet, regulatory gaps, resource constraints, and uneven implementation threaten to stall progress. To fully realize the transformative potential of FNPs, Eswatini must invest in robust policy frameworks, strengthen professional networks, and ensure that APNs are supported not only in education but also in practice. With sustained commitment, FNPs can become the cornerstone providers in a more equitable, resilient, and people-centred health care system.

Bonisile Nsibandze, PhD, MNS-FNP, SRN, SRM is an Educator and the Coordinator of the FNP Program in the Department of Nursing Sciences, Faculty of Health Sciences at the University of Eswatini in Mbabane Eswatini (WHO Africa Region)

Nurse Practitioners Practices in the United States

Background and Country Context

The nurse practitioner (NP) role emerged in the United States in the late 1960s to expand access to high-quality care for all (particularly underserved populations) and to meet the nation's healthcare needs. Since then, advanced practice nursing (APN) has evolved into a graduate-prepared, licensed, and nationally certified profession spanning primary, acute, and specialty care. The framework for the ANP role evolved over time and was formalized in the Consensus Model for APRN Regulation: Licensure, Accreditation, Certification and Education (LACE) developed by the APRN Consensus Work Group [21, 22]. The model identified four APN roles: nurse anesthetist, nurse midwife, clinical nurse specialist, and nurse practitioner. Within each role, they identified population foci including family, adult/gerontology, pediatric, women's health, and psychiatric mental health. Licensure occurs at the role and population foci. For instance, in this vignette, you will read about a pediatric nurse practitioner who works in acute care and an adult/gerontology nurse practitioner who works in primary care. LACE further delineates specialties such as

Oncology, Older Adults, Nephrology, and Palliative Care, but these are specialty certifications beyond the basic education for entry-to-practice APRNs. Implementation of LACE in 2008 standardized requirements for licensure, accreditation, certification, and education throughout the United States and promoted practice to the full scope of educational preparation [23].

Education Advanced Practice Nurses (APNs) are required to complete graduate-level education (MSN or DNP) at an accredited educational institution. The curriculum (didactic and clinical experiences) is competency-based and standardized based on nationally agreed-upon domains of practice [24]. Graduates of an accredited program are entitled to sit for a national board certification exam, which is required for licensure to practice. Ongoing continuing education and recertification are required to maintain clinical competence.

Regulation and Credentialing Nurse practitioner practice is governed by each state's Nurse Practice Act and licensing boards, so authority and processes vary. Broadly, states fall into Full, Reduced, or Restricted practice models, which determine whether NPs practice independently or under required physician collaboration/supervision. Most states require graduate preparation (MSN/DNP), national board certification in the population focus (e.g., PNP or AGNP), and state APRN/NP licensure; many also require specific pharmacology/controlled-substance training for prescriptive authority. In states (or organizations) where collaboration is mandated, written agreements or standardized procedures define scope, prescriptive limits, and supervision ratios. Separate from licensure, hospital credentialing and privileging verify competencies and grant procedure-specific privileges (often with supervision), and renewal typically involves continuing education and maintenance of national certification.

Practice Climate and Impact The NP role and full scope of practice are increasingly supported, especially amid provider shortages, documented health disparities between and within populations, and evidence of improved outcomes. However, barriers remain, such as inconsistent scope-of-practice laws across states, billing limitations, and variable public awareness of the value-added of NP practice. Professional associations such as the American Association of Nurse Practitioners (AANP), National Organization of Nurse Practitioner Faculty (NONPF), and state-level groups advocate for greater recognition. Research has shown that Nurse Practitioners provide high-quality care and increase universal access to health care when and where it is needed [5]. They assess, diagnose, prescribe, perform procedures, and provide holistic and dignified care across the lifespan. Their presence strengthens the use of evidence-based pathways, improves handoffs and transitions, and supports clear communication with families. NPs also lead quality and safety efforts, standardizes protocols, teaches, and tracks outcomes, delivering results comparable to physician-only models while improving throughput and prudent use of resources.

Next steps for nurse practitioners in the United States include harmonizing state scope of practice toward full authority and adopting national standards for credentialing and privileging that clearly delineate procedural competencies in intensive and surgical settings. Priorities include reimbursement parity, portable licensure, and structured transition to practice residencies that build readiness for primary care and high acuity care. The field should expand rigorous outcomes research, embed NP leadership in quality and safety programs, and coauthor evidence-based pathways that reduce variation. Workforce efforts should grow and diversify the pipeline, strengthen mentorship and retention, and deepen interprofessional training with medicine, nursing, respiratory therapy, and pharmacy. NPs are also well-positioned to scale telehealth and hospital-at-home models, advance data-driven care through informatics and AI, and use clear role-specific titles in public communications to improve patient understanding and equity.

Nurse Practitioners in the United States, as a professional cadre, are deeply committed to advancing the health of the nation. They are uniquely well prepared and positioned to make an important contribution to achieving the goal of Universal Health Coverage (UHC). They provide services across all areas where individuals receive the necessary quality health services—from prevention and promotion to treatment and palliative care in a cost-effective way. UHC is a human right, requiring accessible services, financial protection from out-of-pocket costs, and adequate quality of care for everyone, regardless of their background or ability to pay. Nurse practitioners are pivotal players in closing the gap in health care in the United States.

Personal Reflections on my Practice as a Pediatric Nurse Practitioner in Acute Care

As a Pediatric Nurse Practitioner in Acute Care, I provide specialized, evidence-based care to acutely ill infants, children, and adolescents in inpatient hospital settings. My practice spans both pediatric critical care and neurosurgery. I assess and diagnose complex conditions, prescribe treatments, perform procedures, and manage transitions of care. While I collaborate closely with multidisciplinary teams, I also function independently in many aspects of care delivery. Beyond direct patient care, I teach medical, nursing, and advanced practice trainees in both hospital and university settings, mentor new APNs, and contribute to quality improvement initiatives that enhance patient outcomes. I currently practice under standardized procedures and cannot obtain independent practice because I work in a specialty practice. My institutional credentialing includes pediatric-specific procedural competencies, simulation training, and annual evaluations.

Becoming a Pediatric Nurse Practitioner was a leap in scope and responsibility (*Stepping Up: Transitioning into the APN Role*). As an RN, I was deeply engaged in bedside care, but advanced practice required diagnostic reasoning, independent decision-making, and leadership of care plans. My first position was in a well-established hospital program for new APNs with structured onboarding, simulation, and close preceptorship. That scaffolding let me move safely from observation to supervised practice and then to independent practice, with frequent feedback that built clinical judgment and confidence. Over nearly a decade, I have grown into the role, learning to anticipate clinical trajectories, communicate clearly during high-stakes moments, and lead family-centered plans of care.

In daily work, I practice both independently and collaboratively to manage acutely ill infants, children, and adolescents. I evaluate patients, form differentials, order and interpret diagnostics, prescribe medications, and coordinate care with physicians, bedside nurses, and multidisciplinary teams. My procedural practice includes central venous and arterial line access, lumbar puncture, moderate sedation, and endotracheal intubation with ongoing competency verification through privileging and mentoring/supervision. I often serve as the first call for our service, initiating guideline-aligned therapy and setting priorities before morning rounds. Independence has grown with experience, yet practice remains team-based and consultative when complexity demands it (ANP Living It: Practicing Independently and Confidently). I value the rapid huddles with medical residents, fellows, and attending physicians for our patients when needed. These moments strengthen mutual trust and keep the focus on timely, safe decisions.

Progress has not removed all the obstacles to autonomous practice. (*ANP Bounce-back Ability: Facing Challenges*). Practicing in California means navigating a transitional regulatory environment in which requirements for physician oversight and institutional processes can slow decisions even when I am fully capable of proceeding. Specialty inpatient roles like mine still depend on standardized procedures and hospital privileging, which support safety but can create delays during policy updates. Another challenge is conveying the value of advanced practice nursing in inpatient settings where impact is not measured by clinic volume but by timely orders, clear handoffs, coordinated multidisciplinary work, and fewer avoidable escalations. On a personal level, emotional resilience is also essential when working in pediatric neurosurgery and critical care, where outcomes are uncertain and family needs are intense. I rely on debriefs, team support, and reflective practice to sustain empathy while maintaining clinical precision.

Education and communication with families run through all of this work (*ANP Setting in Motion: Driving Improvements Beyond the Bedside*). I prioritize plain language explanations, written plans, and teach back to support understanding during high-stress hospitalizations. It is an honor to be present with children and their families and to care for them during some of their most difficult moments, and the advanced practice nurse's ability to support them is grounded in continuous presence, timely clinical decisions, clear translation of complex information, and coordinated planning that respects culture, values, and goals from admission through discharge.

Beyond direct care, I work to improve how the system functions (*ANP-Setting in Motion: Driving Improvements Beyond the Bedside*). I led a project to standardize neurocritical care practices, updating order sets, checklists, and handoff tools, and tracking outcomes for adherence and complications. I serve on a hospital quality improvement task force focused on neurocritical care initiatives, where I help design workflows that leverage the NP's continuous presence and understanding of both the nursing and medical systems. Teaching and mentorship are central to my role; I precept new APNs and residents, develop simulation scenarios, and offer just-in-time teaching at the bedside. I also contribute to global nursing programs, sharing approaches to pediatric acute care and learning from partners in resource-limited settings. My DNP training prepared me to turn bedside questions into structured projects that test changes, measure results, and spread successful practices. I work with partners around the world to establish and strengthen advanced practice nursing aligned with country and regional priorities. In my role as Nursing Lead for the WHO Collaborating Centre for Emergency, Critical and Operative Care, I champion nursing and advanced practice participation in developing, implementing, and evaluating initiatives in emergency, critical care, and operative care.

Looking back, my journey in advanced practice from dependent practice to increasing autonomy reflects both personal effort and the broader evolution of NP practice in California. Pediatric acute care nurse practitioners have become integral to hospital care for children with complex conditions, providing continuity, accelerating evidence-based therapy, and helping teams function reliably. The landscape continues to change through legislation, credentialing standards, and interprofessional collaboration, and I am committed to advocating for clear role definitions, efficient privileging, and practice environments that let NPs contribute fully and safely. I am proud of this work, and of the collective progress our teams make every day to optimize quality and access to care for our communities' children and their families.

Rebecca Silvers, DNP, APN, CPNP-AC, CCRN, RNFA, is a Pediatric Nurse Practitioner in Acute Care, Nursing Lead for the WHO Collaborating Center for Emergency, Critical and Operative Cae and on faculty at UCSF School of Nursing practicing in the United States (WHO Region of the Americas).

Personal Reflection on my Practice as an Adult/Gerontological Nurse Practitioner in Primary Care

Reflecting on my experiences as a primary care NP, it became clear that my undergraduate education as a nurse was instrumental in shaping who I am and how I practice today as an NP. My clinical experiences as an undergraduate nursing student caring for diverse patients, along with my minor in urban studies, as an undergraduate were eye-opening and highlighted the challenges and opportunities in our health care system. Consideration of these complexities (the social determinants of health) has been a driving factor in my interest in health care disparities. After completing my BSN, I worked as a staff nurse at a large academic teaching hospital on a unit that cared for high acuity patients from diverse socioeconomic, racial, and ethnic groups. This work challenged and inspired me to pursue graduate education as both an adult nurse practitioner (ANP) and a geriatric nurse practitioner (GNP).

Following graduation, I sat for the adult (AANP) and geriatric (ANCC) examinations and was certified in the adult and geriatric nurse practitioner role [25]. This certification was accepted by my state board of nursing, and I am credentialed/licensed in Massachusetts as a Registered Nurse (RN) and Certified Nurse Practitioner (CNP). I also had to apply for prescriptive authority in both my state and the federal government in order to be able to prescribe medications.

My first position as an AGNP was in a geriatric care facility (nursing home) where I was a senior clinician. I found it challenging as a new graduate to be isolated in this setting without colleagues to talk to. (*ANP-Stepping up*) When I did not understand a clinical case or struggled with a differential diagnosis, it was hard for me, a new grad NP, to find a provider to bounce a case by, and it was even more difficult for me to find a provider to come and look at a lesion or examine a patient with me. I worried I was not providing the type of expert care I wanted and felt alone in this position, so when an NP position became available in the outpatient primary care department at the hospital I had worked at as an RN, I quickly accepted this job.

I would work for the next 20 years in this clinic as an NP! I functioned as an NP comanager, sharing patients with physician colleagues and providing complex primary care to diverse patients. Being an NP comanager in my clinic meant that each patient would have a primary care provider (PCP) of record that was a physician, but if the patient needed more than one or two visits a year and had complex health issues like diabetes, hypertension, chronic pain, or other chronic health challenges they would be assigned an NP to also comanage them. The NP would then usually see this patient on an alternating basis from their PCP to manage their health needs through assessment, medication intensification, and health coaching. These visits were performed autonomously, but typically the NP would communicate with the PCP if there was a major change in the patient's health status or care plan. In addition to co-management of chronic illness, NPs in the clinic would also see any patient in the practice for urgent care, which involved assessing patients with a new medical concern or symptoms, ordering tests, making a diagnosis, developing a care plan, and if appropriate prescribing a new medication for this diagnosis. Additional types of clinic visits included health maintenance and prevention visits for common health screening tests like cervical cancer screening, and also post-hospital follow-up visits. (*ANP-Living it*) The clinic had a strong support system, with an on-site faculty preceptor available to us to discuss complex cases or to see patients in real time for consultation during the clinic. Having experienced clinicians on site was an integral resource to me as a new NP, and one that I feel really was invaluable to me as I honed my clinical skills.

In 2024, I made the hard decision to leave this hospital practice where I had grown up as an RN and NP to take on a new challenge. I accepted a position as an NP in a primary care practice at a different large academic teaching hospital in Boston. In my state, NPs had recently been authorized to practice as independent practitioners, and the practice was implementing an innovative model of primary care that recognized NPs as independent providers. The intention of this new mode was to increase access to primary care, an issue that I cared deeply about. Essentially, this new model meant that NPs could carry their own panel of patients just like physicians do. In the co-management model, I contributed to care, but the physician was listed as the primary care provider (PCP). In this independent practice model, I was officially listed as the PCP. This was something I decided I needed to try for my own professional advancement and because I firmly believe we need to try new ways to address the critical gap in access to primary care. In the United States, primary care is still trying to recover from the pandemic and the downstream complexities of our healthcare system. The primary care provider shortage is a daily reality in most primary care practices, and we who are practicing feel the pinch of a smaller workforce, more complex patients, and so much work to be done. There are so many patients catching up from years of missed care during the pandemic. January will be my two-year anniversary in this position, and thinking back, it has been a busy 2 years! I have about 600 patients in my panel that I am responsible for. We have fabulous resources that support me as a PCP, including easy access to consultation for complex diagnostic situations. The clinic also has a wonderful coverage system, so when I have a day off, I know my patients will be managed appropriately. These resources have been important to my success and happiness in this position.

I have also found that continuous professional development has been important to my success and happiness in the NP role. I completed the education to become a Certified Diabetes Care and Education Specialist (CDCES) and was able to become a practice expert on diabetes management and consultation (primarily patients with type two diabetes).

At this point in my career, I would not identify patient management and complex decision-making as challenges for me. *(ANP-Bounce back)* I feel confident practicing in the role and have a good understanding of what I know and what I don't know (and when to ask for help) which I think is important to safe practice. Perhaps the most challenging issue for me practicing independently has been professional recognition and identity. Patients have had a lifetime of being acculturated into a system where the physician is in charge. For some, having an NP for their primary care clinician was a new idea that they were not entirely comfortable with and it took time to trust that they would get the same level of care. Although this has not happened often, it was hard not to personalize, and I had to remind myself that it really was not about me. It was an opportunity to clarify the role, showcase my experience, and forge ahead in the relationship. Another particularly difficult part of being an independent primary care provider is being able to manage the heavy emotion that comes with the job-it's hard to not to be able to fix everything and especially painful when you realize you are the PCP—the one ultimately responsible for care. It can also be difficult to handle the time pressure and myriad competing demands of being a PCP. My schedule is full every day yet there are also many calls from my patients requesting urgent visits or requesting call backs about health concerns. These requests can be difficult to balance during a busy clinic day.

(*ANP-Setting in motion*) In addition to the satisfaction that I get from the clinical aspects of my role, there are a number of activities outside my direct care responsibilities that add value to my work. Teaching/preceptorship has long been a regular part of my daily work which I love. Another indirect care opportunity that I enjoy is quality improvement. As a new NP, I was drawn to improvement science to identify primary care challenges, find root causes, and use data and resources to create system-level improvement that promote health equity. This interest in turn led me to pursue a DNP where my focus was on improving obesity management in my practice. My DNP has also led to my teaching in the academic as well as clinical setting.

Overall, I would say my practice works really hard to support me. I feel like my expertise is valued, and if a patient is not happy about being assigned to me or wants a different PCP this is handled appropriately and fairly by my practice coordinators (and I have started to realize when talking to physician colleagues this is something that seems to happen across the board not just for patients whom are assigned an NP as PCP). I do feel my professional experiences and training have prepared me for becoming an independent primary care provider. I also strongly believe that primary care is in crisis, and we as NPs need to roll up our sleeves and try to help through practicing at the top of our license; our patients and our colleagues are depending on us to do just that.

Maura Moran Brain DNP, ANP, AGNP, CDCES, is practicing in Primary Care in the United States (WHO Region of the Americas).

Key Takeaways and the Way Forward toward Autonomous APN Practice

Taken together, these vignettes offer meaningful insights into the factors associated with practicing autonomously and into the full scope of practice in a variety of roles, countries, and settings. The practice settings that the APNs describe vary widely, including urban, rural, high-resource, resource-constrained, acute care, and ambulatory/community care, but in each setting, the APNs describe practicing with clinical autonomy and to the full scope of practice based on their license and experience. While the roles differ (midwife, nurse anesthetist, acute care NP, primary care NP), they each describe being able to assess, diagnose, and treat patients (tailored to their population and local context), manage unexpected clinical developments, and adjust care in real time to optimize outcomes and patient safety. Perhaps the most salient observation is the confidence with which each of these APNs describes their full scope of practice and the passion they have for their work. Each is an experienced clinician which has been reported to correlate with being more likely to practice with clinical autonomy and likely contributed to the strong stories they told [8].

Mentoring and strong supportive environments emerged as an important influence as these APNs stepped up and moved into their APN roles and clinical responsibilities. This mentoring was both formal and informal and involved APN and interdisciplinary colleagues in the clinical setting. Examples of formal mentoring included the availability of expert resources to provide on-site, real-time consultation around complex cases. The value of role-modeling and hands-on mentoring, of being allowed to see colleagues practice competent, respectful care, was particularly meaningful. In resource-constrained settings, the importance of international partners who could mentor and role-model competent, respectful care was important when the role was new in the country, and they did not have local APN experts to observe. Some APNs noted that despite feeling confident in their ability to deliver autonomous care, they also acknowledged the importance of utilizing the resources in their practice to seek consultation if they had a question or were unsure about how to treat a patient, and the importance of referring patients who needed escalation of care. This highlights the concept that autonomous practice is not divorced from interdisciplinary care, but in fact values peer and mentor input (formal and informal). An interesting aside is the notion that one can practice autonomously in settings where the model is co-management, guided by state regulations, standardized procedures, and/or hospital privileging. Within these regulatory constraints, the APNs reported providing a full scope of practice care during the visit or episode of care. These restrictions (restricted authority to practice) did not limit the APNs' perceived ability to act independently within their scope of practice to admit, treat, and discharge patients or perform procedures. Another value added of informal and formal peer support (debriefing and team support) was that this suppoer served as an important counterbalance to the heavy emotional burden of being responsible for complex care in oftentimes challenging situations, and a contributor to resilience.

In each of the countries discussed in the vignettes, there was a well-established education and regulatory/credentialing framework aligned with international standards and a formally acknowledged APN role and scope of practice. That said, however, in some cases there were policy issues which precluded full role implementation due to regulatory malalignment. In Eswatini, for example, despite an accredited education program that meets international standards, role authorization (scope of practice and licensure), integration within the Eswatini Nursing Council and Ministry of Health, the lack of expanded prescriptive authority and designated role in the country's employment scheme (standardized job description) has hampered role implementation. Full practice authority eludes APNs in some states in the United States and is poorly defined in some countries globally. Professional recognition and identity appeared to be a challenge for each of the APNs who shared their story. Despite gains over the past decade, this is still a relatively new role and ongoing education of the public and our professional colleagues is important in gaining acceptance for the independent role of APNs.

Despite the many challenges discussed in the vignettes, these are stories of resilience. Each APN described the way that they rose to the occasion and mitigated the challenge with solutions across the clinical and policy domains. Challenging environments (refugee communities, remote rural regions, workforce shortages, resource and infrastructure limitations) were met with resolve and commitment to meet the needs and did not seem to limit the APNs' ability to practice autonomously. They felt empowered to act and valued their ability to do so. It is important to acknowledge the reality that meeting these challenges (workforce and resource constraints) was not without stress for the clinician, but it did not appear to limit autonomy and even seemed to bolster it.

The future demands an APN workforce able to meet a complex set of needs and environments and able to articulate a clear profile of the NP role and its significant contribution to the healthcare workforce [26, 27]. The five vignettes presented in this chapter provide a window through which we can view the day-to-day practice of five APNs, shaped by unique experiences, beliefs, and cultural backgrounds, practicing in different roles and in different parts of the world. A common characteristic, pride in mission, was apparent in each of their stories. The origin of the spark that ignited their passion for their work may differ, but each is deeply committed to improving equitable access to evidence-based, quality, safe, dignified, and respectful care when and where it is needed. In their own words, they see APNs as *agents of change, advocates of dignity, guardians of life, courageous, transformative, survivors,* and *resilient.* While there is still work to be done to harmonize APN education, policy, and practice, to gain professional recognition and identity, and to improve the practice environment and gain full practice authority, these stories illustrate the ability of APNs to effectively practice with clinical autonomy and with confidence across a range of settings, populations, and roles. And this, in turn, demonstrates (and comports with recent evidence) the contributions made by APNs around the world to improve universal access to safe, dignified care across the lifespan [5–7].

Literature Cited

1. Lockwood EB, Lehwaldt D, Sweeney MR, Matthews A. An exploration of the levels of clinical autonomy of advanced nurse practitioners: a narrative literature review. Int J Nsg Pract. 2022;29:312978. https://doi.org/10.1111/ijn.12987.
2. International Council of Nurses, Schober M, Lehwaldt D, Rogers M, Steinke M, Turale S, Pulcini J, Roussel J, Stewart D. Guidelines on advanced practice nursing 2020. Geneva: ICN; 2020. p. 1–38. https://www.icn.ch/system/files/documents/2020-04/ICN_APN%20Report_EN_WEB.pdf
3. World Health Organization. Task shifting; rational redistribution of tasks among health workforce groups: global recommendations and guidance. Geneva: WHO Press; 2008. https://iris.who.int/bitstream/handle/10665/43821/9789241596312_eng.pdf
4. Mbouamba Yankam B, Adeagbo O, Amu H, Dowou RK, Nyamen BGM, Ubechu SC, Félix PG, Nkfusai NC, Badru O, Bain LE. Task shifting and task sharing in the health sector in sub-Saharan Africa: evidence, success indicators, challenges, and opportunities. Pan Afr Med J. 2023;46:11. https://doi.org/10.11604/pamj.2023.46.11.40984. PMID: 38035152; PMCID: PMC10683172
5. Poghosyan L, Bettina Maier C. Advanced practice nurses globally: responding to health challenges, improving outcomes. Int J Nurs Stud. 2022;132:104262. https://doi.org/10.1014/j.iinurstu.2022.104262.
6. Wheeler KJ, Miller M, Pulcini J, Gray D, Ladd E, Rayens JK. Advanced practice nursing roles, regulation, education, and practice: a global study. Ann Glob Health. 2022;38(1):42. https://doi.org/10.5334/aogh.3698.
7. Kilpatrick K, Savard I, Audet L-A, Costanzo G, Khan M, Atallah R, Jabbour M, Zhou W, Wheeler K, Ladd E, Gray DC, Henderson C, Spies LA, McGrath H, Rogers M. A global perspective of advanced practice nursing research: a review of systematic reviews. PLoS One. 2024;19(7):e0305008. https://doi.org/10.1371/journal.pone.0305008.
8. Lockwood EB, Schober M. Factors influencing the impact of nurse practitioners' clinical autonomy: a self-determining perspective. Int J Nurs Pract. 2024;71:1375–95.
9. Evans DK, Goldstein M, Popova A. Health-care worker mortality and the legacy of the Ebola epidemic. In: Lancet, vol. 3. Published Online July 9, 2015; 2015. https://doi.org/10.1016/S2214-109X(15)00065-0.

10. Meara JG, Leather AJ, Hagander L, Alkire BC, Alonso J, Ameh EA, Bickler SW, Conteh L, Dare A, Davies J, Merisier ED, El-Halabi S, Farmer PE, Gawande A, Gilles R, Greenberg AL, et al. The lancet commission on global surgery global surgery 2030: evidence and solutions for achieving health, welfare and economic development. Lancet. 2015;386:569–624.
11. International Federation of Nurse Anesthetists. Code of ethics, standards of practice, monitoring, and education. IFNA: International Federation of Nurse Anesthetists; 2016. https://ifna.site/app/uploads/2015/08/IFNA-STANDARDS-2016.pdf
12. International Council of Nurses Guidelines on advanced practice nursing nurse anesthetists 2021 ICN. Geneva: 2021. https://www.icn.ch/sites/default/files/2023-06/ICN_Nurse-Anaesthetist-Report_EN_WEB.pdf
13. Odinkemelu DS, Sonah AK, Nsereko ET, Dahn BT, Martin MH, Moon TD, Niconchuk JA, Walters CB, Kynes JM. An assessment of anesthesia capacity in Liberia: opportunities for rebuilding post-Ebola. Anesth Analg. 2021;132(6):1727–37. https://doi.org/10.1213/ANE.0000000000005456.
14. Dlamini CP, Khumalo T, Nkwanyana N, Mathunjwa-Dlamini TR, Macera L, Nsibandze BS, Kaplan L, Stuart-Shor EM. Developing and implementing the family nurse practitioner role in Eswatini: implications for education, practice, and policy. Ann Glob Health. 2020;86(1):50. https://doi.org/10.5334/aogh.2813. PMID: 32477886; PMCID: PMC7243836
15. Ministry of Health, Kingdom of Eswatini. The National Health Sector Policy 2016–2024: Towards attainment of Universal Health Coverage. Mbabane, Eswatini; 2016.
16. Ministry of Health, Kingdom of Eswatini, 2024. Eswatini STEPS report, 2024. Mbabane: Eswatini. Accessed from Eswatini Steps 2024 Report_Final_23042025 (3)—Copy.cdr
17. Ministry of Health, Kingdom of Eswatini. National health Sector Strategic Plan 2024/2025—2027/2028. Mbabane, Eswatini; 2024. Accessed from: NATIONAL HEALTH SECTOR STRATEGIC PLAN 2024/25—2027/2028 | WHO | Regional Office for Africa
18. Bryant-Lukosius D, Dicenso A. A framework for the introduction and evaluation of advanced practice nursing roles. J Adv Nurs. 2004;48(5):530–40. https://doi.org/10.1111/j.1365-2648.2004.03235.x.
19. Eswatini Nurses and Midwives Act of 1965. Act 16 of 1965. Accessed from Nurses and Midwives Act, 1965—EswatiniLII
20. Eswatini Nursing Council, 2025. Continuing professional development. Accessed from Eswatini Nursing Council on 4th September 2025
21. APRN. Consensus Work Group & the National Council of State Boards of Nursing APRN Advisory Committee. Consensus Model for APRN Regulation: Licensure, Accreditation, Certification & Education; 2008. https://www.ncsbn.org/public-files/Consensus_Model_Report.pdf
22. Stanley JM. Impact of new regulatory standards on advanced practice registered nursing: the APRN consensus model and LACE. Nurs Clin North Am. 2012;47(2):241–50, vi. https://doi.org/10.1016/j.cnur.2012.02.001.
23. American Nurses Credentialing Center. https://www.nursingworld.org/our-certifications/?utm_source=&utm_medium=cpc&utm_campaign=ancc-aprn-competitive%20conquest-certifications_us_search_pros1_leads_idx_google_paid-search&utm_content=competitors&utm_term=aacn&utm_campaign=&utm_source=adwords&u
24. American Association of Colleges of Nursing. The essentials: Core competencies for professional nursing education. AACN; 2021. https://www.aacnnursing.org/Portals/0/PDFs/Publications/Essentials-2021.pdf
25. American Association of Nurse Practitioners. Certification Examinations. https://www.aanpcert.org/certs/program
26. World Health Organization. State of the world's nursing 2025: investing in education, jobs, leadership and service delivery. Geneva: World Health Organization; 2025. License: CC BY-NC-SA 3.0 IGO. https://www.icn.ch/sites/default/files/2025-05/SOWN%202025.pdf
27. Schober M. The future for international NP role development. In: Thomas SL, Rowles JS, editors. Nurse practitioners and nurse anesthetists: the evolution of the global roles. Cham: Springer; 2023. p. 303–10.

Introduction to Legal and Regulatory Accountability

Jessica Matei

Advanced Practice Nurses (APNs) are pivotal in healthcare delivery systems worldwide. APNs typically have an expanded scope of practice in comparison to standard nursing scope of practice, often allowing them to assess, diagnose, treat, and manage various health conditions. While managing different conditions, they may be ordering diagnostic tests, prescribing medications, and making life-saving decisions for their patients. Within their clinical practice, APNs must continuously balance their clinical autonomy and legal oversight. The APN makes independent practice decisions for patient care utilizing their clinical autonomy, standards of care, strategies gained through experience, their scope of practice, and education obtained. APNs must practice within the bounds of legal oversight, laws, regulations, and review processes to assure safe and ethical practice. As the scope of each APN widens and varies globally, it becomes increasingly important to understand their legal and regulatory accountability. Understanding legal and regulatory accountability is necessary for today's APN workforce to fully embrace the legal responsibility that each APN holds in relation to their clinical practice.

Legal accountability refers to the legal responsibility APNs bear for the outcomes of their clinical decisions and professional actions. Legal accountability is grounded in core legal principles such as negligence, informed consent, and duty of care, which assist in creating the legal expectations of APNs in clinical practice.

Regulatory accountability reflects the bodies that define and enforce the standards of practice that APNs must abide by. Regulatory accountability arises from the governance of professional bodies and adheres to licensure requirements and scope of practice regulations.

Legal and regulatory frameworks seek to ensure safe, effective, and ethical healthcare delivery; however, each framework is unique in its sources of authority and enforcement mechanisms. This chapter explores the scope of practice and

J. Matei (✉)
Northern California, San Francisco, CA, USA

A. Kapu et al. (eds.), *A Global View on Clinical Autonomy for Advanced Practice Nurses*, Advanced Practice in Nursing,
https://doi.org/10.1007/978-3-032-21458-4_13

regulatory mechanisms, practice authority, credentialing and privileging, types of liability, and preventative measures that the APN can take to minimize risk. In addition, this chapter will discuss the challenges of a standardized approach to the APN role and the impact this challenge has on APN practice and liability.

Regulatory Constraints Impacting APNs

Scope of Practice and Regulatory Mechanisms

APN, a term known around the world for providing and delivering care, represents four established roles, including clinical nurse specialist (CNS), nurse practitioner (NP), nurse anesthetist, and nurse midwife [9]. In the context of legal and regulatory accountability, the term APN is captured frequently in a global context to reflect the role of the APN regardless of their practice environment. An Advanced Practice Nurse is, "a generalist or specialized nurse who has acquired, through additional graduate education (minimum of a master's degree), the expert knowledge base, complex decision-making skills and clinical competencies for Advanced Nursing Practice, the characteristics of which are shaped by the context in which they are credentialed to practice [4]." The two most commonly identified APN roles are Clinical Nurse Specialist (CNS) and Nurse Practitioner (NP) [9]. Depending on the regulatory body, the terminology "APN" may be adjusted as regulatory requirements vary among countries/provinces/states/etc. For example, in the United States, APNs are Advanced Practice Registered Nurses (APRNs). Though the terminology is defined, globally, the practice environment, education, regulatory mechanism, etc., all differ worldwide.

The practice environments for APNs vary significantly due to global government structures and variations across nurse regulatory bodies. This creates a varied regulatory environment for an APN. Even in countries with defined regulatory requirements, the titling, tasks, roles, education, and practice structures under which APNs can provide care differ [9]. In the United States, e.g., the authority to define the scope of practice resides within individual states, leading to widespread disparities in the scope of care an APN can provide across the same country. Furthermore, practicing in each state varies, with some states granting full practice authority to APNs while others impose collaborative or supervisory requirements. In Canada and other nations with centralized healthcare systems, APNs are regulated at the national or provincial level, resulting in more standardized practice nationwide.

A multinational survey study conducted by Wheeler and colleagues provided an in-depth examination of the global landscape of APN education and regulatory frameworks. Among the countries that responded, all reported the existence of formal education programs, with the vast majority offering master's degrees as the primary academic credential to APN preparation. While widespread education preparation was evident, variations existed in formally acknowledging these roles. In addition, education may be unique to geographic areas and schools offering courses. Approximately half of the countries indicated that APNs were formally recognized by governmental bodies, healthcare institutions, and/or professional organizations. In contrast, the remainder acknowledged the presence of APNs in practice without the support of formal governmental regulation or legislative frameworks [9]. Outside of regulations and legislative frameworks, an APN is at high risk for liability, as there is no clear definition of their scope of practice and responsibilities in the geographic region they work in.

In regions where regulation of the APN practice is reported, oversight most commonly occurred at the federal level. Some countries previously implemented "grandfathering" provisions, allowing experienced practitioners to continue practicing despite not meeting the current, more rigorous education standards [9]. The practice of "grandfathering" may have its own interpretations of legal and regulatory accountability, especially in a situation where the APN works in a capacity outside of that country's borders or regulations.

Regulatory mechanisms extended beyond initial entry into practice. In over half of the responding countries, APNs must obtain some legal recognition, such as licensure, registration, or endorsement through governmental channels, to practice. In addition, maintenance of advanced practice status mostly involved ongoing professional engagement. The maintenance that APNs commonly need to continue their licensure or certification involves meeting specified thresholds in continuing professional development. Continuing professional development activities for APNs may include accruing continuing education units, maintaining clinical practice, or meeting portfolio requirements periodically [9].

Consensus Model

In the United States, the Consensus Model was developed to create consistency in the licensure, accreditation, certification, and education process regulating the use of Advanced Practice Registered Nurse (APRN) throughout the country. The recommendations made through the Consensus Model highlight the requirements suggested for regulating the APRN profession. Based on the model, "APRNs are licensed independent practitioners who are expected to practice within standards established or recognized by a licensing body [1]." APRNs are accountable to the patients, the nursing profession, and their licensing authority, and comply with state nurse practice acts while maintaining the highest standards for advanced nursing care. Operating under state-specific regulatory frameworks, state licensing boards serve as the final authority in recognizing and authorizing APRN practice.

The Consensus Model defines an APRN as one who has completed the appropriate education, passed national certification examinations while maintaining competence relevant to their role, has acquired advanced knowledge and skill, builds on the competencies of registered nurses, and who is both clinically and educationally prepared to obtain and practice as one of the four APRN roles including: certified registered nurse anesthetist (CRNA), certified nurse-midwife (CNM), clinical nurse specialist (CNS), or certified nurse practitioner (CNP) [1].

Certificate/Certification

The American Accreditation Board for Nursing Specialties clarifies the difference between the meaning of "certificate" and "certification." A "certificate" refers to an educational program that awards a certificate after completing the program. A "certification" is an earned credential demonstrating the holder's knowledge, skills, and expertise. A certification is generally awarded by a third party demonstrating the recipient's knowledge, skills, and experience [9].

Title Protection

Title protection is a way to manage the APN practice and to establish clear regulations and the scope of practice. Title protection, "as adapted from the American Nurses Association definition, refers to the restricted use of the title to only those individuals who have fulfilled the requirements for the licensure/recognition in each jurisdiction's legislation/regulations/rules so as to protect the public against unethical, unscrupulous, and incompetent practitioners [9]." While title protection of APN roles is used in some areas of the world, its application is not consistent and lacks global standardization.

In the United States, advocacy is occurring for the consistent use of title protection regarding the APRN role and the type of APRN the individual is. For example, the regulation of the CNS practice was developed through law, and its scope of practice is delineated in regulations [5].

While APN roles may be similar worldwide, there is no single regulatory body globally for all APNs. Within different countries, states, and provinces, there is typically a body that regulates practice, for example, in the United States, each state has a Board of Nursing; there is also a resource that defines the scope of practice, for example, in the US, a Nurse Practice Act. Similar language is often used globally to identify education and credentialing. In several countries, the education and credentialing received by APNs are given to the regulating body for oversight.

Models of APN Regulation and Practice Authority

Models regulating APN regulation vary in scope, structure, and levels of professional autonomy. The variability between the types of APN regulation models worldwide is shaped by each country's legal infrastructure, governing regulatory bodies, and overall healthcare delivery systems. While some nations have adopted national standardization of APN practice, others are more dependent on regional or local oversight. A foundational understanding of why and how regulation is implemented, and an overview of the different models are essential for comprehending global approaches to APN oversight.

There are three dominant models of APN Practice Authority, which are influenced by the models of regulation: full practice authority, reduced practice authority (collaboration/supervision), and restricted practice authority (delegated authority). Country specific professional regulation help guide the APN practice includes the authority to diagnose, authority to prescribe medications, authority to order diagnostic testing and therapeutic treatments, authority to refer clients/patients to other services and/or professional, authority to admit and discharge clients/patients to hospital and other services, title recognition, protection of titles, and legislation and policies from an authoritative entity or some regulatory mechanism explicit to APNs [4].

According to Schmitt and Shimberg, the purpose of professional regulation is to "1. Ensure that the public is protected from unscrupulous, incompetent, and unethical practitioners, 2. Offer some assurance to the public that the regulation individual is competent to provide certain services in a safe and effective manner, and 3. Provide a means by which individuals who fail to comply with the profession's standards can be disciplined, including the revocation of their licenses ([8], as cited by the National Council of State Boards of Nursing)."

In discussions of APN regulation, the scope of practice emerges as a central concept, particularly in relation to practice authority. A 2005 Federation of State Medical Boards reported defined the scope of practice as the "definition of the rules, the regulations, and the boundaries within which a fully qualified practitioner with substantial and appropriate training, knowledge, and experience may practice in a field of medicine or surgery, or other specifically defined field. Such practice is also governed by requirements for continuing education and professional accountability [3]".

APN titling and title protection are not regulated globally; however, advocacy continues for it as it easily identifies nurses with advanced, graduate-level nursing knowledge who can provide care within a specific role [1]. When the scope of practice is limited or unclear, title protection becomes a valuable resource as it assists in defining the background the individual has and the care they may provide within a specific role.

Full Practice Authority

Full practice authority means that APNs can provide care independently without a supervising or collaborating physician. They independently evaluate, diagnose, treat, and prescribe. In most places, these systems recognize APNs as autonomous practitioners who are held accountable to their national/regional/provincial boards. This model supports the full enactment of the APN role as intended by advanced education and clinical training. The benefits of a full practice authority model mean that people have increased access to care, especially in underserved areas. The APN autonomy and scope of expertise can be fulfilled at its highest level, reducing the systemic burdens on physicians and other healthcare members. With APNs functioning at their full scope of practice, there is a greater opportunity for innovation, role development, and advancement within their own independent practice.

While there are many benefits, the full practice authority model does require robust and consistent regulatory oversight, standardized practice standards, and a strong credentialing and licensing infrastructure. Additionally, although this model may alleviate strain on the broader medical workforce, it can encounter opposition from medical associations and/or other professional organizations concerned about changes in professional jurisdiction or liability.

In the United States, full practice authority is supported in part by the LACE framework- Licensure, Accreditation, Certification, and Education. The LACE framework was developed by the APRN Consensus Model workgroup, and it provides a structured approach to defining APN roles. The model describes, "Licensure is the granting of authority to practice. Accreditation is the formal review and approval by a recognized agency of education degree or certification program in nursing or nursing-related programs. Certification is the formal recognition of the knowledge, skills, and experience demonstrated by the achievement of standards identified by the profession. Education is the formal preparation of APRNs in graduate degree granting or post graduate certificate programs [1]."

Reduced Practice Authority

With reduced practice, APNs can perform many clinical functions independently; however, they are required to have some form of formalized linkage to a physician or medical team. This model has the ability to grant full practice authority for some roles and reduced authority for others. There is typically a need for formal collaborative agreements, referral pathways, or specific restrictions on diagnosing or prescribing authority. Reduced practice authority is often linked with supervisory and collaborative models. These models can enhance patient care by supporting a team-structured approach while still allowing moderate APN autonomy.

A reduced practice authority model inherently limits the full use of APN competencies. The requirement for ongoing collaborative agreements can create administrative burdens, may be difficult to obtain, and may be challenging to sustain. Additionally, they can create an uneven power dynamic, where the medical authority holds a type of authority over the APN's scope, regardless of their qualifications. Due to the variability in autonomy, there is also a concern for institutional culture shifts, including the structure and variance as to how these APNs are integrated into clinical teams or supported in leadership roles.

Restricted Practice Authority

In a restricted practice, APNs are legally required to be under direct or indirect physician supervision and cannot practice independently. Additionally, they often have limited rights when it comes to prescribing, diagnosing, and referring patients. Their role is heavily defined by what has been explicitly delegated by a physician or outlined through standing orders. Restricted practice authority can also be seen as a delegated authority type model, where APNs function within the confines of physician-defined parameters.

A restricted practice authority has a hierarchical structure, which may enhance perceived safety and oversight in teams where traditional stakeholders maintain control. These models align with physician-led health systems structures. However, they have the potential to limit access to care, particularly in rural or underserved areas where physicians may not be consistently available. By not utilizing the APN to their full practice authority, these systems risk under-leveraging the significant clinical training and expertise APNs possess.

APNs in restricted models may have reduced job satisfaction, limited career advancement, and higher turnover. The structure can reinforce professional power imbalances, potentially limiting APN's involvement in policy-making, leadership, and clinical decision-making.

Credentialing and Privileging

Healthcare systems are able to validate and authorize the clinical functions of APNs through credentialing and privileging. While the process of credentialing and privileging is well established in many countries, the practices may vary widely internationally and are often shaped by national infrastructure, regulatory oversight, and healthcare delivery models.

Credentialing

Credentialing is the formal process to affirm that an APN has acquired the necessary education, licensure, certification, and experience to safely practice within a defined role. The International Council of Nurses (ICN) defines credentialing as "processes used to designate that an individual, programme, institution, or product has met established standards set by an agent (governmental or non-governmental) recognized as qualified to carry out this task. The standards may be minimal and mandatory or above the minimum and voluntary. Licensure, registration, accreditation, approval, certification, recognition, or endorsement may be used to describe different credentialing processes (Wheeler et al. [9]—difficulty finding original ICN citation)." In several countries, especially with limited regulator capacity, credentialing may be less formalized or reliant on the institution for which an APN is working.

Credentialing practices vary between countries and also within countries. The scope of practice and licensure criteria for APRNs in the United States may differ based on the State Board of Nursing. For APRNs specifically, some APRNs may be able to prescribe medications in one state; however, when relocating, they may lose prescribing rights, although their education or national certification remain the same. These inconsistencies interfere with the flexibility of APRNs to practice in different settings and can impact the ability of APRNs to work with short notice or in the face of care shortages. Several countries now have a more centralized and uniform structure, for example, Australia's Nursing and Midwifery Board, under the Australian Health Practitioner Regulation Agency, ensuring a more regulated environment where APNs may more easily move between geographic regions and healthcare organizations.

Privileging

Privileging defines the clinical services an APN is authorized to perform within a particular institution and is context-specific. When an APN is credentialed, privileges determine the types of clinical responsibilities that the individual APN is permitted to do within a specific practice setting. Privileging is often organization-specific and is reviewed by the organization, looking at the APRN's education, certification, experience, and competencies. Privileging at different organizations typically aligns with the APN scope of practice and facility standards.

An APN may be fully credentialed by a regulatory body; however, based on the privileging where they work, they may only be able to provide a more limited range of services. When institutional privileging is more restrictive than regional/national scope of practice regulations, this can cause tension as APNs are not able to practice to their full scope and highlight discrepancies between legal authorization and practical application.

Globally, the difference between credentialing and privileging can present many barriers, including the ability to utilize the workforce to their highest scope of practice, optimize the role in different settings, and provide efficient healthcare delivery.

Legal Accountability and Liability for APRNs

Defining Legal Accountability for APRNs

Legal accountability is the obligation of APNs to act in accordance with laws, legal standards, and judicial rulings. APNs practicing in different areas of the world will have different practice requirements and authority. Each practicing APN is responsible for legal accountability, ensuring they fulfill the requirements for their licensing and place of work. APNs have a responsibility to patients, professional accountability, and third-party accountability.

A responsibility to patients is seen in an APN's legal duty of care and is defined by their ability to practice safe, competent, and ethical care. APNs must uphold responsibilities pertinent to their line of work that may include items like obtaining informed consent, ensuring confidentiality, and maintaining appropriate documentation. Professional accountability is aligning with the professional code of conduct in a place of work, abiding by standards established by regulating bodies, and aligning with clinical guidelines. Third-party accountability incorporates the APN's responsibility to employers, insurers, and other healthcare providers. Violations of the APN's responsibility to patients, professional accountability, and third-party accountability can result in disciplinary actions by the APN's employer, regulatory body, or legal system.

Types of Legal Liability for APRNs

When reviewing APN accountability and the types of liability associated with different areas of law, understanding the source of laws is essential to navigating the legal landscape. Globally, legal systems vary due to differences in governmental structures, although many share similar foundations. For this discussion, the US legal framework will serve as an example. The sources of US law include constitutional law, statutory law, administrative law, and common law. The types of law APRNs may encounter, which become their legal liability, include criminal law, civil, contract, and tort law. The types of law define and determine the liability for APRNs. The most common types of liability for APRNs include criminal liability, civil liability, contractual liability, administrative/regulatory liability, and indirect liability.

Criminal Liability

Criminal liability begins with understanding the framework of criminal law. "Criminal law is created to provide guidance and protection to those injured by offenses against society. A criminal action by an individual is considered a criminal act against society as a whole, even if the act is directed solely at an individual [2]." The level of proof required for criminal law is beyond a reasonable doubt. Conduct for criminal law can include criminal actions like forgery, burglary, murder, assault, battery, theft, rape, and false imprisonment (Dickenson & Meyer, 2019). Consequences of criminal law typically include fines, imprisonment, and loss of licensure. Examples of criminal law in the context of APRNs and healthcare can include fraudulent billing, drug diversion, patient abuse, not reporting abuse, sexual misconduct, and theft. A healthcare provider can incur both criminal (against society) and civil liability (injury incurred by an individual or entity) [2].

Civil Liability

Civil liability, a type of liability in the context of civil law, includes cases of tort law (negligence). "Civil law is law that applies to the rights of individuals or entities, whereas criminal law deals with offenses against the general public. Under civil law, the remedies for a person or entity involve money or compensation to make the plaintiff whole again [2]." Civil liability typically arises in negligence or malpractice claims. For courts to consider malpractice, four elements must exist: (1) a relationship, or duty, between parties must exist, (2) a breach of care, (3) causation, and (4) harm [7]. APRNs may face civil liability for diagnostic errors, treatment delays, and failure to adhere to protocols. To determine liability, standards of care/community of practice can be benchmarked against what a reasonably prudent APRN would do.

"Tort law is an area of civil law that encompasses negligence, personal injury, and medical malpractice claims. A tort is a wrongful act committed by some individual or entity that causes injury to another person or property. Remedies in tort law attempt to make the injured person "whole" again, usually with compensation in the form of a monetary award [2]."

For APRNs, it is important to understand the differences between professional negligence and ordinary negligence. "Professional Negligence is the failure to act as a reasonably prudent similar professional would under similar circumstances [2]." The professional negligence is specific to the scope of practice of the APRN and their responsibilities; it involves a deviation from the standard of care. For example, inappropriate treatment decisions or omissions in clinical judgement that another APRN would have reasonably avoided. Further examples of professional negligence may include the following: positioning a patient incorrectly during surgery with subsequent paralyzation of a limb, not properly providing care in a timely manner, failing to detect signs of bleeding resulting in a worsening condition, and not properly administering medication in a timely manner.

Ordinary negligence means that a failure to use reasonable care occurred, regardless of training. Ordinary negligence would include examples similar to failing to clean up a spill, forgetting to lock a wheelchair, leaving confidential material out, and using broken equipment.

In the review of liability, there are differences between criminal liability and civil liability, and the potential legal consequences of each. Some consequences may include fines, loss of licensure, and imprisonment.

Contractual Liability

When an APN makes an agreement between individuals or entities to provide services, whether written or oral, the liability the APN may accrue may be based on the inability to perform the duties discussed. Several examples exist in today's healthcare environment, such as collaboration agreements, employment contracts, or even productivity expectations in their current work setting. "There are specific requirements for a contract law to be applicable, these requirements include the capacity to contract, legality, offer, acceptance, and consideration [2]."

Administrative Liability

APNs must keep their licenses, certifications, and necessities to practice for their licensure and the organization or individual they work for up to date. To ensure compliance, regulating bodies for both licensure and the organization may perform licensure audits, competency audits, and continuing education reporting. Breaches are a failure to report unsafe practices or failing to maintain active registration, resulting in administrative penalties. Risks include violating the scope of practice, not meeting continuous education requirements, or violating professional conduct standards.

Indirect Liability

APNs are in situations where they may be supervising another staff member. APNs must be familiar with their scope of practice and the scope of practice of the person to whom they are delegating a task. The task needs to be appropriate for that individual's scope of practice and be able to be completed appropriately and safely. When an APN supervises a task, and it has the possibility to result in harm, the situation could cause indirect liability for the APN.

In addition to indirect liability, APNs who are business owners have a responsibility to their employees to make sure materials are updated through policies and procedures, conduct standards are maintained, hiring practices are fair, education is provided through hiring, and supervision is maintained. Additionally, there should be available documents regarding job descriptions and employee responsibilities. The APN, or employer, becomes responsible for the actions of their employees through the legal theory of "vicarious liability" [7].

Some nurse regulatory bodies have resources that identify what acts are considered violations in the area where the APN practices. Having resources to identify violations leaves less vagueness and creates a specific guideline.

Legal Precedents and Case Law Involving APRNs

Based on the Nurse Practitioner Professional Liability Exposure Claim Report, fifth Edition, the number of claims made against Nurse Practitioners (NPs) has increased. The top three locations where NPs can incur claims are physician office practice, aging services facilities, and nurse practitioner office practice [7]. Claim reports and court cases involving APNs are valuable for the examination of legal outcomes as well as implications for the nursing profession. APNs can review these cases, analyze allegations and injuries, to aid in learning more about where their own liability is and how to take preventative steps from similar occurrences in their own practice. While several of these malpractice reports focus on NPs, the value from reviewing cases and situations can be applied to all APN roles.

In a Nurse Practitioner License Protection Case study presented by the Nurses Service Organization (NSO), the State Board of Nursing investigated a complaint against an NP where negligent treatment and care of an infant may have occurred, resulting in death. The NSO was made aware of this case as a result of a malpractice lawsuit. In this investigation, a 10-month-old female was seen by an experienced NP in a pediatric practice for a "bad cough." The NP assessed the baby, diagnosed bronchitis, ordered a breathing treatment, an albuterol inhaler, amoxicillin, and encouraged the continued use of Tylenol and Acetaminophen. The NP failed to document her assessment findings of wheezing, and later said that this is why she ordered the breathing treatment. After the breathing treatment occurred, there was no post-assessment documentation. When the infant and mother returned home, the mother called the office several times and was given the information to "wait for the meds to take effect" without additional information on what to do in the event that her child continues to decline. During the night, while sleeping, the infant was choking with blue lips. Emergency services were called, and during transport, the infant had a full cardiac arrest. The infant was declared brain dead with respiratory syncytial virus (RSV) and anoxic brain injury being stated as the cause of death.

During the State Board of Nursing investigation, it was noted that the NP documented categories that would have included fever and wheezing as "within normal limits." The NP did not document any abnormal respiratory assessment findings, nor heart rate, oxygen saturation, or respiratory rate in the chart. The State Board of Nursing determined this to be "gross negligence" due to the breach of care. They stated that there were several failures that a similarly competent NP would have taken note of.

In this case, the NP settled the malpractice lawsuit with the family. The State Board of Nursing found several areas in which the NP failed to perform and document outside care standards. In this case, the State Board of Nursing recommended disciplinary action that included probation, with additional conditions needing to be met, including a civil penalty, supervision, ongoing counseling, reports, and several others.

APNs can take proactive measures to minimize legal risk, but the complexity of doing so is heightened by variations in legal systems globally. Due to laws, regulations, and judicial processes differing across states, provinces, and countries, the review and outcomes of legal cases involving APNs can follow different paths. This variability contributes to uncertainty and highlights the importance of APNs staying informed and prepared to navigate the legal landscape within the region in which they practice. Several measures and preventative actions can minimize legal risk.

Managing Legal Risk: Risk Management Strategies and Malpractice Insurance

APNs are in a position where they must continuously evaluate their legal risk, as each decision made can potentially increase or decrease their legal risk. They need to take careful consideration through adherence to standards, their documentation, and clinical decisions to protect themselves against malpractice claims. APNs must maintain the public's trust by ensuring safe care is delivered appropriately and that no negligence in their care can jeopardize outcomes.

To manage their legal risk, APNs must ensure they are following the legal parameters of their scope of practice and their employment while preserving their certifications, licenses, etc. APNs are in a unique situation where they must stay updated on evolving legal frameworks and decisions made by their regulatory bodies that may affect their practice.

With good risk management strategies, APNs are valued members of interdisciplinary care teams and can reduce risk exposure for the institutions they work for. By reducing risk for themselves and therefore the institutions, they can increase their job stability, grow within their field, advance their careers, and contribute to discussions about their role and the future they have.

Risk Management for APRNs

Preventative Practices

APNs are responsible for protecting themselves from legal risk while providing the highest form of safe, ethical, and high-quality patient care. This responsibility is foundational to best practice and serves as a legal safeguard. Minimizing liability begins with proactive, preventative strategies to minimize adverse outcomes and avoid liability. One way APNs can mitigate legal exposure is by conducting regular assessments of an APN's legal and clinical risk within their practice setting. The assessments performed include a clear understanding of their scope of practice as defined by the area in which they work. They must clearly understand their licensure and professional regulatory body, as well as legal parameters set by their state/region/province/country and their current employer.

As regulation and scope of practice continue to change, monitoring the state prescribing laws and any additional laws will need to be reviewed regularly. Regularly reviewing legislation and updates by the board of nursing, state/province health departments, and national regulatory bodies is a way to be prepared for legal situations. Adherence to guidelines can help prevent possible claims.

APNs are also encouraged to review their current job description or contract to make sure their practice is aligned with the role they are employed to fulfil. Instances have occurred where the job description or contract may be different from the abilities they are able to perform through their regulatory body, and which they are credentialed to perform. Similarly, if they function as a part of a larger group, under a collaborative or supervisory agreement, those documents should also be reviewed regularly to ensure they are valid and current.

Additionally, APNs should also be aware of the organization's specific policies, procedures, guidelines, and protocols that may be related to their scope of practice or the care they are providing to patients. APNs must be aware of what requires collaboration with other disciplines in accordance with regulatory requirements, and also when to consult based on patient needs. As privileges may be unique in each area an APN practices, an understanding and written document of privileges will help the APN know expectations and boundaries.

On a daily basis, an APN must engage in ongoing education, evidence-based practice strategies, quality improvement, and reflective practice to manage legal risk. Education can include reviewing new data, simulation training, and peer and self-assessments. Additionally, ongoing education supports the APN in maintaining evidence-based practice recommendations. While conducting regular educational review, documents that pertain to this, for example, continuing education credits or completion certificates, would be beneficial to have as a reference.

In addition to education, meticulous documentation and clear communication are essential. An APN is responsible for the communication that takes place with other interdisciplinary care team members, as well as the patients they care for. Documentation of these interactions helps prevent misunderstandings in the future.

An APN can adopt proactive risk management strategies, such as finding appropriate insurance if they are not automatically covered by their region or organization. In several areas, APNs may also obtain their own private malpractice insurance and that offered by an organization. Organizational coverage assists in covering an APN when they follow all policies and procedures within the organization; however, for deviations, additional coverage may help.

While providing care, an important part of preventative practice includes keeping thorough and accurate patient records. APNs see multiple patients and are involved in several aspects of care. The timely and accurate record keeping of the APN protects both the patient from harm and the APN from risk. In addition to documentation, APNs must focus on the details of the documentation, including documenting their assessments, communications, education given to the patient or family members, and any additional counseling that occurred. When an issue arises with a patient outside of the care provided by the APN, the APN has a responsibility to refer them to an alternative provider, escalate concerns, and report any issues.

The Continental Casualty Company (CNA) and NSO Nurse Practitioner Professional Liability Exposure Claim report: fifth Edition, reviews an analysis of diagnosis-related allegations. An APN can review these allegations proactively to further educate themselves on potential failures that may arise. The most frequent allegations include failing to refer a patient to other services. In order to help improve the diagnostic process, the CNA and NSO have laid out additional questions that an APN may ask while considering potential unintended consequences of pursuing a specific diagnosis, including (1) Are factors present that do not align with the diagnosis? (2) Are there elements that cannot be explained? (3) Are there symptoms that are inconsistent with the current diagnosis? (4) Why are these symptoms not indicative of another diagnosis? (5) Is there a life-threatening condition with similar symptoms that hasn't been considered? (6) Is it possible that there are multiple issues ongoing? [7].

Effective communication is an essential component of preventive practice for an APN. The APN communicates with members of the interdisciplinary teams, patients, family members, and more. They must ensure that they communicate accurately and effectively to avoid misunderstandings and possible errors. APNs must become skilled in effective communication strategies that they can routinely employ with team members. For their patients, APNs must use effective communication and resources available, including translation services, services for the hearing impaired, etc., to ensure they communicate effectively and receive appropriate, informed consent when applicable.

Malpractice Insurance

APNs have a professional accountability to manage their own legal risks; however, regulatory bodies, institutions, and private insurers take additional forms of risk management. Legal risk management varies globally and is influenced by regulatory structure, liability coverage, malpractice insurance access, and role regulation. Titling and a formal definition of the APN role have become increasingly important when discussing liability and coverage.

In many countries, APNs are regulated by nursing bodies, state scope of practice, licensing, professional standards, etc., that serve as the first line of preventative practices, making sure that all APNs are able to practice safely in their roles. Countries like Canada, with the Canadian Nurses Protective Society, and the United States, with their LACE documents, have structured frameworks that assist in mitigating risk while standardizing their approach to certification, education, and credentialing.

Depending on the area where the APN is practicing globally, they must understand the liability they take within their role, be aware of government and organizational support, search out additional malpractice insurance, and also be aware of the risks of not carrying insurance. Practicing preventative strategies will be essential in all aspects of the APN's practice.

Globally, malpractice coverage looks different. In some countries, the APN is required to have indemnity coverage or professional liability protection. Some countries have APNs purchase insurance privately, and some are covered by the government. Internationally, many employers offer some form of legal protection; however, this is varied and may not cover all aspects. When employers offer legal services, in many areas, APNs may continue to purchase their own in addition to employer coverage.

Institutional vs. Personal Insurance

Several institutions offer generalized protection for APNs working within their facilities. The coverage owner of these insurances is usually the institution or healthcare organization that the APN is employed by. These aim to protect the organization and, by doing so, aid employees working within their scope of practice. Representation from the institution is typically in the organization's best interest. If the APN is acting outside their scope of practice, coverage from their employer may not cover the liability. While coverage may be in hospital policies and documents, practicing APNs may not have detailed access to what the coverage looks like or what may/may not be supported. The cost of this coverage is typically free for the APN.

There are nuances associated with this coverage. Typically, organizational coverage only applies when working at that organization and not outside it. For example, suppose an APN works at Hospital A and Hospital B. In that case, the coverage may differ, and Hospital A will typically not cover the nurses if something occurs while working at Hospital B. Coverage is typically only for working employees and may not cover the APN before their start date or after their employment.

APNs who carry their own personal malpractice insurance typically purchase the coverage to protect themselves as individuals, outside of any organizations they work for. Globally, the ability to choose the type of insurance, purchase their own insurance, or find privately covered malpractice insurance may vary, especially for an APN who may work across borders or spend time working in multiple countries. Coverage is specified by the insurer as to what the APN is approved for. For example, it can be based on their license only, regardless of where they work, or at an approved place of work, or any place of work/contract work, or volunteering, etc. Coverage typically protects the APNs' full scope of practice, with the APN retaining control over their policy decisions. When personal insurance is covered for the APN and their license, regardless of job changes, the same policy can remain in effect. APNs typically pay for their own personal policies, meaning that the cost may vary by state, country, scope of practice, and the carrier of insurance. With private insurance, there may be the ability to add on additional roles that the APN may take on, like consulting or volunteering, whereas with an institution-based coverage, these additional roles outside the organization are often excluded.

Malpractice insurance can protect the APN against claims that arise from professional errors or omissions. Coverage specificity may be unique, especially with such variance in titling and roles across the world. Coverage specificity would hopefully include the role and practice setting. Coverage may vary and may include both professional liability and license protection. It is important to have this independent practice because institutional coverage may not always extend, depending on the type of legal scenario or jurisdiction.

The importance of carrying malpractice insurance can include an APN's livelihood, their ability to work and obtain income, and have practice implications for future APNs. The cost of a malpractice claim, additionally, can be a reason to carry it. In the United States, the average cost of nurse practitioner malpractice claims in 2022 was $332,137 compared to $300,506 in 2017 [7]. The cost is not only associated with the lawsuit but also with any fines associated with nurse practitioner license protection matters.

Global Variability in Level and Regulatory Expectations for APRNs

As the regulatory disparities and frameworks for regulatory expectations vary significantly across countries, APNs face challenges imposed by these disparities. These include increased legal risk and professional liability, particularly for APNs who practice internationally or who move across borders to practice. Due to the lack of regulatory alignment, the ability for an APN to relocate within a country or from one country to another can be hindered. This variability not only affects the APNs themselves but also impacts the populations they serve. Regulatory inconsistency limits patient access to timely and quality care.

The International Council of Nurses (ICN) and World Health Organization (WHO) have important roles in advocating for the standardization of the APN role. The ICN advocates for countries to adopt clear and consistent regulatory frameworks for practicing APNs across countries. The WHO focuses on ensuring that APNs are a part of global strategies to assist in meeting healthcare needs and workforce demands. Together, these organizations help advance the APN profession and support the establishment of legal recognition, regulatory guidance, and patient safety initiatives.

Mobility and Cross-Border Practice

With the need for APNs increasing globally, many find opportunities to practice in different settings and across borders. Practical, legal, and regulatory challenges may limit this ability, often stemming from the definition and titling of the role itself. Discrepancies between borders are highlighted by variability in the scope of practice, different credentialing standards, and inconsistent legal and regulatory laws, including immigration law and licensure regulations. Regulatory gaps between countries can possibly delay emergency staffing or response to disasters.

Many countries have taken steps to overcome the obstacles to disparities and are attempting to support the practice of role standardization. The European Union's Directive on the Recognition of Professional Qualifications (Directive 2005/36/EC) attempts to regulate health professionals for their qualifications to be used across the EU. The downside to what is currently occurring in different areas is that adoption is limited. APN roles are still often excluded or subject to limitations, which continues to restrict full mobility and access.

Barriers to Legal and Regulatory Progress for APRNs

Barriers to legal and regulatory progress for APNs occur at a variety of stages, in local governments (ex, state level), countries, and globally. When there is a lack of standardization of titling, role, and practice, the APN is limited in their ability to meet healthcare needs. Practitioners must collaborate across borders, communicate using standardized terminology, and engage in dependable research that evaluates the profession's scope and outcomes of care [9]. While the legal and political obstacles exist globally, there may also be additional institutional resistance, public perception, and misconceptions of the role.

Global Level Barriers

The APN practice is affected by disparities in healthcare systems, a lack of global regulation of the APN role and professional standards, and differing global laws. There is a lack of consensus on the legal recognition of APN roles, including education preparation, titles, and scopes of practice. In addition, licensing and credentialing vary within and between countries, leading to the APN having to overcome many hurdles to practice internationally. In developing countries, the APN may be more vulnerable to legal action and have greater liability due to a lack of clarity of the role and scope. In these situations, the APN may have less formal legal protection. In addition to the potential for a lack of formal legal protections, not all countries have nursing organizations that affect the current regulation of the role and promote future development of the role.

When nurses attempt to work internationally, even where demand exists, there are also geopolitical and immigration restrictions that the APN must overcome. The APN may experience visa and work permit limitations, especially in the context of credential evaluation, as each country has its own regulations and recognition systems. In some countries, APNs may often end up in a process that lasts several years before being recognized as an APN in a different country, which includes redoing clinical hours or coursework.

State/Province/Local Level Barriers

Although practice may vary significantly within many countries, the legal authority to regulate the APN practice is typically at the state, provincial, or territorial level.

In the United States, adoption of the APRN consensus model, which aims to unify licensure, accreditation, certification, and education (LACE) standards, is inconsistent across states. As a result, APRN titling may lack legal protection. This means that individuals without the proper education and credentials could use protected titles, which has the potential to risk patient safety as well as professional credibility. At the state level, there is variation in the scope of practice laws, with different states granting different practice authority.

Additionally, dynamics between nursing boards and medical boards have the potential to create barriers. While each board regulates its own profession, in some states, medical boards may have influence over nursing practice by having representatives from both regulatory bodies. The influence of medical boards in nursing practice has the potential to lead to policy conflicts and resistance to APN roles.

Institutional Resistance

Institutional resistance is a significant barrier to APN recognition and integration. The resistance can potentially slow or block APN advancement. Understanding the challenges that arise from institutional resistance, identifying barriers, and working toward overcoming these are crucial to advancing APN roles. Reviewing these challenges can serve as a prevention mechanism for liability, as an APN can be aware of issues that come up and take steps proactively.

The incongruence between regional law and healthcare organization policies may limit APN privileges, creating more restrictive practice environments. These healthcare policies are often created from internal risk aversion and liability concerns.

Physician opposition to APN practice may exist. There are concerns about scope encroachment, power dynamics, and income protection. For example, as APNs diagnose and prescribe, concerns about scope encroachment, patient loads, and income may exist. Between physician and nurse groups, there may be confusion about roles and a lack of understanding of advanced practice capabilities. "Physicians were the first health professionals to obtain legislative recognition and protection of their practice authority [6]." When other healthcare professions sought legislative recognition, they were seen as claiming the ability to do tasks that were already included in the universal and implicitly exclusive authority of medicine. This dynamic has fostered a view of the scope of practice that is conceptually faulty and potentially damaging [6]. These interprofessional misunderstandings can create institutional resistance, which leads to a lack of understanding as to the APN preparation and capabilities. This affects not only administrators, nurses, and physicians, but also patients.

Public Perception and Misconception

The general public often misunderstands what APNs do and what distinguishes the different APN roles. Patients may be unaccustomed to APNs practicing as independent providers, including providing their care and managing prescriptions. The difference in understanding the APN role can make patients reluctant to accept care and ultimately affect patient trust. In addition, when a patient visits multiple settings or multiple countries, the scope of practice and privileging may differ, further leading to confusion.

The lack of consistent titling is another significant contributor to the public's confusion about the role. Additionally, several media sources portray an outdated hierarchical system by consistently framing nurses as subordinate to physicians. This framing minimizes the expertise of APNs, despite their extensive training and advanced degrees, often at a master's or doctoral level.

Future Directions: Reform and Advocacy for APRNs

APNs must remain advocates for their profession. APNs are faced with a complex legal and regulatory landscape globally. They will need to work continuously alongside legislators and regulatory bodies to improve the standardization of their practice, which will lead to increased patient access to care. Achieving the APN's full scope of practice and defining what this means globally means working in a partnership with legislators at the state/provincial level, where licensure and practice laws differ. Globally, this means continued advocacy for legislation and a shared view of the APN practice.

When working, APNs must be aware of the legal and regulatory framework in which they are working, as the governmental structure, regulation, and law may vary considerably, impacting the legal liability of the APN. APNs must be able to thoughtfully navigate and articulate the legal expectations within their setting. Additionally, the availability of professional protections, like country-sponsored or private malpractice insurance, can vary by location, further influencing their legal exposure and the need to protect themselves against liability.

Ongoing research, global case studies, and analysis of malpractice claims are critical to understanding legal accountability in advanced practice. In addition to reviewing global legal claims, continued research in APN practice globally will be needed to obtain ongoing data about the similarities and differences across countries. Publishing and widely disseminating this information supports the development of APN practice, informs future legislation, and helps APNs understand their liability and mitigate legal risk.

Education for APNs on legal and regulatory accountability in their practice may be an important part of advanced practice nursing education or continuing education as the number of APNs practicing rises and the number of claims increases.

Conclusion—Recap and Call to Action

APNs are a part of the solution for protecting their license, legal liability, and regulatory oversight. Advocacy of APNs for their own practice needs to continue with global goals of aligning APN practice through accreditation models, titling, role consistency, and educational preparation. Additional areas where APNs need to continue advocating for their profession include aligning institutional privilege with regulatory credentials.

APNs need to stay current on health policy and the legal liabilities in the context of their work. Based on their role and population, APNs can join professional organizations and advocacy groups. By joining advocacy groups, they can improve legal and regulatory systems to support APNs and their opportunity to practice at their full scope. APNs also need to continually evaluate their risk and take proactive, preventive measures.

References

1. APRN Consensus Work Group, & National Council of State Boards of Nursing APRN Advisory Committee. Consensus model for APRN regulation: licensure, accreditation, certification & education. American Association of Colleges of Nursing; 2008. https://www.aacnnursing.org/Portals/0/PDFs/Teaching-Resources/APRNReport.pdf.
2. Dickinson J, Meyer A, editors. Legal nurse consulting: principles and practices. 4th ed. Routledge; 2019. https://doi.org/10.4324/9780429283642.
3. Federation of State Medical Boards. Assessing scope of practice in health care delivery: critical questions in assuring public access and safety. Federation of State Medical Boards; 2005.
4. International Council of Nurses (ICN). Guidelines on Advanced Practice Nursing. 2020.
5. National Association of Clinical Nurse Specialists. Statement on clinical nurse specialist practice and education. 3rd ed; 2019. https://members.nacns.org/store/viewproduct.aspx?id=19695699.
6. National Council of State Boards of Nursing. Changes in healthcare professions' scope of practice: legislative considerations. National Association of Clinical Nurse Specialists; 2012. https://nacns.org/wp-content/uploads/2020/12/3A-Scope_of_Practice_2012.pdf.
7. Nurse Service Organization. Nurse practitioner professional liability exposure claim report. 5th ed. NSO; 2022. Retrieved July 29, 2025, from https://www.nso.com/Learning/Artifacts/Claim-Reports/Nurse-Practitioner-Claim-Report-5th-Edition.
8. Schmitt K, Shimberg B. Demystifying occupational and professional regulation: answers to questions you may have been afraid to ask. Council on Licensure, Enforcement and Regulation; 1996.
9. Wheeler KJ, Miller M, Pulcini J, Gray D, Ladd E, Rayens MK. Advanced practice nursing roles, regulation, education, and practice: a global study. Ann Glob Health. 2022;88(1):42. https://doi.org/10.5334/aogh.3698.

Economic and Reimbursement Challenges

Jamie Wiggins

Introduction and Setting the Context

The global economics of Advanced Practice Nursing is shaped by the healthcare system and fiscal resources utilized to deliver care to the population served. Healthcare economics analyzes how scarce resources are used to improve the health of a population.

A common indicator of a country's investment in healthcare is to quantify the percentage of gross domestic product (GDP) spent on healthcare services. The World Bank Group notes, in 2022, the world spent 9.89% of the global GDP on healthcare goods and services—approximately 9.8 trillion US Dollars [1]. This does not include capital investments for buildings, machinery, information technology, or vaccines for outbreaks. The value delivered from the fiscal investment is often assessed by reviewing morbidity and mortality, life span, and disease burden of a specific population.

The fiscal resources to deliver healthcare continues to increase in cost related to a worldwide aging population, increased chronic disease, workforce challenges, and technology. As populations continue to live longer, their utilization of healthcare services also increases, with a significant increase near the end of life. Diseases that were once synonymous with short life expectancy have benefited from the evolution of treatments that either cure or mitigate morbidity, leading to increased consumption of healthcare in addition to longer term utilization of healthcare services. Across the globe, there are workforce challenges through either misdistribution of

J. Wiggins (✉)
Arkansas Children's, Little Rock, AR, USA

School of Nursing Louisiana State University Health Sciences Center—New Orleans, New Orleans, LA, USA

Department of Health Policy and Management, College of Public Health, University of Arkansas for Medical Sciences, Little Rock, AR, USA

A. Kapu et al. (eds.), *A Global View on Clinical Autonomy for Advanced Practice Nurses*, Advanced Practice in Nursing,
https://doi.org/10.1007/978-3-032-21458-4_14

labor where needed, lack of educational programs to adequately train healthcare providers, or limited number of people pursuing highly technical healthcare positions. Technology and innovation continue to advance at warp speed; with new treatments, pharmaceuticals, and diagnostic tools available to improve disease diagnosis and management.

Understanding how healthcare is financed is critical for APNs who seek to establish or improve reimbursement for healthcare services they deliver. There are many different types of healthcare systems across the world. Universal coverage, national health systems, and private industry, or a combination of government and private insurance are all in place as a method of paying for the healthcare of a population. In all models of healthcare financing, there is a consistent drive to achieve value by improving population health outcomes at a lower cost. Some countries manage health with a significant investment in primary care and prevention of disease, while other countries focus on disease treatment.

Background and Conceptual Framework

Advanced Practice Nurses' understanding of the healthcare economic landscape including basic economic principles, healthcare funding processes, and high-quality care frameworks allow APNs to quantify their impact to patient care and advocate for their unique contributions to patient care.

Healthcare System Financing

Across the globe, there are several types of financial models used to pay for healthcare. Single-payer, public insurance, private insurance and self-pay are all models used to finance healthcare [2].

Single-payer: In a government model, taxes or other revenue streams are used to either directly pay for healthcare services or provide supplemental payments for healthcare services. Often referred to as The Beveridge Model, where publicly available healthcare services are free at point of service and healthcare providers are salaried. These types of systems have lower overall costs because the single payer controls what providers do and what they can charge. The Beveridge Model, or variations of the model, can be found in Great Britain, New Zealand, Hong Kong, and Cuba.

Public Insurance: Social insurance where the government withholds part of wages that is shared between the employee and employer. May also be called The Bismarck Model that uses non-profit insurance systems, and everyone must be covered. The Bismark Model is found in Germany, France, Belgum, the Netherlands, Japan, and Switzerland.

Private Insurance: Operated by private insurance companies where individuals regularly pay a premium. Most private insurance companies are for profit organizations that seek to control costs to improve health. Depending on the coverage, there may be payment required at the site of service.

Self-Pay: When healthcare services are sought after and paid for by the person receiving care.

Economic Concepts

In basic markets, the price for a good or service is related to supply and demand in the marketplace. Supply is the amount of goods or service available in the marketplace and demand is how much interest there is in a specific good or service. When supply is low and demand is high, the cost will be higher than it would be in a situation where the demand is low and the supply is high. Healthcare does not follow normal market conditions for many reasons.

Healthcare Is Inelastic

Healthcare demand is usually inelastic; in most markets as prices rise, the demand usually decreases. People usually do not have the ability to shop for the best price. When a person is suffering from an acute event, they typically seek care without much consideration for price.

Demand Is Provider Driven

There is some truth to the saying, "if you build it, they will come." Having a piece of technology available, like an x-ray machine for example, may mean a provider gets more x-rays than they would have if the technology was not available, despite that the evidenced based treatment plan may not require a chest x-ray to provide appropriate care.

Supply Is Constrained by Regulation

Establishing or opening new healthcare organizations and services is often governed by regulation, licensing, and increased cost burden to enter a market. In most other markets, suppliers of goods and services can enter the market quicker.

The variation in healthcare financing often prevents the individual from encumbering the total cost of care. When healthcare services are provided at reduced or nominal costs relative to the actual cost of care, individuals do not make decisions about healthcare consumption with a total understanding of the cost of care received.

Healthcare Quality Frameworks

The goal of healthcare economics is to allocate finite resources to improve the health of the population. There are many models used to determine the value of healthcare, which is most often referred to as the healthcare outcome divided by the cost. Developed by the Institute for Healthcare Improvement (IHI), The Quintuple Aim is a framework of healthcare delivery that focuses on five key goals [3]:

Improving the Patient Experience—the overall patient experience should be enhanced based on their individual needs including communication, access to care, and patient satisfaction.
Improving the Health of the Populations—promoting health and well-being of entire communities, addressing social determinants of health, and implementing preventative measures to improve overall population health outcomes.
Reducing Per-Capita Cost of Healthcare—lowering the cost of healthcare services for individuals and society as a whole, focusing on efficiency and value-based care models to ensure sustainable healthcare spending.
Improving the Experience of the Providers—healthcare providers' well-being is critical to achieving the other three aims. This goal focuses on enhancing the work experience of healthcare professionals, reducing burnout, and fostering a supportive work environment.
Advancing Health Equity—improving health worldwide requires a focus on equity of access to quality care and outcomes.

The World Health Organization notes that quality of care is the degree in which healthcare services for individuals is based on the likelihood of desired health outcomes —cure, decreased suffering, increased life expectancy. High quality healthcare services should be as follows [4]:

Effective—ensuring the provision of evidence-based healthcare services to those who need them.
Safe—avoiding harm to people for whom the care is intended.
People-centered—care that meets the individual needs and preferences.

High-quality healthcare services must be as follows:

Timely—reduce waiting times and harmful delays.
Equitable—eliminate quality-care variation due to gender, ethnicity, geographic location, and socioeconomic status.
Integrated—provide a full range of healthcare services throughout the life course.
Efficient—maximize the benefit of resources and avoiding waste.

Provider Payment Systems

There are many ways that healthcare providers are paid for services. While historically, provider payment was directly related to the volume of patients seen or procedures being completed, increasingly, there is a desire to align provider payment incentives to drive lower cost care and share in the goal of lowering the cost of care.

Volume-based payments are also referred to as fee-for-service where there is a charge for each visit or service that is provided. In volume-based payments, the financial incentive is to see more patients and do more procedures.

Value-based models of care seek to incentivize healthcare outcomes and control costs. Reimbursement is based on quality metrics, patient outcomes, and cost savings. Value based models require effective data collection systems and are complex.

Capitation models pay a provider a fixed amount per month, or other interval off time, to cover the costs of caring for a patient regardless of the services that are provided. The goal is to control costs; however, it may also incentivize underutilization of healthcare services.

In all payment systems, the care provided by the APN is aimed at improving healthcare outcomes. While it may be possible for the APN to bill for the services rendered in some models of care, it is not true everywhere.

Current Landscape

Advanced Practice Nursing (APN) reimbursement is challenging due to variation across the globe in APN practice and utilization. Differences in healthcare delivery and funding mechanisms impact opportunities for reimbursement for healthcare services delivered [5] (see billing practices table). Advanced Practice Nursing continues to augment healthcare delivery in meeting complex patient needs and healthcare system demands. Further, more APNs are assuming roles in leadership, education, and advocacy. In the face of increased utilization of APNs, there are barriers to billing and reimbursement for services. Regulation, practice limitations, role ambiguity, physician resistance, and local funding mechanisms all contribute to challenges for billing for services. In some cases, APNs can bill for services, but at a lower rate than if services were provided by a physician, while in other countries direct billing for direct services is not allowed.

Future Considerations

Global efforts to standardize the scope of practice for APNs, along with continued research to quantify their financial and clinical impact, will be required to advancing APN autonomy and securing reimbursement for services provided. As healthcare systems worldwide face growing provider shortages, aging populations, and rising costs, APNs are increasingly vital to meeting the complex health needs of the populations served. Regulatory reform and payment strategies will be crucial in improving access to care, optimizing health outcomes, and ensuring the sustainability of healthcare delivery systems.

Billing Practices for Advanced Practice Nurses (APNs) Across the Globe

Region/country	Billing model	Key notes	References
United States	Independent billing under National Provider Identifier; reimbursed at 85% of physician rate. Incident to billing allows 100% reimbursement	Widely established, with ongoing debate over complexity of incident to billing rules	[6, 7, 8]
Canada	Provincial models; NPs may bill directly in some provinces (e.g., Ontario). In others, salaried through health authorities	Significant interprovincial variation; NP-led clinics unique in Ontario	[9–11]
United Kingdom	NHS salaried contracts; no independent billing	NP/APN roles integrated into NHS workforce planning, not separate billing	[9, 11, 12]
European Union (general)	Mixed models: mostly salaried, with pilots for direct billing in select countries (e.g., Netherlands, Switzerland)	Evolving regulatory and reimbursement structures	[11, 13, 14]
Australia	NPs register as Medicare providers; eligible for item numbers, independent billing	Strong national framework, though scope of reimbursable services is limited	[11, 15, 16]
New Zealand	NPs funded through PHARMAC and primary care contracts; independent billing in some contexts	Limited prescribing rights compared to Australia	[15, 16]
Sub-Saharan Africa (e.g., South Africa, Ghana, Malawi)	Mostly salaried; independent billing rare or absent	Reimbursement often tied to pilot programs or donor-funded projects	[17–19]
Asia (Hong Kong, Singapore, Japan)	Primarily salaried; limited or no independent billing. Some pilot initiatives in Singapore	Developmental stage; legislation and funding vary	[9, 20, 21]

Case: Correct Billing

Scott is a primary care pediatric nurse practitioner in a private practice clinic in the Midwest United States. Scott is an independent practitioner and bills for his services. In a fast-paced environment, Scott will see 25–30 patients per day. Scott is also a Pediatric Primary Care Mental Health Specialist (PMHS) and assists his clients with early identification, intervention, and collaboration of care for children and adolescents with mental and behavioral health concerns.

Scott will often have children visit him for a mental health consultation. These consults include an extensive patient history reviewing the present illness, family history, environmental assessment, suicide risk, health screening tools, and individual interviews with the patient and their family. During these visits, Scott provides education on medical management, sleep hygiene, and any medications that are prescribed. Total face-to-face visit time is 60 minutes and an additional 30 minutes for documentation and reviewing charts and screening tools. In the course of treatment, Scott will routinely complete screens for physical and emotional health status and adjust plans of care to meet the client's individual needs.

For the success of Scott's clients and economic reality of running a private practice, it is critical that Scott understand the correct billing codes to ensure accurate reimbursement for services rendered. The complexity of Scott's clients' needs exceeds what can be adequately addressed in standard primary care visits. To ensure Scott is accurately reimbursed for services, he has identified the correct billing codes to ensure accurate payment from insurance companies. The long-term financial stability of Scott's primary care practice, requires effective billing practices that accurately reflect the care he provides, comply with regulatory requirements, and are covered by the client's insurance company.

References

1. World Bank Group. Current health expenditure 2025. Available from: https://data.worldbank.org/indicator/SH.XPD.CHEX.GD.ZS?most_recent_value_desc=false
2. Program PFANH. Health care systems – four basic models 2009. Available from: https://www.pnhp.org/single_payer_resources/health_care_systems_four_basic_models.php
3. Institute for Healthcare Improvement. Improvement topic: quintuple aim. Cambridge: Institute for Healthcare Improvement; 2022.
4. World Health Organization. Quality of care 2025. Available from: https://www.who.int/health-topics/quality-of-care#tab=tab_
5. Mackavey C, Henderson C, de Zwart van Leeuwen E, Maas L, Ladd A. The advanced practice nurse role's development and identity: an international review. Int J Adv Pract. 2024;2(1):36–44.
6. Medicare Payment Advisory Commission (MedPAC). Improving Medicare's payment policies for advanced practice registered nurses and physician assistants. Washington, DC: MedPAC; 2022.
7. Ulmer E, Harris A. Billing for non-physician provider services to support the delivery of physician care. FPM. 2023;30(1):13–7.
8. Barney L, Nicoletti B, Savarise M. Billing for services performed by nonphysician practitioners. Bull Am Coll Surg 2014;99(5):36–38.
9. Kilpatrick K, Savard I, Audet LA, Costanzo G, Khan M, Atallah R, et al. A global perspective of advanced practice nursing research: a review of systematic reviews. PLoS One. 2024;19(7):e0305008.
10. van Soeren M, Micevski V. The role of nurse practitioners in Canada: overview, context, and future prospects. Rev Lat Am Enfermagem. 2013;21(1):38–46.
11. Brownwood I, Lafortune G. Advanced practice nursing in primary care in OECD countries: recent developments and persisting implementation challenges. Paris: OECD; 2024.
12. Torrens C, Campbell P, Hoskins G, Strachan H, Wells M, Cunningham M, et al. Barriers and facilitators to the implementation of the advanced nurse practitioner role in primary care settings: a scoping review. Int J Nurs Stud. 2020;104:103443.
13. Gysin S, Sottas B, Odermatt M, Essig S. Advanced practice nurses' and general practitioners' first experiences with introducing the advanced practice nurse role to Swiss primary care: a qualitative study. BMC Fam Pract. 2019;20(1):163.
14. Maier CB, Batenburg R, Birch S, Zander B, Elliott R, Busse R. Health workforce planning and the role of nurses. Health Policy. 2018;122(10):1053–8.

15. Wheeler KJ, Miller M, Pulcini J, Gray D, Ladd E, Rayens MK. Advanced practice nursing roles, regulation, education, and practice: a global study. Ann Glob Health. 2022;88(1):42.
16. Adams S, Komene E, Wensley C, Davis J, Carryer J. Integrating nurse practitioners into primary healthcare to advance health equity through a social justice lens: an integrative review. J Adv Nurs. 2024;80(10):3899–914.
17. Mtengezo J, Atuhaire C, Cumber SN, Ndirangu E, Anney A, Nalwadda G, et al. Development of advanced practice nursing in sub-Saharan Africa: a scoping review. BMC Nurs. 2023;22:240.
18. Porat-Dahlerbruch J, Ratz S, Ellen M. Development of a taxonomy of policy interventions for integrating nurse practitioners into health systems. Int J Health Policy Manag. 2024;13:8194.
19. World Health Organization. State of the world's nursing 2020: investing in education, jobs and leadership. Geneva: WHO; 2020.
20. Sheer B, Wong FKY. The development of advanced nursing practice globally. Geneva: International Council of Nurses; 2020.
21. Pulcini J, Jelic M, Gul R, Loke AY. An international survey on advanced practice nursing education, practice, and regulation. J Nurs Scholarsh. 2010;42(1):31–9.

Cultural and Professional Pushback

Ruth E. Zielinski, Nora Drummond, Kathryn N. Nelson, and Veronica Millicent Dzomeku

Introduction

What is in a name? Nurse practitioners, nurse anesthetists, clinical nurse specialists, and nurse-midwives have a long history of being referred to by terms other than what they are: Advanced Practice Nurses. Terms such as "mid-level providers," "physician extenders," and "non-physician provider" have all been used to categorize APNs. Despite repeated calls from APN professional organizations over more than a decade, these terms continue to be used today [1]. These terms serve to "other" APNs as less than their physician counterparts by literally categorizing APNs as under physicians, in value and importance. APNs, including nurse-midwives, nurse practitioners, clinical nurse specialists, and nurse anesthetists represent a diverse group of autonomous healthcare providers. While using terms such as "physician extender" may seem a small matter, the use of outdated and hierarchical terms perpetuates misconceptions both culturally and professionally. If APNs are to gain footing and status globally, use of language that acknowledges APNs as equal and valuable members of healthcare teams is essential.

Factors contributing to challenges in recognizing APNs as valued members of the healthcare workforce are rooted in historical representations and current disrespect for nursing and midwifery that then extend to APNs. While there is widespread recognition of a global shortage of healthcare providers, APNs encounter significant barriers to addressing these gaps. These challenges stem not only from resistance within the medical profession but also from cultural norms that view

R. E. Zielinski (✉) · N. Drummond · K. N. Nelson
University of Michigan School of Nursing, Ann Arbor, MI, USA
e-mail: ruthcnm@umich.edu; noradrum@umich.edu; kathrynn@umich.edu

V. M. Dzomeku
School of Nursing and Midwifery, Kwame Nkrumah University of Science and Technology, Kumasi, Ghana

A. Kapu et al. (eds.), *A Global View on Clinical Autonomy for Advanced Practice Nurses*, Advanced Practice in Nursing,
https://doi.org/10.1007/978-3-032-21458-4_15

nursing and midwifery as "helping" roles rather than autonomous professionals; a patriarchal perception that persists across high-, middle- and lower-income countries. The culture of nursing historically has added additional barriers to APN practice through lack of consensus about nursing titles, scope of practice, and level of education [2].

The authors of this chapter are all APNs and as such, have experienced pushback to our profession and autonomy in at least one instance. For this reason, we felt it important to include positionality statements at the chapter's end to contextualize to the text included and disclose how we relate to the content. While we made every effort to remain unbiased, we wish to provide transparency of how we are positioned within the topic of autonomy for APNs.

Historical Context

Nursing has long struggled to be recognized as a profession [3]. In the US annual Gallup poll, nurses have been ranked as the most "trusted" profession for the past 23 years indicating they are considered honest and ethical [4]. This trust, however does not mean that as a profession nurses are respected or recognized as autonomous, valuable members of the healthcare team. Nurses have long been considered to be the handmaidens of physicians. "Doctors and Nurses" (are grouped together) not as partners but as people in charge on the one hand and their "handmaidens" on the other [5]. The relationship works well as long as nurses go along with the decisions made by physicians and "follow orders." [6] When nurses question or push back against physician orders, they are considered insubordinate [6].

Consistency in Education, Role, and Title of APNs

The concept of Advanced Practice Nurses was first introduced in the US in early 1960s although nurse-midwives and nurse-anesthetists existed prior to this [7]. Since then other countries have recognized APNs, however recognition of the role they play in healthcare is often not well understood [8]. The education, scope of practice and titles vary widely both within countries and between countries [9]. While the entry level for APNs is recognized as a master's degree, there are barriers to achieving that in many contexts, particularly in countries where generalist nursing education is still progressing [10].

Case Study—Implementing an APN Program in the Context of a Low- or Middle- Income Country (LMIC)

An anonymous donor funded a nurse-midwifery master's education program in Haiti, coordinated by three US-based faculty with volunteer support from US and Haiti-based faculty. The program was designed in a hybrid format to accommodate available resources as well as student and faculty schedules. Initially planned as midwifery only, it shifted to a dual-track curriculum (midwifery and family nurse practitioner [FNP]) when applicants expressed greater interest in nurse practitioner training due to midwifery's lower status in Haiti.

The program faced multiple challenges, including language barriers, sociopolitical instability in Haiti, and the onset of the global COVID-19 pandemic. The move to a fully online program due to COVID became a barrier for six of the twenty students, who dropped from the program and another left Haiti. Despite further challenges with internet reliability, thirteen completed the program including clinical immersions at health facilities in Haiti.

Post graduation, securing positions proved difficult given Haiti's instability and the novelty of the FNP role. Coordinators obtained funding to subsidize graduate salaries for one year, enabling three non-governmental organizations to hire them. Evaluations at 6 and 12 months showed outstanding results, leading to the hiring of two more graduates. Community health outcomes, patient satisfaction, and physician support have been highly positive, though insecurity still limits wider placement.

This case underscores the need for regulatory frameworks, role recognition, and scope of practice before launching APN programs in LMICs to ensure sustainability and impact.

Systems Barriers to APN Autonomy

Despite a global need for healthcare providers, barriers exist to APN practice that often disproportionately affect marginalized communities. In a recent US survey of APNs, restrictions included obtaining hospital privileges, providing homecare, ordering durable medical goods, and requiring physician supervision for care within the APNs scope of practice [11]. An example comes from the Aotearoa/New Zealand context where incorporation of APNs, in a model of healthcare that includes Māori health models, could positively impact healthcare outcomes, however barriers exist to developing and expanding the APN role [12].

Within institutional systems, barriers exist that restrict APNs practice; for example, requiring APNs to admit patients under the name of a "supervising physician" or limiting the procedures they can perform, or medication they can prescribe. Hospitals may block APNs from being credentialed and having any hospital privileges [13]. In healthcare systems where the medical model is prevalent, the autonomy of APNs remains fragile. Sustaining a level of autonomy requires vigilance that can be fatiguing and can ultimately lead to APNs seeking alternative practice settings [13].

Case Study—When Nurses Aren't at the Table

It is common for nurses worldwide to face challenges with representation. When nurses are absent from decision-making forums within communities, hospitals, or governments, their voices go unheard. One country where nurses have struggled to have a voice is Mongolia. Mongolia has a nurse-to-physician ratio that is significantly lower than in most other countries. Historically, there have been more physicians than nurses in Mongolia, with recent estimates of 1.09 physicians for every nurse [14]. *Nursing in Mongolia has made significant progress over the past decade, with a handful of Mongolian nurses now holding terminal degrees. These emerging nurse leaders are training the next generation and providing leadership for the profession. Although nursing is now represented within the Ministry of Health and other key organizations in Mongolia, this representation is new, and much work remains to fully integrate nurses into all levels of healthcare leadership. In this context, where establishing nursing leadership and representation at the national level is the focus for the profession, it is not surprising that APN roles do not yet exist. How often does this happen globally? When nursing is not well-respected within society, and nurses frequently lack representation in decision-making forums, APN roles tend not to exist because nurses are not present to advocate for the positive impact they could bring.* [14]

Physician Opposition to APN Autonomy

Significant opposition to APN autonomy comes from physician groups. This represents a major barrier to APNs practicing to the full extent of their training as physician organizations such as the American Medical Association actively lobby against APN autonomy in the US citing "scope creep" as endangering patient safety [15]. According to the AMA, they have successfully lobbied to defeat 150 state scope of practice bills thus far in 2025 [15]. One of several examples is their opposition to expanding the Enhanced Nurse Licensure Compact (eNLC) to include APNs. States that have adopted the eNLC recognize the license of nurses licensed in other states eliminating the need to apply for a license specifically in that state. As of 2025, 41 states have enacted legislation to join the eNLC. The Enhanced Nurse Licensure Compact for APNs was introduced in 2020 and to date only four states (Utah, South Dakota, North Dakota, and Delaware), have enacted legislation recognizing the eNLC for APNs [16]. The American Medical Association opposes the eNLC, claiming it will undermine physician-led care and "allow all four types of Advanced Practice Registered Nurses [as recognized in the US]—including nurse anesthetists, nurse-midwives, nurse practitioners, and clinical nurse specialists—to practice without any physician involvement." [17]

Opposition to APN autonomy is not limited to the US. In 2022, the Canadian organization "Doctors of BC" formally stated "NPs cannot replace doctors and they do not provide better care." [18] Fortunately, the Canadian government has taken action to ensure that patients have access to NPs within the national health system and midwifery service was included in healthcare plans as of 2024 [19]. The outcome from physician opposition in these two countries underscores the influence of lobbying by professional organizations such as the AMA and how that has repeatedly restricted APN autonomy.

Who Can Call Themselves "Doctor"

With an increasing number of APNs in the US earning doctoral degrees, and some specialties, such as CRNAs, now requiring a doctorate for entry into practice, the use of the title "Doctor" has become a topic of debate. Physician groups have advocated for legislation in several states restricting the use of the title to individuals with MD or DO degrees [20]. In California and Georgia, laws have been enacted that prohibit non-physician providers from using the title "Doctor" in clinical settings [20]. The California law is currently being challenged by nurse practitioners, who argue that it violates free speech and that their academic credentials entitle them to the honorific [20]. Other states have adopted less restrictive measures, requiring nurse practitioners to clearly state their credentials and avoid using "Dr" without specifying their qualifications [20].

The actual harm to patients from nurse practitioners using the title "Doctor" is not well established. Physicians have cited isolated cases of poor management by nurse practitioners as justification for restricting the title [21]. However, if one were to argue that a single case of physician error should disqualify MDs from using the title, the flaw in this reasoning becomes evident. Rather than a concern for patients, physicians concern over the use of the title "Doctor" represents another form of resistance to the expanding role of APNs.

Ruth Zielinski: Positionality Statement—Respect for the Profession of Nursing

I have been a nurse-midwife for 30 years, first in full scope practice and then as faculty in midwifery education in the US. I began nursing school in 1985 and as students we were told that nurses were expected to "stay in our place;" to literally give up our seat to physicians. We were explicitly told nurses don't diagnose, charting "patient resting with eyes closed" as "sleeping" was considered a diagnosis beyond the scope of nursing practice.

After completing a Master's degree in midwifery, I believed those early experiences of being viewed as a handmaiden were behind me. With advanced education, clinical experience, and a changing healthcare landscape, I expected to gain respect as a nurse–midwife.

Yet 20 years later, I found myself in a board room being informed that as nurse–midwives, we would no longer be permitted to care for patients with a history of cesarean birth. This decision was not based on adverse outcomes related to midwifery care, but rather an arbitrary mandate from physicians I had once considered colleagues. When we challenged the decision, the Medical Director stated, "This hospital is here for the physicians and their decisions stand."

Nora Drummond: Positionality Statement: An Uncertain Success Story

I have been a nurse–midwife for 7 years and a family nurse practitioner for six. I currently work in a midwifery-led practice that provides care in both ambulatory and hospital settings. I have been unusually lucky in my career to have worked with physicians and a hospital system that reflects the positive possibilities of collaborative care between Advanced Practice Nurses and physicians.

Several factors contribute to this collaborative environment, but three stand out in supporting our success. Though state-law requires that our group of Advanced Practice Nurses have a collaborating physician, our team has the autonomy to hire our own collaborating physician. By selecting our physician from a pool of internal candidates—often individuals we have previously worked with—we ensure alignment in philosophy and practice. We also have the authority to replace this physician, if necessary, which protects our professional autonomy and mitigates the undue influence a single physician could exert. The hospital recognizes the collaborating physician as a leadership role, and many who have served in this capacity have advanced within the organization, bringing their positive experiences with our team into broader institutional decision-making.

Second, our organization supports us in defining our own scope of practice, and all providers including Advanced Practice Nurses and physicians are held to the same standards set by evidence-based guidelines. As a group, we have developed protocols based on our training and standards set by the American College of Nurse–Midwives. This allows us to effectively delineate which patients we manage autonomously, co-manage, or refer to physicians. These guidelines promote clarity and consistency, while exceptions remain possible based on clinical judgment. Both midwives and physicians are held to national standards and evidence-based practices, fostering a shared approach to patient care.

Finally, while we have a designated collaborating physician, we work continuously alongside all physicians on the labor and delivery unit. This 24/7 collaboration improves unit efficiency, facilitates real-time trust-building, and strengthens mutual respect through shared patient care and outcomes. This integration allows us to capitalize on each provider's strengths—such as calling on surgical expertise for obstetric emergencies or leveraging midwifery skills to optimize vaginal birth outcomes.

These factors have contributed to outstanding patient outcomes. Our hospital's cesarean birth rate is significantly below national and state averages, with our group maintaining a cesarean birth rate between 8–11% and a vaginal birth after cesarean rate of 88%. Despite these successes, our practice remains vulnerable as we lack full practice authority in our state. Our roles depend on the trust and goodwill we have cultivated with our colleagues and administration, and changes in leadership or policy could jeopardize what we have built over the past 15 years.

Kathryn Nelson: Positionality Statement—Organizational Challenges to Autonomy

I have worked as a pediatric nurse practitioner for 20 years. My APN experience includes roles with pediatric cardiac surgery, newborn hospitalist services, and a pediatric hospitalist service in various settings, from a large academic medical center to a small community hospital. One of my favorite aspects of each nurse practitioner role has always been collaboration with interprofessional colleagues, including physicians. I have consistently enjoyed positive working relationships with my physician colleagues. Working closely with them, I have built trusting and collaborative relationships and have rarely encountered pushback in the context of these one-on-one working relationships.

Instead, when I have faced situations where I felt neither trusted nor valued as a nurse practitioner, they have typically originated from the organization and lacked a clear explanation. For example, several years ago, the organization where I worked implemented changes to its electronic health record that required physicians to co-sign everything an APN entered into the medical record. This extended beyond Billable Notes, such as Admission Notes, Discharge Notes, and Progress Notes, to include minor note entries as well. This meant that bedside nurses and nursing assistants had more autonomy to communicate within the medical record than I did as a nurse practitioner. This conveyed to me that, as an APN, I was not trusted or valued by the organization.

Veronica Dzomeku Positionality Statement: Pushback Within Nursing and Midwifery

I am a nurse–midwife with over 30 years of professional experience spanning clinical practice, education, and research. My academic journey has taken me through advanced nursing and midwifery studies, culminating in doctoral training and scholarly contributions that seek to advance maternal and neonatal health, strengthen nursing and midwifery education, and influence health policy within Africa and beyond.

My positionality is shaped by both privilege and struggle. On the one hand, I have had the opportunity to obtain advanced academic credentials in nursing and midwifery and to serve in leadership and research roles. On the other hand, my trajectory has not been without resistance. Throughout my career, I have encountered some professional pushback not only from other disciplines but also from within nursing and midwifery itself. In my early professional years, I was met with dismissive questions such as, "What will you use your degrees in nursing and midwifery for?" and belittling remarks suggesting that, regardless of my education, I would "still serve bedpans."

These experiences reflect broader societal and institutional hierarchies that devalue nursing and midwifery, especially in African contexts where power dynamics within health systems often marginalize these professions. Such attitudes have both challenged and strengthened me. They have pushed me to reimagine nursing and midwifery not merely as technical or subordinate roles but as intellectual, leadership, and advocacy professions capable of shaping health outcomes, policy, and systems of care.

As a clinician, I carry with me the lived realities of mothers, newborns, and families navigating fragile health systems. As an educator, I mentor the next generation of nurses and midwives to see themselves as innovators and leaders. As a researcher, I position myself within the global academic space while remaining deeply rooted in African realities.

My positionality is therefore one of resistance, advocacy, and transformation. I acknowledge the structural inequities and stereotypes that have historically undermined nursing and midwifery, while also recognizing my responsibility to disrupt them. I see my role as leveraging my academic credentials, professional experience, and lived challenges to shift narratives: from bedpans to boardrooms, from undervaluation to evidence-driven influence, and from silence to systemic change.

Conclusion

Progress in expansion of APNs globally will continue to be hampered by cultural and professional barriers unless individuals and organizations work to break down those barriers. Organizations such as the American Association of Nurse Practitioners are actively working to achieve full scope practice for APNs in the US and globally. Organizations such as the International Council for Nursing established the Nurse Practitioner/Advanced Practice Nurse Network (NP/APN Network) as an affiliate more than 20 years ago.

While evidence consistently shows that patients are highly satisfied with care received by APNs [22, 23], there is a lack of knowledge in what APNs are and what they do leading to confusion and mistrust [24]. Leveraging social media as an educational tool provides an opportunity to counter misinformation, highlight the rigorous preparation and scope of APNs, and ultimately strengthen recognition and acceptance of their critical role in improving health care delivery globally.

References

1. What Should You Call Us? | ASH Clinical News | American Society of Hematology. https://ashpublications.org/ashclinicalnews/news/1958/What-Should-You-Call-Us. Accessed 9 Sept 2025.
2. Torrens C, Campbell P, Hoskins G, et al. Barriers and facilitators to the implementation of the advanced nurse practitioner role in primary care settings: a scoping review. Int J Nurs Stud. 2020;104:103443. https://doi.org/10.1016/j.ijnurstu.2019.103443.
3. Karnick PM. The elusive profession called nursing. Nurs Sci Q. 2014;27(4):292–3. https://doi.org/10.1177/0894318414546422.

4. Inc G. Americans' Ratings of U.S. Professions Stay Historically Low. Gallup.com. January 13, 2025. https://news.gallup.com/poll/655106/americans-ratings-professions-stay-historically-low.aspx. Accessed 9 Sept 2025.
5. Chapman C. Report of the Committee on Nursing, Chairman: Professor Asa Briggs, Cmnd. 5115, HMSO, London, 1972. x+327 pp. £1.90. J Soc Policy. 1973;2(3):286–8. https://doi.org/10.1017/S0047279400003123.
6. Holder VL. From handmaiden to right hand—the infancy of nursing. AORN J. 2004;79(2):374–90. https://doi.org/10.1016/S0001-2092(06)60614-5.
7. Sheer B, Wong FKY. The development of advanced nursing practice globally. J Nurs Scholarsh. 2008;40(3):204–11. https://doi.org/10.1111/j.1547-5069.2008.00242.x.
8. Almukhaini S, Weeks LE, Macdonald M, et al. Advanced practice nursing roles in Arab countries in the eastern Mediterranean region: a scoping review. JBI Evid Synth. 2022;20(5):1209–42. https://doi.org/10.11124/JBIES-21-00101.
9. Heale R, Rieck BC. An international perspective of advanced practice nursing regulation. Int Nurs Rev. 2015;62(3):421–9. https://doi.org/10.1111/inr.12193.
10. Schober M. International Council of Nurses Guidelines on advanced practice nursing. Published online 2020. https://www.icn.ch/system/files/documents/2020-04/ICN_APN%20Report_EN_WEB.pdf. Accessed 23 May 2025.
11. Kleinpell R, Myers CR, Schorn MN. Addressing barriers to APRN practice: policy and regulatory implications during COVID-19. J Nurs Regul. 2023;14(1):13–20. https://doi.org/10.1016/S2155-8256(23)00064-9.
12. New Zealand Nurses Organization. Position statement on advanced. Nurs Pract. 2020; www.nzno.org.nz
13. Brassard A, Smolenski M. Removing barriers to advanced practice registered nurse care: hospital privileges. AARP Public Policy Institute; 2011:12. chrome-extension://efaidnbmnnnibpcajpcglclefindmkaj/. https://digirepo.nlm.nih.gov/master/borndig/101576355/insight55.pdf. Accessed 21 Sept 2025.
14. Dovdon B, Park CSY, McCarley N. Nursing policy and practice in Mongolia: issues and the way forward. Int Nurs Rev. 2022;69(3):265–71. https://doi.org/10.1111/inr.12773.
15. Advocacy in action: fighting scope creep. American Medical Association March 11, 2025. https://www.ama-assn.org/practice-management/scope-practice/advocacy-action-fighting-scope-creep. Accessed 16 Sept 2025
16. About. APRNCOMPACT. https://www.aprncompact.com/about.page. Accessed 16 Sept 2025.
17. How the APRN compact would undermine physician-led care. American Medical Association. June 27, 2024. https://www.ama-assn.org/practice-management/scope-practice/how-aprn-compact-would-undermine-physician-led-care. Accessed 16 Sept 2025.
18. Statement: Nurse practitioners cannot replace doctors | Doctors of BC. https://www.doctorsofbc.ca/health-promotion/2022/statement-nurse-practitioners-cannot-replace-doctors. Accessed 28 Sept 2025
19. Brown C. Canadian government says primary care by non-physicians must be publicly funded. BMJ. 2025;388:r156. https://doi.org/10.1136/bmj.r156.
20. Sanjabi S. Can a nurse practitioner be referred to as a doctor? Sermo December. 2024;13. https://www.sermo.com/blog/insights/why-non-physicians-should-not-use-doctor-in-their-title/. Accessed 28 Sept 2025
21. Gaddis G. Nurses with a doctorate in nursing practice (DNP) should not call themselves "doctor" in a clinical setting. Mo Med. 2022;119(4):314–20.
22. Htay M, Whitehead D. The effectiveness of the role of advanced nurse practitioners compared to physician-led or usual care: a systematic review. Int J Nurs Stud Adv. 2021;3:100034. https://doi.org/10.1016/j.ijnsa.2021.100034.
23. Midwifery care during labor and birth in the United States. Am J Obstetr Gynecol. https://www.ajog.org/article/S0002-9378(22)00799-2/fulltext. Accessed 16 Sept 2025.
24. American Medical Association. National Survey: patient sentiment on scope of practice. Published online. 2021; https://www.ama-assn.org/practice-management/scope-practice/advocacy-action-fighting-scope-creep. Accessed 16 Sept 2025

Educational Barriers and Global Impact

Ann-Chatrin Linqvist Leonardsen
and Benjamin A. Smallheer

Introduction and Setting the Context

Advanced Practice Nurses (APNs) represent a vital and growing force in global healthcare systems. These highly trained professional nurses, most notably including Nurse Practitioners (NPs), Clinical Nurse Specialists (CNSs), Certified Nurse–Midwives (CNMs), and Nurse Anesthetists (NAs), are uniquely equipped to deliver expert, patient-centered care across a wide range of clinical settings. Often serving in underserved, rural, or complex care environments, APNs bring advanced clinical knowledge, diagnostic acumen, and a holistic approach to care that is essential for improving health outcomes and addressing disparities.

Central to the effectiveness of APNs is the promise of clinical autonomy; the ability to independently assess, diagnose, treat, and manage patient care. Autonomy empowers APNs to fully leverage their training, exercise leadership, and collaborate meaningfully within interdisciplinary teams. It is not merely a professional privilege but a cornerstone of high-functioning healthcare systems that rely on distributed expertise and agile decision-making. Yet, despite the growing recognition of APNs and their contributions, educational barriers continue to hinder their development and practice across the globe. These barriers are not solely academic in nature; they are deeply rooted in systemic challenges such as political interference, limited access to high-quality educational programs, insufficient funding for nursing education, and a lack of formal recognition of APN roles in many countries. These

A.-C. L. Leonardsen (✉)
Faculty of Health, Welfare and Organization, Østfold University College, Halden, Norway

Faculty of Health and Social Sciences, University of Southeastern Norway, Borre, Norway
e-mail: ann.c.leonardsen@hiof.no

B. A. Smallheer
Duke University School of Nursing, Durham, NC, USA
e-mail: benjamin.smallheer@duke.edu

A. Kapu et al. (eds.), *A Global View on Clinical Autonomy for Advanced Practice Nurses*, Advanced Practice in Nursing,
https://doi.org/10.1007/978-3-032-21458-4_16

obstacles restrict the ability of APNs to achieve clinical autonomy and, in turn, limit their impact on health systems and population health.

This chapter explores the global landscape of educational barriers facing APNs, examining how these challenges affect their professional growth, scope of practice, and integration into healthcare systems. By analyzing the intersection of education, policy, and practice, we aim to illuminate the broader implications for global health equity and the urgent need to support and invest in the APN workforce worldwide.

Background and Conceptual Framework

The educational preparation and regulatory recognition of APNs vary widely across the globe, creating a fragmented landscape that directly impacts their ability to practice autonomously and contribute meaningfully to healthcare systems. Even within high-income regions, inconsistencies persist. For example, only a minority of European countries have enacted national legislation establishing minimum educational requirements for APNs [1]. These structural complexities hinder the scalability and sustainability of APN education. Understanding these disparities is essential to contextualizing the barriers APNs face and the broader implications for global health.

Global Variability in APN Education

Across countries, the educational pathways for APNs range from rigorous, graduate-level programs to informal or ad hoc training models. In the US, APNs are prepared through graduate-level education, most commonly a Master of Science in Nursing (MSN) or a Doctor of Nursing Practice (DNP). Programs are accredited nationally and include rigorous clinical training, didactic coursework, and certification exams. The LACE model (Licensure, Accreditation, Certification, and Education) guides standardization across states, although implementation varies. Nurse Practioners, CNSs, Certified Nurse-Midwives, and Certified Registered Nurse Anesthetists (CRNAs) are all recognized APN roles.

Canadian APNs also complete graduate-level education, often through Master programs in nursing with a focus on advanced clinical practice. Regulation and accreditation are managed provincially, and scope of practice varies by province, which can create administrative challenges. Programs emphasize primary care, chronic disease management, and rural health service delivery. In Canada, dual regulatory systems, one for professional regulation and another for educational accreditation, have created financial and administrative burdens, particularly during periods of fiscal constraint [2].

Australia offers APN education through Master-level programs, with a strong emphasis on clinical leadership and evidence-based practice. The NP and CNS roles are nationally regulated, and candidates must demonstrate advanced clinical skills and complete a recognized program. The Australian Health Practitioner Regulation

Agency (AHPRA) oversees credentialing and scope of practice for NPs. Clinical Nurse Specialists (CNSs), are regulated by the Nursing and Midwifery Board of Australia (NMBA), which works with the AHPRA. Nurse Anesthetist (NAs) are not recognized or have an equivalent independent role in Australia. Anesthesia is provided by specialist anesthetist doctors, with nurses acting in an assisting role, not a primary, independent one. Australian nurses in this field work as anesthetic or sedation nurses who assist the anesthetist.

In the UK, the role of a NA as defined in the US does not exist. The UK has "Anesthetic Nurses." but their scope of practice and level of autonomy are different from a NA, and they operate under the supervision of anesthetists. An Anesthetic Nurse is a nurse with a specialization in anesthesia, but their role is more akin to that of an assistant or equipment technician compared to a NA. They do not typically administer anesthesia independently and work under the supervision of a consultant anesthetist. Midwifery is a distinct, regulated profession, separate from nursing, not a sub-specialty of nursing like the American "nurse–midwife" model. While it is possible for a registered nurse to become a midwife, most midwives in the UK follow a direct-entry path.

Nurse Practitioners (NPs) in the UK are known as Advanced Nurse Practitioners (ANPs) or Advanced Clinical Practitioners (ACPs), though the role and its standardization are still developing compared to countries like the US. Advanced Nurse Practitioners (ANPs) pursue a Master's degree in Advanced Clinical Practice, which aligns with the NHS framework for ACPs. These programs include modules on leadership, research, education, and clinical practice.

Regulation is evolving, and while APNs are increasingly integrated into primary and acute care settings, title protection and scope of practice remain inconsistent. They are regulated by the Nursing and Midwifery Council (NMC), have prescribing authority, and can work autonomously, but the profession has faced challenges with inconsistent education and a lack of a separate register. Recent efforts, such as the Centre for Advancing Practice, are working to standardize the definition and education of ACP roles across the country.

India's APN education is relatively new with the first pilot postgraduate programs launched in 2012. These pilot programs, such as the Nurse Practitioner in Critical Care (NPCC) are overseen by the Indian Nursing Council. These are diploma programs designed to address workforce shortages in intensive care units. Expansion is slow due to limited recognition, regulatory ambiguity, and resistance from other healthcare sectors. Nurse- midwives are recognized in India with the "Nurse Practitioners in Midwifery" (NPMs) being trained to meet International Confederation of Midwives (ICM) standards and provide midwifery-led care. This initiative aims to formalize and professionalize midwifery, complementing the work of existing nurses, including Auxiliary Nurse-Midwives (ANMs), and improve maternal and infant care outcomes across the country.

South Korea offers APN education through Master programs, particularly in specialized areas, such as anesthesia, midwifery, and psychiatric nursing. In February 2025, the country's first Nursing Act was passed to regulate roles like physician assistants (PAs) to enhance nursing autonomy and address healthcare shortages.

While APNs have existed for decades and are legally recognized, their scope of practice is limited and tightly regulated. They are not permitted to diagnose or prescribe medications, and the profession faces challenges with a lack of clear recognition and reimbursement within the healthcare system. The country has made strides in integrating APNs into hospital systems, though primary care roles are less developed.

Norway provides APN education through Master-level programs with national regulation and clear scope of practice. Nurse Practitioners (NPs) are integrated into primary care and community health, and their roles are supported by legislation. Norway serves as a model for countries seeking to formalize NP roles within universal health systems, with authorization from the Norwegian Directorate of Health. However, the role is still in the early stages of implementation in Norway, with a lack of formal role protection and standardized descriptions. Also, regarding other APN roles, the hospitals themselves assess whether the education is sufficient to practice as NA or CNS. Nurse-midwives are recognized in Norway and must hold an authorization status granted by the Norwegian Directorate of Health after meeting their approval or authorization requirements.

In contrast, many low-resource settings lack formalized programs, standardized curricula, or qualified faculty to deliver advanced practice education. This disparity undermines the consistency and quality of APN preparation globally.

Regulatory Challenges and Credentialing Gaps

The lack of cohesive regulatory frameworks further compounds educational challenges. In many countries, APNs face unclear or restrictive title protection and scope-of-practice laws, which limit their ability to practice independently—even when they possess advanced training. The US LACE consensus model, while intended to unify APN standards, has introduced its own set of challenges, including variability in implementation across states and confusion around role delineation.

Credentialing gaps and inconsistent recognition of APN qualifications prevent seamless integration into healthcare systems. Without clear regulatory support, APNs may struggle to gain professional legitimacy, secure appropriate roles, or advocate for expanded practice authority.

Political Challenges

Political and institutional dynamics play a significant role in shaping APN education and practice. In countries such as Kenya and several European nations, the absence of national policies or standardized regulations has stymied the development of APN roles. Even where regulations exist, they often impose restrictive scopes of practice that prevent APNs from working to their full potential [2, 3].

Oversight of APN roles is frequently fragmented, with governance left to individual institutions or regional bodies. This decentralization leads to inconsistent standards and role ambiguity [3, 4]. Moreover, increasing involvement of non-nursing stakeholders in regulatory processes has introduced additional barriers, often prioritizing institutional or political interests over clinical efficacy and workforce development [4]. In low-resource settings, financial constraints and inadequate infrastructure further limit the expansion of APN roles. For example, in Kenya, the lack of funding and institutional support has significantly hindered the establishment of formal APN education programs [5].

Impact on Clinical Autonomy

These educational and regulatory barriers have a direct impact on APNs' clinical autonomy. Without robust preparation and legal recognition, APNs may be restricted in core functions such as prescribing medications, diagnosing conditions, and leading care teams. These limitations not only diminish the professional scope of APNs but also reduce their effectiveness in addressing healthcare gaps—particularly in rural and underserved communities where their expertise is most needed.

Global Health Implications

The underutilization of APNs due to educational barriers has significant consequences for global health. APNs are critical to achieving universal health coverage, addressing workforce shortages, and managing the growing burden of chronic disease. Countries that have invested in APN education and autonomy—such as Canada, the United States, and Australia—demonstrate improved patient outcomes, enhanced access to care, and greater cost-effectiveness.

Task-sharing, driven by physician shortages and evolving health needs, has prompted many nations to adopt APN roles. However, the success of these initiatives depends heavily on governance models, which vary widely and affect implementation outcomes [3, 6]. To overcome these challenges, policy recommendations include harmonizing educational and practice standards, updating legislation regularly, and ensuring national-level regulation and support for APN roles.

Current Landscape: Where We Are Now

In 2020, the International Council of Nurses (ICN) defined an APN as "a generalist or specialized nurse who has acquired, through additional graduate education (minimum of a Master's degree), the expert knowledge base, complex decision-making skills, and clinical competencies for Advanced Nursing Practice, the characteristics of which are shaped by the context in which they are credentialed to practice [7]. The current landscape of APN education reflects notable advancements, yet several obstacles hinder its comprehensive integration into global healthcare systems. These challenges include disparities in educational pathways, issues with standardization and accreditation, faculty shortages, and regulatory difficulties. The global diversity in APN education complicates international recognition due to varying qualification levels. Regulatory inconsistencies further impede APN education and practice, particularly in decentralized governance systems, underscoring the need for robust national policies. Nations undergoing task-shifting require supportive legislative frameworks to enable comprehensive APN practice. APN programs universally require entrants to be registered or generalist nurses with academic degrees, typically demanding a minimum of two years of nursing experience, with some requiring up to seven years [8]. These variations contribute to uncertainties regarding APN education, roles, and scope of practice.

The CNS education is defined as "graduate program (Master's or Doctoral degree) education from an accredited school/university or department of nursing. Educational preparation is built on the educational foundation for the generalized or specialized nurse in the country in which the CNS will practice." The same counts for NPs, however the guidelines also specify that "All-purpose or nonspecific Master's degree nursing programs are not a recommended pathway for NPs. Master's degree education related to nursing management, nursing research, or nursing education alone is not considered sufficient preparation for NPs. Existing Master's-level programs may be adapted to include additional skills specific to NP practice including advanced physical assessment, advanced clinical reasoning and diagnostic decision-making, pharmacology/pharmacokinetics, clinical and professional leadership, and practice-based research." [7] The minimum standard for the educational preparation of NAs is also a Master's degree. However, for some countries, this is an aspirational goal, as country-specific issues currently prevent this minimum standard for Master's-level education from being realized. It has been suggested that countries, "Make available a level of advanced education that is realistic considering the country's needs and availability of human and financial resources." [9] The pathway to become a midwife can be by either following initial education as a nurse, or "direct entry" into a midwifery education program. There is a growing call for the minimum education of midwives and nurses to be standardized at the bachelor degree level [10].

The evolving landscape of APN education highlights significant progress, yet persistent barriers challenge its full integration into global healthcare systems. These educational obstacles primarily consist of disparities in educational pathways, standardization and accreditation issues, faculty shortages, and regulatory hurdles. The global diversity in APN education, with countries offering varying levels of qualifications, complicates international recognition and standardization. For example, Canada and the US provide comprehensive credentials for APNs, including Doctoral degrees, whereas countries like Ghana, Israel, and Spain offer lower-level certifications [2, 8, 11]. The Nordic and Baltic countries demonstrate a more homogenous approach, aligning with the competencies recommended by the ICN guidelines [12], even if there are variations here as well. While mandating a Master's degree for APNs, countries like France lack a national strategy for APN role implementation [13]. Wheeler et al. [8] surveyed the global status of APN scope of practice, education, regulation, and practice in 26 countries. Table 1 gives an overview of the variations between countries regarding APN education.

Table 1 shows that program length varies from 18 months to 5 years according to program type and degree, with most reporting programs that require 2–3 years of

Table 1 Overview of education characteristics for APNs

Country	*N*	Formal education, no. of programs	Education credential	Types of education for NPS/APNS[a]	Program details	Student requirement details
Australia	5	Yes, >10	Doctorate, Master's	a-m	2 year full time/3 year part time 300 dedicated clinical, 5000 hours before endorsement as NP Funding by government and/or student.	Registration as RN/ generalist nurse Academic degree Minimum 2 years as RN in specified clinical field and2 years of current advanced nursing practice in same clinical field
Botswana	2	Yes, <10	Master's, baccalaureate, advanced diploma	a, d, f, g, j, k, l, m	2 year full time 500 clinical hours Funding by government and/or student	Registrationas a RN/ generalist nurse Academic degree Minimum 2 years as RN/ generalist nurse
Canada	85	Yes, >10	Doctorate, Master's, baccalaureate, certificate, advanced diploma	a-m, n (anesthesia/ anesthetist, neonatal, primary care)	Program length varies according to school and degree Clinical hours vary according to school and degree Funding by government, private funding, and/or student	Registration as a RN/ generalist nurse Academicdegree Minimum of 2 years as RN/ generalist nurse
Chile	3	Yes, <5	Master's	m, n (degree generic, considered = to MSN)	2 year full time 500–800 clinical hours Funding by student	Registration as a RN/ generalist nurse Academic degree Minimum of 3 years as RN/ generalist nurse

(continued)

Table 1 (continued)

Country	*N*	Formal education, no. of programs	Education credential	Types of education for NPS/APNS[a]	Program details	Student requirement details
Ecuador (role not established outside US agencies)	1	No	N/A	N/A	N/A	N/A
Finland	4	Yes, <5	Master's, certificate, advanced diploma	a, b, g, i, l, m	Program length varies according to school and degree Clinical hours vary according to school and degree Funding by government or employer	Registration as aRN/generalist nurse Academic degree Minimum of 3 years as RN/generalist nurse, more if they will be a prescriber
France	4	Yes, <5	Master's, advanced diploma	b, e, k, l, n (oncology, nephrology)	Program length varies according to school and degree No response to clinical hours question Funding by government	Registration as a RN/generalist nurse Academic degree Minimum of 3–5 years as RN/generalist nurse, depending on school and degree
Germany	3	Yes, <5	Doctorate, Master's, baccalaureate, no credential is granted	b, c, e, g, h, k, l, m	2–3 year, depending on school and degree No response toclinical hours question Funding by government and/or student.	Registration as a RN/generalist nurse Academic degree Minimum of 1–2 years as RN/generalist nurse, depending on school and degree
Ghana	3	Yes, <5	Baccalaureate, advanced diploma	a, f, g, l, m, n (general nurse practitioner)	2–3 year full time Noresponse to clinical hours question Funding by student	Registration as a RN/generalist nurse Academic degree Minimum of 3 years as RN/generalist nurse

Hungary	1	Yes, <5	Master's	a, c, e, k, n (anesthesiology, perioperative)	18 mo. Full time 1490 clinical hours No response to source of funding	Registration as a RN/ generalist nurse Academic degree Minimum of 3 years as RN/ generalist nurse
Israel	1	Yes, <5	Certificate	No response	No response.	No response.
Italy	1	Yes, <5	Doctorate, Master's	d, e, g,	2 year full time 500 clinical hours Funding by student	Registration as a RN/ generalist nurse Academic degree
Jamaica	1	Yes, <5	Master's	d, f, g, j, l, m	2–3 year full time No response to clinical hours question Funding by student	Registration as a RN/ GeneralistNurse Academic degree Minimum of 2 years as RN/ generalist nurse
Kenya	2	Yes, <10	Master's	b, j, k	No response regarding program length, clinical hours or funding	Registration as aRN/ generalist nurse Academic degree Minimum of 2 years asRN/ generalist nurse
Netherlands	39	Yes, >10	Master's, baccalaureate, certificate, advanced diploma	a-m, n (other: Five APN types-acute, preventive, intensive, chronic and mental health. Soon only general healthcare and mental healthcare. GYN skills transferred to nurse specialists)	2 year, though one program 3 year Unclear response to clinical hours question Funding by government, private funding, student and/or other	Registration as a RN/ generalist nurse Academic degree. Minimum of 2 years as RN, generalist nurse

(continued)

Table 1 (continued)

Country	*N*	Formal education, no. of programs	Education credential	Types of education for NPS/APNS[a]	Program details	Student requirement details
New Zealand	4	Yes, <10	Doctorate, Master's, baccalaureate, certificate, advanced diploma	All except midwife. Midwives are not considered APNs.	2–5 year full time 300–500 clinicalhours Funding by government, private funding, and/or student	Registration as a RN/ generalist nurse Academic degree Minimum of 4 years as RN/ generalist nurse
Portugal	3	Yes (for clinical specialist, specialist nurse), <10	Master's, certificate	a, d, f, i, j, k, l, m, n (rehabilitation)	18 mo. No response to clinical hours question No response to funding question	Registration as a RN/ generalist nurse Academic degree
Republic of Ireland	5	Yes, <10	Master's, advanced diploma	a-m	2 year FT 500 clinical hours +100 hours prescribing question Funding bygovernment or other.	Registration as a RN/ generalist nurse Academic degree Minimum of 3 years as RN/ generalist nurse
Singapore	3	Yes, <5	Master's	a, b, c, d, e, f, g, h, i, k, l	2 year plus 1 year internship, under review to reduce to 18 mo. 800 clinical hours, increasing to 1200 in 2020, 12 mo. Internship Funding by government and/or other	Registration as a RN/ generalist nurse Academic degree Minimum of 5 years as RN/ generalist nurse
Spain	10	Yes, <5	Doctorate, Master's, certificate, advanced diploma	a, b, d, e, f, h, i, j, k, l, m, n (emergency nurse anesthetist)	2 year full time No response to clinical hours question Funding by government and/or student	Registration as a RN/ generalist nurse Academic degree

Tanzania	1	Yes, <5	Doctorate, Master's	j, l,	2 year full time Noresponse to clinical hours question Funding by government and/or student	Registration as a RN/ generalist nurse Academic degree Minimum of 1 years as RN/ generalist nurse, though 3 preferred
United Kingdom	41	Yes, >20	Doctorate, Master's, baccalaureate, certificate, advanced diploma, no credential is granted, other (unspecified)	All & n (neonatal)	2–3 year full time 500–1000 clinical hours according to school and degree Funding by government, private funding, student and/or other	Registrationas a RN/ generalist nurse Academic degree Minimum of 2–7 years as RN/generalist nurse
United States	103	Yes, >20	Doctorate, Master's, baccalaureate, certificate, advanced diploma	a-m, n (nurse anesthetist)	18 mo. To 4 years depending on school and degree 500–1200 clinical hours according to school and degree Funding by government, private funding, student and/or other	Registration as aRN/ generalist nurse Academic degree Number of years of experience as RN/generalist nurse varies according to school and program

[a]a = Hospitalist/acute care NP/APN, b = specialty care specific to disease or illness NP/APN, c = specialty care specific to an age group or population NP/APN, d = family NP/APN, e = geriatric/gerontologic NP/APN, f = pediatric NP/APN, g = adult NP/APN, h = adult gerontologic NP/APN, i = women's health NP/APN, j = midwife, k = community health NP/APN, l = mental health NP/APN, m = clinical nurse specialist, n = other

full-time studies. Several programs report a minimum of 500 clinical hours, though some require considerably more (e.g., 800, 1000, 1200, or 1490), or additional internships (e.g., 1 year long; another as long as 5000 h).

The shortage of clinical training sites poses significant challenges to the practical training of APNs. The exponential growth in health professions education has intensified competition for clinical training sites [14]. This shortage adversely affects APN education by limiting essential hands-on experience, which is crucial for developing clinical expertise. The shortage of sufficiently trained and/or experienced educators further compounds this issue, leading to deferred admissions and reducing the number of qualified APNs entering the workforce [15]. As such, implementing innovative solutions, such as utilizing teaching assistants within APN programs, have been suggested to mitigate faculty shortages and enhance educational capacity [15].

Countries like Spain and Mexico underscore the need for organizational and institutional support to overcome educational barriers. In Spain, challenges such as the predominance of medical specialization models and regional approaches complicate the integration of APN education [11]. Similarly, Mexico's nascent development of APN roles necessitates government support for advanced training, role establishment, and solid regulation [16]. Moreover, regulatory inconsistencies continue to impede APN education and practice. Countries with decentralized governance systems exhibit disparities in APN practice levels, suggesting the necessity for robust national policies as essential components for overcoming these challenges [3]. Countries experiencing task-shifting require supportive legislative frameworks to enable APNs to practice comprehensively [6].

Several solutions have been suggested to decrease these variations and to remain quality education for APNs, including targeted interventions and collaborative efforts among policymakers, educators, and healthcare administrators to standardize educational pathways, expand faculty capacity, and establish robust regulatory frameworks [1, 4].

Case Studies or Exemplars

Norway: A High-Income Exemplar of APN Development

For several decades, Norway has maintained educational programs for APNs, encompassing specialties such as NAs, midwives, and CNSs, including operating room nurses, pediatric nurses, critical-care nurses, and cancer-care nurses. Initially, these programs were hospital-based with significant variability in duration. In 1999, a national framework was established to standardize these programs (known in Norwegian as "rammeplaner"), and by the early 2000s, they were integrated into the university sector. These educational programs originally consisted of 90 ECTS credits, with 45 of those credits allocated to clinical studies and practical experience. Transitioning around 2012, the programs evolved into Master's degree tracks comprising 120 ECTS credits.

In 2019, the Norwegian government initiated a national guideline for the education of "advanced clinical general nursing" (known in Norwegian as "avansert klinisk allmennsykepleie") aligning closely with the international education for NPs. This guideline, legislated in 2020, also entailed a 120 ECTS requirement. The development of this initiative was driven by political motives, with the Minister of Health emphasizing that it would bolster the recruitment of specialist nurses within municipal healthcare settings. However, this provoked challenges in defining the professional roles for graduates and sparked debates in national media between the Norwegian Nurses Organization and the Norwegian Medical Association.

Further legislative actions were taken with the establishment of guidelines for education programs for NAs, pediatric nurses, critical care nurses, operating room nurses, and cancer care nurses, effective January 1, 2022. These programs also adhered to the 120 ECTS credit structure. Nevertheless, the government demanded that students who completed 90 ECTS credits—consistent with the previous non-Master's degree format—should still qualify to work as APNs.

In August 2023, guidelines governing the education of midwives were legislated, exclusively requiring a Master's degree and encompassing 120 ECTS credits. This has inadvertently created a discrepancy between midwifery and other nursing specialties such as NAs and critical care nurses, which have a longstanding presence within Norwegian healthcare and clearly defined advanced practice roles.

The rationale for limiting certain programs to 90 ECTS credits remains ambiguous, particularly considering these fields have a more established history. Informal feedback suggests economic reasons may play a role, citing the extended duration and associated costs of educating APNs to the full 120 ECTS level. Consequently, students compelled to conclude their studies after 90 ECTS credits face difficulties in attaining their program completion, as they are prematurely integrated into the workforce. This truncated educational approach compromises students' ability to obtain internationally recognized and transferable competencies—a Master's program is fundamentally structured from its inception rather than initiated midway, following 90 ECTS credits.

Kenya: A Lower-Middle-Income Exemplar of APN Development

Kenya presents a compelling case study in the development of APN within a resource-constrained and politically complex environment. Unlike Norway, which benefits from a well-established, nationally regulated APN framework supported by universal healthcare and robust educational infrastructure, Kenya's journey toward APN integration is marked by fragmented governance, emerging policy frameworks, and significant educational and regulatory challenges.

In 1949, the Nurses, Midwives and Health Visitors Council was created under Ordinance No. 16, marking the first legal step toward nursing regulation in Kenya. This council laid the groundwork for a self-regulating profession, adapting procedures from British models. By 1952, the Nursing Council of Kenya (NCK), the regulatory body for nursing and midwifery education and practice, was established.

The Examination Sub-Committee held its first formal exams for Assistant Enrolled Nurses Grade I and II, and the King George Hospital (now Kenyatta National Hospital) launched the first Kenya Registered Nurse training program. This program included a structured 3½-year curriculum with both theoretical and clinical components, setting a precedent for formal nursing education in the country.

The NCK was later codified under the Nurses Act Cap 257 of the Laws of Kenya, giving it the legal mandate to regulate nursing and midwifery education and practice. Its responsibilities include approving training institutions, setting curricula, conducting examinations, maintaining professional registers, and advising the government on nursing matters. Over the decades, the NCK has evolved into a central authority for nursing regulation, playing a pivotal role in Kenya's efforts to professionalize and expand its nursing workforce.

The development of the APN framework is being guided by institutions such as Aga Khan University, which offers Master of Science in Nursing programs focused on advanced practice and midwifery. However, access is limited, and national regulation is still emerging. The National Nursing and Midwifery Policy (2022–2032) is Kenya's first comprehensive policy guiding nursing and midwifery development. This document formally introduced the Scope of Practice for Nurse Practitioners, providing a framework for APN roles in Kenya. This marks a significant step toward institutionalizing APN practice, and includes provisions for strengthening education, regulation, leadership, and service delivery, aligned with WHO's strategic directions, and aims to standardize education and expand APN roles, but challenges include faculty shortages, funding constraints, and lack of infrastructure.

As of 2022, when this policy was implemented, NPs are not recognized in Kenya. However, Nurse Anesthetists are recognized under the designation of Kenya Registered Nurse Anesthetists (KRNAs), who are regulated and licensed by the Nursing Council of Kenya and represented by the Kenya Registered Nurse Anesthetists (KRNA) association. Kenya Registered Nurse Anesthetists (KRNAs) undergo specific training and possess a defined scope of practice, enabling them to provide safe anesthesia care and perform a critical role in the country's healthcare system, particularly in surgical procedures and childbirth. Nurse-midwives are formally recognized in Kenya, regulated by the Nursing Council of Kenya (NCK) and required to be licensed to practice. Kenya also approved its first national policy recognizing and incorporating midwifery in 2022, further strengthening the profession's status. Nurse–midwives operate at various qualifications, from certificate to degree levels, and serve a critical role in the nation's healthcare system.

Kenya has made strides in establishing graduate-level APN education, with universities such as Aga Khan University offering Master of Science programs in Advanced Practice Nursing and Midwifery. However, access to these programs remains limited, and the number of trained APNs is still relatively small. Faculty shortages, lack of clinical training sites, and limited funding for students pose significant barriers to scaling these programs nationally.

Until recently, Kenya lacked a comprehensive national policy guiding the development of nursing and midwifery professions. The National Nursing and Midwifery Policy 2022–2032 now provides a long-term framework to strengthen education, regulation, workforce management, and leadership. This policy aims to align Kenya's nursing development with global standards, including the WHO's strategic directions for nursing and midwifery.

Despite this progress, regulatory clarity around APN roles remains elusive. Title protection, scope of practice, and credentialing are inconsistently applied across counties, and oversight is often decentralized. This fragmentation limits APNs' ability to practice autonomously, even when they are well-trained.

Political will and stakeholder alignment are critical to APN role development. In Kenya, external influences—including resistance from the medical profession and lack of interprofessional collaboration—have slowed APN integration. Financial constraints and infrastructure gaps further hinder the expansion of APN roles, particularly in rural and underserved areas.

In contrast, Norway has a nationally unified APN framework supported by legislation, standardized curricula, and strong professional recognition. Advanced Practice Nurses (APNs) in Norway enjoy broad clinical autonomy, integrated roles in primary and specialized care, and clear pathways for career progression. Kenya's model, while promising, is still in its formative stages and requires sustained investment, policy enforcement, and stakeholder engagement to reach similar levels of maturity.

Challenges and Barriers to Clinical Autonomy

The fragmentation in regulatory frameworks for licensing and practice across countries poses significant barriers. In many instances, there is no clear pathway for credentialing APNs, which complicates their professional practice. The development and implementation of supportive policies for APNs are often hindered by a lack of political will or understanding of these roles' contributions to healthcare. This can result in underdeveloped legislative frameworks that fail to fully utilize advanced nurses' potential to improve health outcomes. Yet even here, variations exist, notably in prescribing competencies. The lack of prescribing authority in certain programs can limit the scope of practice for APNs, impacting their ability to operate independently and efficiently in healthcare teams. Also, recognition and regulation of APN roles vary markedly across different regions, which further complicates the establishment of APN roles at an international level. Wheeler et al. [8] noted that formal recognition of APNs by governmental bodies is inconsistent, with nearly half reporting some form of recognition and others operating without formal regulations. The absence of a unified regulatory framework creates barriers to broad acceptance and integration of APNs in healthcare systems, impacting their ability to practice at the top of their license.

Most countries with some sort of APN practice report more than one advanced role. Though most used the titles NA, NP, CNS, or midwife, other titles have been listed, such as nurse in advanced practice, expert nurse, nurse specialist, and others. In some countries the term *CNS* (or a similar title) referred to nurses who function more as NPs, or vice versa (i.e., providers titled NP but who functioned more as

CNSs). Some countries report that midwives are commonly educated at the registered/generalist level or as a non-nurse, while other countries report educating midwives at a post registered/generalist nurse level. Title protection as APN has been reported in Australia, Botswana, Canada, France, Hungary, Israel, Jamaica, the Netherlands, New Zealand, Portugal, Republic of Ireland, Singapore, and the US. Similar title protection is not reported in Chile, Finland, Germany, Ghana, Italy, Kenya, Spain, Tanzania, or the UK [8].

In most countries, the basis for development of the APN role has been due to a need for providers in rural or underserved areas, specifically physician shortage issues in neonatal care or psychiatry, or policy changes that limited work hours of residents or junior doctors. Development of APN roles has been advocated by various sources; government, international organizations, individual nurses, individual physicians, consumers, insurance companies, universities, media, and/or in-country nursing, physician, non-governmental/non-profit institutions or private institutions. In contrast, physician organizations, individual physicians, individual nurses, and governments also have opposed such role development [8].

The common barriers to APN role implementation include a lack of recognition of roles at national levels, role ambiguity, lack of clear scope of practice, resistance from male physicians, low involvement of nurses in policy-making, and low status of nursing as a profession [6]. As such, a Swedish study from 2010, found that APNs and GPs expressed confidence and trust in the APNs' new role, noting that initial resistance from some GPs and other colleagues was eventually overcome. The APN role emerged as distinctly separate from that of physicians, and APNs were perceived as an additional resource for both GPs and nurses, enhancing patient care availability. However, the authors stated that clearly defining and delineating the APN role concerning responsibilities and interprofessional relations was necessary. Moreover, they claimed that for advancing this role further necessitates granting APNs the authority to prescribe medication and order treatments, alongside a comprehensive evaluation from patient, organizational, and interprofessional perspectives [17]. In Finland, nurse leaders highlighted the critical role of APNs within their organizations. Advanced Practice Nurses (APNs) operated with greater autonomy and independence compared to registered nurses, serving as vital resources for managing chronic diseases and acute health issues. Advanced Practice Nurses (APNs) significantly contributed to the advancement of evidence-based nursing and enhanced healthcare service accessibility for patients. Implications for nursing management included the responsibility of nurse leaders to establish sustainable structures and organizational support systems to facilitate APN practice [17]. Ten years later, a Norwegian study showed that nurse leaders and GPs generally exhibited a positive disposition toward NPs; however, they encountered challenges in defining the roles of NPs and integrating them into existing work models. This difficulty was attributed to economic pressures, diverse departmental needs, and the dynamics of shift work. Both nurse leaders and GPs concurred that NPs should not supplant physicians but should instead fulfill the responsibilities associated with advanced practice nursing with greater expertise. Furthermore, nurse leaders expressed a desire for NPs to serve as a resource for registered nurses. Establishing trust in the new role among not only GPs but also registered nurses was deemed crucial. Implications for practice emphasize the necessity of a proactive implementation team that seeks to establish an appropriate model for the integration process. Early clarification of the roles, tasks, and responsibilities of NPs during the initial stages of implementation could significantly facilitate this process [18].

Also, in Switzerland, the development of the APN role is in its nascent stages, with several unresearched pilot projects underway. A 2019 study aimed to investigate the experiences of APNs and GPs involved in integrating the APN role into Swiss primary care. Participants viewed themselves as pioneers developing new primary care models (pioneering spirit). Both nurses and doctors acknowledged the additional value of the APN role in enhancing care quality and flexibility. However, participants stressed the importance of seeking advice for diagnostic and treatment uncertainties. A noted barrier was the lack of understanding among GPs about the APN role. As such, the introduction of APNs in Swiss primary care is marked by diverse, small-scale initiatives led by pioneering GPs and APNs who recognize the benefits and limitations of APNs amid a lack of governance and understanding among GPs [19].

Strategies, Innovations, and Best Practices

Advanced Practice Nurse (APN) has emerged as a pivotal force in global healthcare, offering a spectrum of roles that bridge critical gaps in healthcare delivery, particularly in underserved or complex settings. These highly trained professionals provide expert care and have the potential to transform healthcare systems through clinical autonomy, educational advancement, and systematic integration.

Clinical autonomy is fundamental for APNs to exploit their training fully, especially concerning decision-making, leadership, and collaborative care. It is the freedom to enact expert judgment and implement healthcare strategies independently, often improving patient outcomes in diverse settings. Autonomy enables APNs to lead care teams, customize patient care, and prescribe medications, contingent upon their comprehensive training. However, the promise of autonomy becomes unattainable without systematic support through robust educational frameworks and recognition of the profession at national and global levels.

Globally, the education and regulation of APNs are fraught with variability and inconsistencies. Educational preparation ranges starkly from one country to another, with the US typically providing Master's-level programs while other countries may lack standardized curricula or qualified faculty. Such disparities hinder APNs' ability to gain universally recognized credentials, impacting their mobility and practice autonomy across borders. In Canada, dual regulatory processes create financial and administrative burdens for APNs, while European countries struggle with the absence of national legislation establishing minimum educational requirements. These educational barriers not only restrict the professional growth of APNs but also contribute to workforce shortages, thereby compromising healthcare delivery, especially in regions with limited resources.

Political challenges further compound the difficulties in APN role development. The lack of national policies in countries like Kenya and fragmented oversight in Europe impede recognition and development of APN roles. Often, stakeholders external to the nursing profession influence regulatory measures, adding layers of complexity to practice autonomously. This scenario restricts the APN's ability to function optimally, particularly in resource-constrained settings where their roles could substantially impact healthcare accessibility.

The consequence of educational inadequacies and political constraints is manifest in the compromised clinical autonomy of APNs. With insufficient support, APNs encounter limitations in prescribing, diagnosing, and leading healthcare teams—components crucial to clinical autonomy. This restriction diminishes the effectiveness of APNs, especially in addressing healthcare gaps in rural or underserved areas, thus impeding their contribution to global health goals, such as universal health coverage.

Educational barriers and restrictive regulatory frameworks hinder the optimal utilization of APNs in achieving universal health coverage and tackling workforce shortages. Countries that have invested robustly in APN education and autonomy, including Canada, the US, and Australia, present improved patient outcomes, enhanced cost-effectiveness, and broader healthcare access. Task-shifting strategies, driven by physician shortages and the chronic disease burden, underscore the necessity for APN roles, yet the inconsistent governance models across countries affect implementation success.

Despite notable advancements in APN education, the international landscape remains plagued by disparities in educational pathways, accreditation issues, and faculty shortages. Countries like Canada and the US have comprehensive credentialing systems, whereas others offer lower-level certifications, affecting global recognition. Faculty shortages and competition for clinical training sites further compound the practical training of APNs, limiting their clinical expertise development. This calls for innovative solutions such as utilizing teaching assistants to mitigate faculty shortages and enhance educational capacity.

Regulatory inconsistencies present formidable obstacles to the integration of APNs. In countries with decentralized governance systems, disparities in practice levels necessitate robust national policies to resolve these issues. Task-sharing demands supportive legislative frameworks to enable APNs to practice comprehensively, yet not all countries have succeeded in establishing such structures. Universal prerequisite requirements for APN program entrants, demanding experience as registered/generalist nurses, highlight the stringent preconditions for advancing into APN roles. These conditions vary globally, contributing to uncertainties regarding educational roles and scope of practice, thereby necessitating targeted interventions and collaborative efforts among stakeholders to standardize educational pathways, expand faculty capacity, and establish robust regulatory frameworks.

Globally, the integration of APN roles is marked by varied success, providing instructive case studies. In Sweden, APNs have gained trust and overcome initial resistance from colleagues, emerging as indispensable resources in healthcare teams. Contrastingly, Finland's nurse leaders underscore the need for sustainable structures to support APN autonomy, emphasizing their contribution to evidence-based nursing and healthcare accessibility. In Norway, nurse leaders advocate defining APN roles clearly and integrating them into existing work models. Trust-building among healthcare teams is deemed crucial for APN role success. Switzerland's pioneering efforts to introduce APNs in primary care amid governance and understanding barriers reflect the complexities faced by APNs in gaining recognition and establishing practice.

Fragmentation in regulatory frameworks remains a significant barrier to APN practice. Lack of clear credentialing pathways complicates professional advancement, while limited political understanding restricts policy development. Prescriptive authority varies across regions, affecting APN practice autonomy. Without formal recognition by governmental bodies, APNs struggle to practice at the zenith of their expertise, impacting healthcare systems' efficiency. Advanced Practice Nurse (APN) roles, although diverse, face common challenges, including role ambiguity and lack of clear scope of practice. Resistance from medical hierarchy, low involvement in policymaking, and nursing's professional status further hinder the integration and recognition of APNs. Overcoming these barriers necessitates strategic advocacy by governments, insurance companies, international organizations, and other stakeholders.

Advanced Practice Nurse (APN) presents a transformative opportunity for global healthcare systems, yet its potential is curtailed by educational barriers, political interference, and regulatory inconsistencies. Addressing these challenges requires a concerted effort toward harmonizing education and practice standards, updating laws regularly, and ensuring national-level regulation. Through strategic interventions and collaborative efforts, APNs can achieve true clinical autonomy, thereby optimizing their role in delivering quality healthcare and advancing global health objectives.

Future Considerations and Directions

The future of APNs lies in a coordinated global effort to dismantle educational and regulatory barriers while advancing policies that empower nurses to practice to the full extent of their training. The World Health Organization's *Global Strategic Directions for Nursing and Midwifery* (2021–2025) provides a critical framework for guiding this transformation. It outlines four strategic policy areas—education, jobs, leadership, and service delivery—that collectively support the optimal contribution of nurses and midwives to health systems worldwide [10].

Education: Building a Competent Workforce

Education is the cornerstone of a strong nursing and midwifery workforce. The WHO emphasizes the need for competency-based education that equips nurses and midwives with the skills required to meet evolving population health needs. This includes expanding access to graduate-level programs, integrating interprofessional education, and ensuring curricula are aligned with global health priorities. Faculty development is also critical, as many countries face shortages of qualified educators capable of delivering advanced practice content. By investing in high-quality education, countries can prepare nurses to take on expanded roles in clinical care, leadership, and policy.

In addition to initial training, the WHO advocates for lifelong learning and continuing professional development. As healthcare systems become more complex and technology-driven, nurses must be supported updating their skills and knowledge throughout their careers. Digital platforms, simulation-based learning, and international partnerships can help overcome geographic and resource limitations. Ultimately, a well-educated nursing workforce is essential for achieving universal health coverage and responding effectively to public health emergencies, chronic disease management, and health inequities.

Jobs: Creating and Sustaining Employment

The WHO calls for the creation of sustainable, well-supported jobs for nurses and midwives, recognizing that workforce shortages and poor working conditions undermine health system performance. Countries must develop policies that ensure fair compensation, safe work environments, and career-progression opportunities. These measures are essential not only for retaining skilled professionals but also for attracting new entrants into the profession. In particular, APNs require clearly defined roles and deployment strategies that allow them to work to the full extent of their training, especially in underserved and rural areas.

Ethical recruitment and international mobility management are also key components of this strategic area. Many low- and middle-income countries face the challenge of losing trained nurses to higher-income nations due to better pay and working conditions. World Health Organization (WHO) encourages countries to adopt ethical recruitment practices and to invest in domestic workforce development to reduce dependency on foreign-trained professionals. By creating meaningful employment opportunities and managing migration responsibly, countries can build resilient health systems and ensure equitable access to care.

Leadership: Strengthening Influence and Advocacy

Leadership development is essential for empowering nurses and midwives to shape health policies and drive innovation. The WHO urges countries to integrate nurses into decision-making bodies at all levels of the health system—from local governance to national ministries. This includes creating leadership pathways within clinical, academic, and regulatory settings. Advanced Practice Nurses (APNs), with their advanced training and systems-level perspective, are particularly well-positioned to lead initiatives that improve care delivery, promote health equity, and respond to emerging health threats.

The strategy also emphasizes the importance of gender equity and diversity in leadership. Given that nursing is a predominantly female profession, elevating women into leadership roles is both a matter of justice and a strategic imperative. Mentorship programs, leadership training, and institutional support can help nurses build the confidence and skills needed to advocate for their profession and influence policy. By strengthening nursing leadership, countries can ensure that health systems are guided by those with frontline experience and a deep understanding of patient needs.

Service Delivery: Enabling Full Scope of Practice

Service delivery focuses on creating environments where nurses and midwives are empowered to provide safe, high-quality care. The WHO advocates for removing restrictive scope-of-practice laws and clarifying role definitions to enable nurses—especially APNs—to practice autonomously. This includes granting authority to diagnose, prescribe, and lead care teams, particularly in primary care and community health settings. When nurses are allowed to work to the full extent of their education and training, health systems become more efficient, responsive, and equitable.

To support optimal service delivery, countries must invest in infrastructure, technology, and supportive supervision. This includes access to electronic health records, telehealth platforms, and clinical decision support tools. Interprofessional collaboration and team-based care models are also essential for maximizing the impact of nursing services. By enabling full scope of practice and providing the necessary resources, health systems can better meet the needs of diverse populations and improve outcomes across the continuum of care.

Monitoring and Accountability

The World Health Organization's Global Strategic Directions for Nursing and Midwifery (2021–2025) places strong emphasis on data-driven decision-making and accountability as foundational elements for effective policy implementation and workforce development. This emphasis is operationalized through a monitoring and accountability framework that supports countries in tracking progress, identifying gaps, and making informed decisions about investments and reforms in nursing and midwifery [10].

At the heart of this framework is the data-dialog-decision-making continuum, which encourages countries to collect and analyze workforce data, engage in intersectoral policy dialog, and use evidence to guide strategic actions. The World Health Organization (WHO) leverages existing reporting mechanisms from Member States to ensure consistency and comparability across regions. This approach not only promotes transparency but also enables countries to align their nursing and midwifery strategies with broader health system goals, such as achieving Universal Health Coverage (UHC), responding to public health emergencies, and addressing workforce shortages in rural and underserved areas. By aligning national strategies with WHO's global directions, countries can unlock the full potential of APNs to advance health equity, strengthen primary care, and respond to emerging health challenges. The path forward requires bold leadership, sustained investment, and a shared commitment to empowering nurses as central agents of change.

Policy priorities of the WHO include the following:

Policy priority: Design education programs to be competency-based, apply effective learning design, meet quality standards, and align with population health needs.

Competency-based education as an outcomes-based approach to curricula design and implementation can contribute to the health of the community when context-specific health issues are used to determine the desired competencies.

Education accreditation, while primarily an accountability mechanism to ensure institutions meet quality standards, also serves to identify and address areas to improve the competencies and numbers of faculty, admissions criteria, and students' competencies through updated and contextually relevant curricula. Accreditation standards should reflect emerging trends in health services, which will influence future health practice, including changing burdens of disease, health systems redesign, interprofessional team-based care, disaster preparedness, patient safety, and the use of technologies.

Action: In collaboration with health and education stakeholders, define the outcomes of curricula as aligned with the health needs and roles of midwives and nurses working within people-centered, integrated, team-based health and care settings. Ensure an appropriate foundation of knowledge to enable the provision of best practices in care provision and appropriate preservice clinical learning opportunities. Require the accreditation of all nursing and midwifery education programs, including private for-profit, to support high-quality education. Collaborate with accreditation organizations to identify and redress quality issues. The Framework for action to strengthen midwifery education is a guide to develop high quality, sustainable pre and in-service midwifery education with a seven-step action plan for stakeholders [10]

Policy Priority: Ensure that faculty are properly trained in the best education methods and technologies, with demonstrated expertise in content areas. Increasing the number while ensuring the quality of faculty will require advanced training or coursework in educational processes and methods, as well as engagement with clinical settings to identify expert clinicians to mentor or supervise students in these settings. It will also require increased investment in digital technologies and infrastructure and training of faculty in the use of digital technology for remote learning, clinical simulations, and engagement with clinical mentors and students in remote or rural areas. Educators must be able to maintain clinical competence, as well as developing and strengthening clinical and didactic teaching and research skills.

Action: Use accreditation findings to determine where investments must be made in faculty recruitment, retention, and development. Investments may be needed in information technology or equipment and to increase access to digital technology for students and faculty in rural or remote areas Develop processes to reward or promote high-performing faculty. Encourage the use of bridge programs (for example, baccalaureate completion) or programs to increase the number of expert clinicians eligible to enroll in graduate schemes that prepare faculty in leadership, systems management, and the conduct of clinical research, including postgraduate coursework Networks of academics and researchers and international faculty exchange programs have been effective in building research capacity among educators [10].

Policy priority: Align the levels of education with optimized roles within the health and academic systems. Reviewing the relevance of program levels with respect to an optimized skill mix of health professionals may indicate a need to adapt or upgrade entry or completion requirements for nursing and midwifery education programs. A key consideration is maintaining a wide array of entry points to education programs, while elevating the status of nursing and midwifery through higher education degrees that bring greater responsibilities in health settings, as well as career advancement opportunities. However, these must match with the institutional capacity for new programs and an ability to absorb graduates into the health and academic systems.

Enabling actions: Assess whether entry-level nursing and midwifery education programs prepare graduates to assume roles in health system and academic settings that utilize the full extent of their education and training. Consider "bridge" programs and other mechanisms to upgrade the education credentials of students and how advanced education can correspond with greater responsibility in the workplace and commensurate remuneration. Explore the geographic harmonization of entry and completion requirements, including opportunities for interprofessional education, to prepare students for multidisciplinary teamwork once in service delivery settings [10].

References

1. De Raeve P, Davidson PM, Bergs J, Patch M, Jack SM, Castro-Ayala A, et al. Advanced practice nursing in Europe-results from a pan-European survey of 35 countries. J Adv Nurs. 2024;80(1):377–86.
2. Staples E. The tension between regulation and the pursuit of quality in Canadian nurse practitioner education programs. Policy Polit Nurs Pract. 2022;23(1):41–7.
3. Maier CB. The role of governance in implementing task-shifting from physicians to nurses in advanced roles in Europe, U.S., Canada, New Zealand and Australia. Health Policy. 2015;119(12):1627–35.
4. Ainslie M, Collins AF, Hebert D, Moore J, Schriefer SP, Venzke MH. Overcoming barriers to healthcare reform: a call to action. Policy Polit Nurs Pract. 2024;25(4):254–9.
5. Ndirangu-Mugo E, Kimani RW, Onyancha C, Mutwiri BD, May B, Kambo I, Tallam E, Koech N, Mukuna A, Henderson C, Shumba CS. Scopes of practice for advanced practice nursing and advanced practice midwifery in Kenya: a gap analysis. Int Nurs Rev. 2024 Jun;71(2):276–84.

6. Almukhaini S, Weeks LE, Macdonald M, Martin-Misener R, Ismaili ZA, Macdonald D, et al. Advanced practice nursing roles in Arab countries in the eastern Mediterranean region: a scoping review. JBI Evid Synth. 2022;20(5):1209–42.
7. International Council of Nurses. Guidelines on advanced practice nursing 2020. 2020.
8. Wheeler KJ, Miller M, Pulcini J, Gray D, Ladd E, Rayens MK. Advanced practice nursing roles, regulation, education, and practice: a global study. Ann Glob Health. 2022;88(1):42.
9. International Council of Nurses. Guidelines on advanced practice nursing- nurse anesthetists. Geneva: Switzerland; 2021.
10. World Health Organisation. Global strategic directions for nursing and midwifery. 2021.
11. Galao-Malo R. Advanced practice nursing, critical care, and Spain: a point of view. Enferm Intensiva (Engl Ed). 2025;36(1):100491.
12. Sulosaari V, Blaževičienė A, Bragadóttir H, Bäckström J, Heikkilä J, Hellesø R, et al. A comparative review of advanced practice nurse programmes in the Nordic and Baltic countries. Nurse Educ Today. 2023;127:105847.
13. Colson S, Schwingrouber J, Evans C, Roman C, Bourriquen M, Lucas G, et al. The creation and implementation of advanced practice nursing in France: experiences from the field. Int Nurs Rev. 2021;68(3):412–9.
14. Kayingo G, Gordes KL, Fleming S, Cawley JF. Thinking outside the box: advancing clinical education in an era of preceptor shortage. J Physician Assist Educ. 2023;34(2):135–41.
15. Baker O, Sparks H, Dalley CB, Everson M, Crowell N, Eshkevari L. Examination of a nurse anesthesia program's teaching assistant model and its impact on increasing nurse anesthesia education capacity. AANA J. 2023;91(3):211–7.
16. Nigenda G, Lee G, Aristizabal P, Walters G, Zárate-Grajales RA. Progress and challenges for advanced practice nursing in Mexico and the United Kingdom. J Nurs Manag. 2021;29(8):2461–9.
17. Fagerström L, Glasberg AL. The first evaluation of the advanced practice nurse role in Finland—the perspective of nurse leaders. J Nurs Manag. 2011;19(7):925–32.
18. Holm Hansen E, Bomann E, Bing-Jonsson P, Fagerstrom LM. Introducing nurse practitioners into Norwegian primary healthcare-experiences and learning. Res Theory Nurs Pract. 2020;34(1):21–34.
19. Gysin S, Sottas B, Odermatt M, Essig S. Advanced practice nurses' and general practitioners' first experiences with introducing the advanced practice nurse role to Swiss primary care: a qualitative study. BMC Fam Pract. 2019;20(1):163.

Challenges and Solutions for Autonomous Practice

Maria Kidner

Introduction

Clinical autonomy among Advanced Practice Nurses (APNs) is shaped by both regulatory environments and real-world conditions, especially in low-resource settings. Practicing independently requires more than clinical expertise; it requires adaptability, critical thinking, and professional courage. This chapter explores the lived experiences of one nurse practitioner whose journey from rural Wyoming to international impact reveals essential lessons for APNs working in resource-limited environments. Her story illustrates how full practice authority, ongoing education, and team-based collaboration foster autonomy, professional identity, and meaningful patient outcomes.

Defining Clinical Autonomy in Context

Advanced Practice Nurses (APNs) practicing in low-resource settings often face clinical, logistical, and cultural barriers that can either restrict or refine their ability to work independently. Clinical autonomy refers to the authority to assess, diagnose, treat, and manage patients within one's full scope of practice. But autonomy is not just regulatory; it is also personal [1]. It is developed through experience, confidence, and the ability to advocate effectively for patients, even amid doubt or adversity. Globally, the World Health Organization (WHO) projects persistent and geographically uneven health worker shortages; optimizing APN roles is a central strategy to expand access, particularly in primary care and rural areas [2]. The

M. Kidner (✉)
Team Heart, Inc, Rotary International, Knoxville, TN, USA

A. Kapu et al. (eds.), *A Global View on Clinical Autonomy for Advanced Practice Nurses*, Advanced Practice in Nursing,
https://doi.org/10.1007/978-3-032-21458-4_17

International Council of Nurses (ICN) emphasizes graduate education, complex decision-making, and context-sensitive scope as defining features of APN practice—features that depend on and reinforce clinical autonomy [3].

Practitioner Reflection "To become an excellent APN in a low-resource setting requires having a positive nursing identity, optimizing continual education, and developing professional credibility. These activities do not take money or equipment; they take time and introspection. How do you know what you're going to do as an Advanced Practice Nurse? How do you know that you will make an impact, or understand the diagnostics, pharmacokinetics, pathophysiology, or hospital policies that will allow you to become your best? Well, you don't need to know before you try! Yet, you do need resources available to help you make clinical decisions until your knowledge and experience can guide your management strategies."

Building Clinical Autonomy in Rural Practice

Practicing in remote areas requires APNs to maximize their clinical judgment and innovate with limited resources. In Wyoming, a US state with vast geography and sparse population, nurse practitioners must become "generalized specialists," collaborators, and often the sole provider in emergency care because there are rarely physicians or specialists nearby. Research indicates that nurse practitioners in rural settings experience greater clinical autonomy compared to their urban counterparts, often managing independent patient panels and prescribing medications with less (or no) physician oversight [4]. To practice with full autonomy as an APN in low-resource settings for complex patients requires a personal paradigm of ethics, scientific knowledge, and understanding your nursing scope of practice that become your foundation of trust, integrity, justice, and fortitude that drive APN behavior [5]. Advanced Practice Nurse (APN) autonomy will significantly enhance your capabilities, resilience, and commitment to helping others.

Practitioner Reflection "We found ourselves in a remote town of 1000 people that served approximately 7000 farmers and ranchers. I spent much of my time as an APN student at the local clinic under two physicians who felt that if I was awake and breathing, I should be in their clinic. They stressed the importance of learning an excellent history and conducting a fine-tuned physical exam as the cornerstone of rural healthcare. The lesson I learned was the critical need to pay attention to details in low-resource settings where there are no CT scanners, MRI machines, or fancy lab tests. A detailed history and physical provide all the clues needed to make correct clinical decisions while building trust with the patient. Providing the detailed history and physical also builds trust and respect from other healthcare providers. Learning to obtain an excellent history and physical is the cornerstone of providing excellent and high-quality care in rural and underserved areas. Asking the correct questions, listening to the patient (words and with a stethoscope), and touch will guide your differential diagnosis and clinical decisions."

Rural Autonomy, Preparedness, and Systems

Standardized emergency training such as ATLS, ACLS, and PALS provides a shared language and algorithms for non-specialist teams, improving trauma and resuscitation readiness across settings [6]. Simple, context-tailored protocols and checklists—along with prepacked kits and trauma algorithms—reduce variation and support safe, rapid, team-based execution in small facilities. Where connectivity allows, telehealth and teleconsultation enhance triage, chronic disease management, and care coordination; deliberate investment in broadband and clear regulatory frameworks maximizes these benefits [7, 8].

The absence of trauma systems or protocols (or understanding the process) in rural settings can challenge early-career clinicians. Practicing without specialty backup or immediate transport options requires autonomy and rapid decision-making. Structured trauma education programs, such as the Advanced Trauma Life Support (ATLS) course, have been shown to enhance provider competency and improve patient outcomes in low-resource settings [6, 18].

Case Insight "This was my first trauma as a provider (with no formal education in trauma) and it changed my practice. Two teenage girls were traveling down a remote road and hit a tree. The ambulance crew called and reported one had a fractured pelvis, and the other had a small upper right quadrant laceration. I knew they would require transport to a hospital. Once in the ER, we quickly obtained X-rays, stabilized the pelvis, and I called the receiving surgeon who accepted the patients. We only had one ambulance; thus, we put both girls in the same ambulance. Unfortunately, the second girl had a liver laceration and hemorrhaged en route. We had not implemented trauma transport recommendations and did not place two large-bore IVs or provide oxygen. Both girls survived because of the talented surgeon who received them."

Practitioner Reflection "That experience led me to pursue the physician-only Advanced Trauma Life Support (ATLS) course. The first time I took the course I was not able to be certified because I was an APN... Eventually, I became part of the ATLS training team and helped develop mass casualty protocols not only in my critical access facility and state, but I also used them in Guyana to help an airport gain international status."

Medication Management and Full Prescriptive Authority

Another critical component of the APN role is to have full prescriptive authority to order, manage, and supervise all medication plans from simple to complex. This is most important in rural settings where cumbersome collaborative practice rules can hinder patient care and delay medication management to improve health outcomes of the community.

Practitioner Reflection "I love pharmacokinetics. Understanding how a medication works, its onset, its half-life, and how best to manage to help a patient become their best is a passion of mine. In the decades that I provided cardiology care, I loved the time it took for complex care management of profound heart failure patients. Understanding the education required for the patient to implement complex plans came into clear focus with one very special patient. I was doing my inpatient hospital rotation and came into a room with a patient in tears. The cardiologist had just left the room after informing her that her heart was only functioning 10% and she should get ready for transplant. Her history included a recent mild viral illness; however, this virus attacked her heart.

After some time of patient education, I convinced her to work with me on a heart failure medication plan and told her, with patience and perseverance, together we could create a medication plan that could help her heart. Thus, after her discharge I saw her every other day for 2 weeks, then weekly until she was stable. We slowly uptitrated the required four medications to start her heart failure treatment plan. Implementing slow titration, excellent patient education on how each medication worked, when to take the medication, diet, and how to self-monitor fluid management, she was slowly able to start walking in her house without profound shortness of breath. At her one-month echo, her heart had improved to over 15%. By her six-month echo, she was well over 45%, and at 1 year, her ejection fraction was almost 60%. To achieve this success, I required full authority to prescribe, manage, and provide the education to this patient and her family to help her become her best. Gaining the knowledge of multimedication plans only requires time and diligence to read about each medication and gaining insight on pharmacokinetics. This type of care should be provided in all rural settings and is truly an excellent role for all APNs. We should not be afraid of complex plans but rather embrace them and be the ones evaluating each and every medication to be appropriate and the best for that patient. Medication management is a time for patient advocacy."

Ethics, Autonomy, and End-of-Life Decisions

Clinical autonomy also entails honoring patients' values and preferences, especially in end-of-life care. In low-resource settings where documentation may be lacking, the risk of acting against patient wishes is heightened.

Case Insight "An 87-year-old man presented after a fall with facial lacerations. He was very hard of hearing, frail, and unbalanced. After I completed the complex facial suturing, I suggested that he be admitted for the night to be observed. Within a few hours he became comatose and required immediate transport to a hospital. I failed to obtain a detailed history. Later, I learned this was not his first fall and that he had previously refused care and resuscitation (thus the likely diagnosis was a subdural hematoma). His wife requested full care, so he was intubated, transported, and yet later died. The surgeon reminded me that honoring DNR orders is vital."

Practitioner Reflection "It first reinforced the need to pay attention to details, especially in low-resource settings where all documentation may not be electronic. Second, it taught me integrity and the value of documentation. His children filed a wrongful death suit—but my detailed notes, consistent across all my charts, helped close the case with no legal action."

Respect for autonomy requires diligent history-taking, verification of prior directives, and clear, culturally sensitive communication, particularly where paper records or family-mediated decisions are common. In some contexts, surrogate decision-making may dominate; APNs should balance patient preferences, local norms, and legal standards while documenting decisional capacity, risks, and goals of care [9]. Standardized code status forms and prompts embedded in intake workflows reduce omission and legal risk [19].

Innovation in Low-Resource Trauma Response

Innovation is a hallmark of autonomy in remote practice. The ability to devise or adapt protocols using available resources often determines clinical outcomes. Implementing cost-effective solutions, such as using fish tank flutter valves for chest decompression, exemplifies resourcefulness in low-resource settings [24]. A clinic with few resources does not mean you provide poor care; it means that APNs need to be creative and develop inexpensive pathways that provide safe and high-quality care and trusting relationships with receiving facilities/physicians.

Practitioner Reflection "I was charged with building the ER care processes in our clinic. During a continuing educational activity for providing ER care, I learned that for a collapsed lung, a fish tank flutter valve, costing $2.00, could be used and proven safe. We implemented this technique to provide transport care after needle decompression, whereas before we did not have a safe transportation process due to lack of equipment. We created posters with trauma protocols and developed trauma history sheets to communicate clearly with air transport teams. These sheets had typical medications for that trauma. Beside each medication was the rationale, dose, how to deliver, the rates of delivery, and major side effects. Thus, we could work as a team and increase our efficiency through practice and experience."

Technology, Telehealth, and Data

Low-cost devices, point-of-care tools, and digital health can extend APN reach and autonomy when paired with training and infrastructure. Telehealth improves triage, chronic disease management, and specialty access, but rural connectivity gaps require deliberate broadband investment and regulatory facilitation (licensure, cross-border practice, reimbursement) [7]. Electronic health records (EHRs) and registries enable proactive panels, track outcomes, and generate evidence for quality improvement and policy advocacy. Digital literacy and protected time are essential for uptake [8].

Team-Based Care and Role Respect

True autonomy is not isolation; it thrives in collaborative environments. When all team members—from nurses to custodial staff—are respected and engaged, care improves. Effective teamwork and role clarity are essential for delivering high-quality care in rural settings [9]. In low-resource settings, care is typically provided by few people. Trauma can quickly overwhelm unprepared staff. The autonomous APN in these settings can use the tools of detailed practice and effective interpersonal trust relationships. Dividing the tasks of trauma care into small parts/roles and mentoring others to complete the role with 100% success builds trust and encourages others to recognize their importance in the clinic (ATLS, ACLS).

Practitioner Reflection "A motorcycle crash left a woman with multiple fractures (both arms and both legs) and her husband with a pelvic injury. Our ER team included me, one nurse, a lab tech, a kitchen helper, and our janitor. In 22 minutes, we obtained the histories, physical exams, treated for shock, and stabilized both patients for air transport—splints, two large-bore IVs, oxygen and airway protection, antibiotics, X-rays, and documentation completed. Even our janitor ensured the space was safe. Everyone carried out their assigned roles just as we had practiced. That's what teamwork looks like."

"Building your clinical team requires you to teach, support, and mentor the nurses, technicians, and even cleaning staff. People who feel valued also trust you to lead them. One of the most effective ways is to compliment those you see doing a great job/task and thank your staff for their work."

Collaboration expands, rather than erodes, autonomy: Interprofessional collaboration improves outcomes and efficiency and is linked to stronger APN autonomy through trust and role clarity [10]. Structured communication practices such as SBAR, team huddles, shared goals, and feedback loops reinforce reliability and coordinated action. In addition, virtual communities of practice and mentorship help offset rural isolation and sustain continuous learning and professional growth [8–11].

Wisdom from Rural APNs

1. Provide education to every patient on why you are using a specific medication, ordering a test, or implementing a change in their plan of care. This builds trust and increases your plan success rate.
2. Recognize every patient as a unique person first.

3. Use the patient's name when you speak to them.
4. Find your country's protocols for specific diseases or trauma processes and use them.
5. Create your patient room to have a sense of safety so your patients can speak freely about their concerns. Safety is built upon trust.
6. If possible, write down your plan of care with your patient so they can better remember when and how to take medications, or what lifestyle management they need to be working upon, based upon your plan. Also include any sign or symptom in which they should return to your clinic.
7. Patient education is just as important as your plan.
8. Support all staff members and encourage them to let you know if they have any concerns about your patients, no matter how small the concern may be. Empowering your staff builds trust, and trust improves the clinic.
9. It is OK to leave the exam room to review a reference, guideline, or call for advice before making your final diagnosis and plans. Let the patient know why you are leaving the room, and you will explain the results when you return. Honesty builds trust.
10. When patients follow the designed plan, congratulate and support the patient. Recognition of success improves outcomes and increases trust.
11. Good communication is the key to success. Know how to refer a patient effectively and to whom you shall make the referral, and provide all information needed or an SBAR.

Professional Identity and Transitioning to Specialty Practice

The shift from registered nurse (RN) to Advanced Practice Nurse (APN)—and later, generalist to specialist—requires building a new identity [16]. This transition can be particularly complex in rural regions where roles are not always well-understood or supported. Engagement in professional organizations and continuous education are pivotal in shaping and reinforcing professional identity [15]. Developing your autonomous professional identity requires introspection and understanding your personal values that drive your behavior and determination to succeed [16]. The role transition from RN to APN and from generalist to specialist is typically stressful, turbulent, and challenges one's self-confidence [12].

Am I an Imposter?

For many APNs, the first experience practicing in a rural setting as a primary care provider—or in a specialty area without significant medical support—creates a period of personal chaos and uncertainty, alongside a process of self-awareness regarding professional identity and the requirements for full practice authority in rural contexts. This period can be a defining moment in the transition into rural practice. An APN's personal and professional identity, self-concept, and personal efficacy and perseverance serve as critical supports during the first 1–2 years, as accumulating experience develops into the wisdom needed to build a sustainable rural practice [5].

Imposter phenomenon commonly occurs when an APN student becomes a practicing APN or when an APN changes roles. It arises when the APN feels like an impostor—believing they should not be providing care due to perceived gaps in understanding or experience. This often involves shifts in self-concept and personal efficacy, with difficulty recognizing workplace successes despite competent patient care [22]. Imposter phenomenon is documented among medical trainees and APNs and should be anticipated when any APN begins practicing in a rural setting with limited support systems [20, 22, 23].

Successful transition to full practice authority (FPA) in rural settings is non-linear and depends on prior preparation as an APN, the individual's skills and knowledge, and the capacity to adapt to change and manage stress through self-understanding as both a person and an APN [21]. To mitigate imposter phenomenon—or when recognizing negative self-talk—APNs can review personal achievements, seek a trusted colleague to discuss current experiences in autonomous practice, and use honest dialogue to reframe doubts. Practical strategies include posting a list of ten personal strengths, reviewing recent clinical activities (accurate diagnoses, appropriate test interpretation, effective lifestyle counseling, and sound medication plans), and seeking additional support when needed. These steps help APNs progress toward becoming highly successful clinicians in any practice location [5].

Practitioner Reflection "A personal challenge that I experienced from the beginning of my rural full practice authority practice was impostor syndrome. I was a new nurse practitioner working in both primary care and the emergency room, and every patient had a different differential diagnosis list. Ultimately, I left every patient room to go consult my books to help me make the final diagnosis and develop my plan. I remember standing in the part of our clinic that had samples of medications for hypertension and wondering which medication I should start with as I was overwhelmed by all of the options! Another provider came into the room and informed me just to choose one and return to the patient to explain that one medication, and over time I would gain a greater understanding of hypertension management. Yet, he assured me that my patient would still have good care that I would provide. Plus, he shared that you get to review your plans of care in all follow-up appointments. I took that message to heart and provided the medication, then went home and did intensive reading on the pharmacokinetics of antihypertensive medications until I could devise a patient education tool and explain in simple terms why I chose each medication for the patient. This took time, and as time went by I gained wisdom through my experiences and lost the feeling that I was an impostor and realized that I was a good APN providing safe and high-quality care to my patients."

Practitioner Reflection "When I interviewed for a cardiology position, I asked, 'Why me?' The physician said his wife, a nurse educator, remembered how detailed my shift reports (history and physicals) were years ago. That reputation got me hired. With introspection I know my core values are integrity, innovation, and perseverance. These values helped me to be successful in my outpatient and inpatient cardiology clinics, acute-care cardiothoracic surgery rotation, teaching for Duke University, providing education for a year in Rwanda, led a rheumatic heart disease initiative in sub-Saharan Africa, and opened my acceptance on boards at local, national, and international levels."

"Often people ask me how I went from a rural practice to making a difference in international settings. My lesson learned is to say 'yes' if you are asked to try something new. Often it is other people who see your true abilities and they ask you to do something out of your comfort zone. Thus, I said yes to live in Guyana, South America for 6 months to help a school of nurses (I built the history and physical assessment curriculum) and yes to a year in Rwanda, Africa. I believe that APNs in low-resource settings are already dedicated to finding creative ways to provide care for those in need with the supplies they have and these activities make one innately innovative and resourceful."

Globally, variability in APN education and regulation contributes to uneven readiness for autonomous practice, particularly in low- and lower-middle-income countries [3, 13]. Solutions include aligning graduate education with ICN standards and embedding critical thinking, leadership, and cultural humility [3]; providing postgraduate consolidation through residencies or fellowships with robust preceptorship and longitudinal mentorship to stabilize the transition [12]; and fostering lifelong learning to sustain clinical judgment in dynamic, resource-constrained settings [10].

Academic Growth and Systems Change

Advanced degrees, such as the Doctor of Nursing Practice (DNP), empower NPs to lead quality improvement initiatives. Scholarly projects rooted in local data can highlight gaps in care and lead to systemic change. For instance, research has shown that full practice authority for NPs is associated with increased access to care in underserved areas [18] and decreases in 30-day mortality [14]. Not every APN can return to an academic setting for a DNP, yet every APN can read research and make a clinical impact to save lives and improve wellness.

Practitioner Reflection "In cardiology my passion was caring for women. In 2012, I read new research concerning the need to obtain the OB/GYN history to correctly risk-stratify women for potential cardiovascular disease (CVD). I learned that women with abnormal menstrual cycles, complications during pregnancy or delivery have a drastically higher risk for CVD due to endothelial cell dysfunction that will persist throughout the woman's life. I pushed for OB/GYN history to be part of every cardiac intake on women—though my male colleagues resisted. I kept encouraging my resisting colleagues and ten years later, the OB/GYN history requirement is in the guidelines for providing cardiovascular care to women. Yet, sadly many male cardiologists still choose not to ask the OB/GYN history and thereby delay treatment to protect women. Advanced Practice Nurses (APNs) can make a difference and save lives through providing education, support, lifestyle management, and medications to women at high risk due to their OB/GYN history. We can use research to make an impact from a small rural clinic to worldwide guidelines."

Professional Advocacy and Organizational

Impact Participation in national organizations can amplify the voice of rural APNs and support professional growth. Advocacy work also shapes the public's understanding of the NP role. Engagement in professional organizations has been linked to enhanced professional identity and leadership development among NPs [15]. In rural settings, many APNs can feel isolated. Yet, through professional organizations and technology an NP peer is only a WhatsApp or Zoom away.

Practitioner Reflection "I felt isolated for eight years of my rural practice as I did not even know the American Association of Nurse Practitioners (AANP) existed. After joining AANP, I received support and mentorship that led me to represent my rural state for thirteen years, then was elected to the board of directors. Often, I was the sole voice of the rural practitioner and explained that in rural settings we do not have access to equipment, specialty labs/testing, and even specialists. Rural healthcare is centered on the patient's history, physical exam, and use of available diagnostics. Through AANP I saw how even a small group of APNs could make a difference in local, state, and national policy. I learned to impact policy. Every APN worldwide can and should be active in their country's policies for the APN role. Advanced Practice Nurses (APNs) working together develop networks that are now impacting nursing worldwide. Nurses can change the world and save lives. Now I have colleagues (dear friends) around the world I can reach out to share experiences, ask questions, learn, and receive guidance with a simple WhatsApp message, call, or Zoom. Being active in a professional organization was a career-change event for me."

Regulation is the bedrock for practice; enabling policy that permits APNs to autonomously evaluate, diagnose, order and interpret tests, and prescribe is foundational to equitable access and system resilience. Frameworks for education, regulation, and titling create scope clarity, portability, and shared understanding across professions. Without such alignment, the benefits of advanced training, teamwork, and technology cannot fully translate into better patient care.

Navigating Role Conflict and Patient Expectations

Autonomous NPs often encounter skepticism—from both physicians and patients. Responding with excellence and empathy can transform these interactions. Patients want their story heard and they want to trust their provider. Advanced Practice Nurse (APNs) are not physicians. The philosophy APNs use is a biopsychosocial model in which each patient is seen as unique and requires a tailored approach to care. In low-resource settings, skepticism can be removed through the detailed H&P and patient-centered education and shared-decision plans.

Practitioner Reflection "New cardiac patients would say, 'I thought I was seeing a cardiologist.' I'd reply, 'If you'd like, I'll do today's visit and schedule you with the physician tomorrow.' After a thorough history, complete physical exam, medication explanation, and shared decision-making for the plan, no one ever asked to switch."

Advocacy During Conflict: Standing Your Ground

Autonomy also means standing up for patients—even when it's uncomfortable. Early-career experiences shape the NP's resolve to lead ethically. Advocating for patient care, even in the face of hierarchical challenges, is a testament to professional integrity and commitment [9, 17]. Many barriers and facilitators of autonomous APN role implementation involve professional judgment, working autonomously, and interprofessional and intraprofessional relationships [1, 17].

Practitioner Reflection "A young woman had a cold, pale foot. A cardiologist delayed her angiogram twice. I called a vascular surgeon who immediately intervened and saved her foot. The cardiologist berated me in front of staff and patients telling me I had no right to contact the vascular surgeon and that I was only a stupid nurse. I cried. But I knew I did the right thing. I would do it again and again over my twenty years in cardiology as a patient advocate despite what a physician would say or do. Trust your decisions, care, and be your patient's advocate."

Systems that foster psychological safety enable APNs to voice concerns and escalate care without fear of retribution—behaviors linked to lower adverse events and improved outcomes. Shared governance and inclusion of APNs in policy and quality councils democratize decision-making and align with clinical autonomy. Leadership development for APNs (coaching, change management) equips them to advocate effectively across professions and systems [1, 16].

Conclusion

The ability to fully use APN autonomy to the full scope of practice and personal ability rapidly increases over the first 3 years of practice [16]. Autonomy is not a destination—it is a journey shaped by lessons, relationships, and courage. In low-resource settings, the ability to practice independently depends not only on regulation but on adaptability, humility, persistence, and the continued educational process of seeking new information to put into clinical practice and developing innovations to implement in low-resource settings.

Practitioner Reflection "These reflections of the past all built my capacity and shaped my identity as an APN in a low-resource setting. None cost money or equipment, yet all were critical to my autonomous APN practice in cardiology, built upon my values to grow trust relationships and my technical knowledge I used to impact care locally, nationally, and internationally." "However, you must also reach out when you're uncertain. Document it. Talk about it. Learn from it. Your education gives you a base, but your experience builds your wisdom. You'll find your identity, and with it, your impact."

A Blueprint for Action in Low-Resource Settings

- Enable clinical autonomy with standardized education and regulation aligned to ICN guidelines ensuring scope clarity, portability, and patient safety [3].
- Invest in graduate education and structured consolidation with mentorship; embed critical thinking, leadership, and cultural humility [10, 12, 13].
- Build telehealth and digital infrastructure to extend reach and enable data-driven improvement [8].
- Institutionalize team-based care, IPE, and shared governance to normalize collaboration and psychological safety [9, 11].
- Measure and communicate APN outcomes (access, quality, cost, equity) to sustain policy and funding support [10].

Key Takeaways

- Full practice authority supports growth, especially in underserved areas.
- Narrative competence, history-taking, and the physical exam are critical diagnostic tools and they build trust.
- Collaboration and mutual respect and trust enable effective team-based care.
- Clinical APNs can translate research into clinical practice changes to improve care and well-being.
- Professional identity develops over time through trials and triumphs.
- Know your values and be introspective.
- Nurse practitioners can—and do—change systems, save lives, and lead globally.

References

1. Piedrahita Sandoval LE, Sotelo-Daza J, Morales Viana LC, Aviles Gonzalez CI. How does professional habitus impact nursing autonomy? A hermeneutic qualitative study using Bourdieu's framework. Nurs Rep. 2025;15(3):88. https://doi.org/10.3390/nursrep15030088.
2. World Health Organization. Health workforce: overview and projections to 2030. Geneva: WHO; 2020.
3. International Council of Nurses. Guidelines on advanced practice nursing. Geneva: ICN; 2020.
4. Smith LB. The effect of nurse practitioner scope of practice laws on primary care delivery. Health Econ. 2022;31(1):21–41. https://doi.org/10.1002/hec.4438.
5. Kidner M. Successful advanced practice nurse role transition: a structured process to developing professional identity through role transition. Cham: Springer; 2022. https://doi.org/10.1007/978-3-030-53002-0.
6. American College of Surgeons. Advanced trauma life support (ATLS) student course manual. 10th ed. Chicago: ACS; 2018.
7. World Health Organization. Global strategy on digital health 2020–2025. Geneva: WHO; 2021.
8. Adler-Milstein J, Holmgren AJ, Kralovec P, Worzala C, Searcy T, Patel V. Electronic health records and care quality: a decade of evidence. Health Aff (Millwood). 2021;40(6):887–96. https://doi.org/10.1377/hlthaff.2020.01454.
9. Poghosyan L, Liu J, Shang J, D'Aunno T. Nurse practitioner autonomy and relationships with leadership affect teamwork in primary care practices: a cross-sectional survey. J Gen Intern Med 2016;31(7):771–7. https://doi.org/10.1007/s11606-016-3652-z.
10. Swan M, Ferguson S, Chang A, Larson E, Smaldone A. Quality of primary care by advanced practice registered nurses. Int J Qual Health Care. 2015;27(5):396–404. https://doi.org/10.1093/intqhc/mzv054.
11. Reeves S, Pelone F, Harrison R, Goldman J, Zwarenstein M. Interprofessional education: effects on practice and outcomes. Cochrane Database Syst Rev. 2013;(3):CD002213. https://doi.org/10.1002/14651858.CD002213.pub3.
12. Barnes H, Faraz Covelli A, Rubright JD. Development of the novice NP role transition scale. J Am Assoc Nurse Pract. 2021;34(1):79–88. https://doi.org/10.1097/JXX.0000000000000566.
13. Oldenburger D, Cassiani SHB, Bryant-Lukosius D, Valaitis R, Baumann A, Pulcini J, et al. Advanced practice nursing in low- and middle-income countries: an integrative review. Int Nurs Rev. 2017;64(3):389–99. https://doi.org/10.1111/inr.12385.
14. Rao AD, Kumar A, McHugh M. Better nurse autonomy decreases the odds of 30-day mortality and failure to rescue. J Nurs Scholarsh. 2017;49(1):73–9. https://doi.org/10.1111/jnu.12267.
15. Goolsby MJ, DuBois JC. Professional organization membership: advancing the nurse practitioner role. J Am Assoc Nurse Pract. 2017;29(1):17–23. https://doi.org/10.1002/2327-6924.12483.
16. Lockwood EB, Schober M. Factors influencing the impact of nurse practitioners' clinical autonomy: a self-determining perspective. Int Nurs Rev. 2024;71:375–95. https://doi.org/10.1111/inr.12948.
17. Torrens C, Campbell P, Hoskins G, et al. Barriers and facilitators to the implementation of the advanced nurse practitioner role in primary care settings: a scoping review. Int J Nurs Stud. 2020;104:103443. https://doi.org/10.1016/j.ijnurstu.2019.103443.
18. Xue Y, Kannan V, Greener E, Smith JA, Brasch J, Johnson BA, Spetz J. Full scope-of-practice regulation is associated with higher supply of nurse practitioners in rural and primary care health professional shortage counties. J Nurs Regul. 2018;8(4):5–13. https://doi.org/10.1016/S2155-8256(18)30131-4.
19. American Nurses Association. Nursing: scope and standards of practice. 4th ed. Silver Spring: ANA; 2021.
20. Ares TL. Role transition after clinical nurse specialist education. Clin Nurse Spec. 2018;32(2):71–80. https://doi.org/10.1097/NUR.0000000000000357.
21. Duchscher JB. A process of becoming: the stages of new nursing graduate professional role transition. J Contin Educ Nurs. 2008;39(10):441–50.

22. Gottlieb M, Chung A, Battaglioli N, Sebok-Syer SS, Kalantari A. Impostor syndrome among physicians and physicians in training: a scoping review. Med Educ. 2020;54(2):116–24. https://doi.org/10.1111/medu.13956.
23. Mullangi S, Jagsi R. Imposter syndrome: treat the cause, not the symptom. JAMA. 2019;322(5):403–4. https://doi.org/10.1001/jama.2019.9788.
24. Deeb AP, Phelos HM, Peitzman AB, Billiar TR, Sperry JL, Brown JB. Disparities in rural versus urban field triage: risk and mitigating factors for undertriage. J Trauma Acute Care Surg. 2020;89(1):246–53. https://doi.org/10.1097/TA.0000000000002690.

Global Case Studies and Exemplars

Brigitte Woo, María Consuelo Cerón-Mackay,
Salma Almukhaini, Franziska Geese, and Isabelle Savard

Introduction

Advanced Practice Nurses (APNs) are increasingly recognized worldwide for their vital role in providing accessible, cost-effective, and high-quality healthcare services [35]. Advanced Practice Nurses (APNs), with their advanced clinical education and training at the master's or doctoral level, are uniquely positioned to deliver independent and comprehensive patient care, particularly in underserved or resource-constrained settings [9]. Much of the literature traditionally associates low-resource healthcare environments with low- and middle-income countries (LMIC). It is increasingly recognized that resource limitations also exist within high-income countries. Examples where these healthcare inequities manifest are in rural, remote, Indigenous, migrant, and economically disadvantaged communities [42].

B. Woo (✉)
Ng Teng Fong General Hospital, Singapore, Singapore
e-mail: brigitte_woo@nuhs.edu.sg

M. C. Cerón-Mackay
School of Nursing, Universidad de los Andes, Santiago, Chile

Canadian Centre for Advanced Practice Nursing Research (CCAPNR), Hamilton, ON, Canada

Asociación Chilena de Enfermería de Práctica Avanzada (ASOCHEPA), Santiago, Chile
e-mail: maceronm@uandes.cl

S. Almukhaini
Canadian Centre for Advanced Practice Nursing Research (CCAPNR), Hamilton, ON, Canada

College of Nursing, Sultan Qaboos University, Seeb, Oman
e-mail: Sallamah@squ.edu.om

A. Kapu et al. (eds.), *A Global View on Clinical Autonomy for Advanced Practice Nurses*, Advanced Practice in Nursing,
https://doi.org/10.1007/978-3-032-21458-4_18

For this chapter, "low-resource settings" are operationally defined as healthcare environments characterized by significant constraints in financial resources, workforce availability, infrastructure, medical technology, and supportive policy frameworks. Recent literature emphasizes that low-resource settings should not only be identified by economic criteria, rather must consider healthcare workforce capacity, infrastructure quality, and sociopolitical contexts [89]. This broader understanding recognizes healthcare inequities across various global settings, including high-income countries [89]. Low-resource settings serve vulnerable populations, including those who are socioeconomically disadvantaged, geographically isolated, or systematically underserved due to structural barriers. Thus, identifying and addressing diverse factors contributing to resource constraints are essential to ensure equitable access to healthcare across different populations and contexts.

Clinical autonomy, the authority of APNs to independently perform clinical assessments, diagnose health conditions, prescribe treatments, initiate referrals and manage comprehensive patient care, is a fundamental element of effective healthcare delivery, especially in low-resource settings [46]. Enhanced clinical autonomy empowers APNs to respond swiftly and effectively to local health needs, eliminating unnecessary delays in delivery of care often associated with hierarchical approval processes [93]. This capability significantly improves healthcare accessibility, particularly in remote or underserved regions, by enabling APNs to operate at the full scope of their practice and training. Having clinical autonomy further facilitates timely clinical interventions, promotes continuity of care, and reduces the reliance on limited physician availability, thereby optimizing resource use and enhancing overall health system efficiency [46].

Moreover, clinical autonomy has direct implications for patient outcomes and healthcare quality. Autonomous APNs are able to implement evidence-based interventions swiftly, thereby improving management of chronic diseases, reducing preventable hospital admissions, and increasing patient satisfaction and adherence to care plans. Evidence has consistently demonstrated that greater APN autonomy correlates with improved health outcomes, including better chronic disease management, reduced emergency care visits, and higher rates of preventive care utilization

F. Geese
Canadian Centre for Advanced Practice Nursing Research (CCAPNR), Hamilton, ON, Canada

Departement of Social Care, Institute of Nursing and Interprofessionalism, Lucerne University of Applied Sciences, Lucerne, Switzerland
e-mail: franziska.geese@hslu.ch

I. Savard
Canadian Centre for Advanced Practice Nursing Research (CCAPNR), Hamilton, ON, Canada

Universite du Quebec en Outaouais (UQO), Gatineau, QC, Canada

Institut universitaire de première ligne en santé et services sociaux (IUPLSSS), Sherbrooke, QC, Canada
e-mail: isabelle.savard@uqo.ca

[35, 97]. These improvements are particularly vital in low-resource settings, where healthcare demands often outstrip available resources, necessitating efficient and proactive healthcare delivery models. Enhanced APN autonomy thus not only meets immediate clinical needs but also contributes to longer-term health system sustainability and resilience.

Despite their potential, APNs frequently encounter barriers to achieving full clinical autonomy. These barriers include lack of or restrictive legislation, inconsistent regulatory frameworks, institutional resistance, limited professional recognition, and inadequate policies on education, funding, and employment [11, 86]. Moreover, cultural perceptions and interprofessional dynamics within healthcare teams often hinder APNs' ability to practice independently and at the full scope of their expertise [78].

This chapter aims to demonstrate, through selected global exemplars, how APNs navigated these challenges and contributed significantly to healthcare delivery across diverse low-resource settings. The exemplars from Singapore, Switzerland, and Québec (Canada), Chile included in this chapter illustrate that resource constraints and clinical autonomy are not solely issues for LMICs but are universally relevant across varied economic and healthcare contexts. Each case study highlights unique strategies and initiatives that support APNs in assuming expanded roles, overcoming systemic barriers, and delivering high-quality care despite significant challenges.

Each case study within the chapter adheres to a structured format comprising a country profile, description of APN roles and scope of practice, examination of specific barriers to clinical autonomy, exploration of innovative strategies and best practices, and a summary of measurable impacts and lessons learned. Through detailed comparative analysis, the chapter identifies common themes, such as the critical importance of supportive policy environments, robust educational pathways, interprofessional collaboration, and strategic use of technology and digital health solutions to enhance APN practice and clinical autonomy.

These global exemplars will underscore the importance and feasibility of enhancing APN autonomy in diverse low-resource settings. Strengthening APN roles through policy, professional education, and advocacy will not only optimize healthcare delivery but also significantly advance global efforts toward equitable healthcare access and improved patient outcomes.

Country Case Study: Advanced Practice Nurses in Singapore

Country Profile and Healthcare System

Singapore is an urban, high-income city–state with a population of approximately 6.0 million [19]. Its healthcare system is characterized by a strong state presence and a mix of public and private provision. The MoH in Singapore is the principal policymaker, funder, and regulator. In response to shifting healthcare demands, driven by population ageing, rising multimorbidity, and a focus on chronic disease management, the MoH has progressively expanded the roles of nurses and other healthcare professionals [55].

Advanced Practice Nursing was introduced in Singapore in 2003, originally as a strategy to enhance the professional status of nursing and to improve the retention of experienced nurses in clinical practice [95]. Advanced Practice Nurses (APNs) are legally recognized and regulated by the Singapore Nursing Board. They must complete an 18-month Master of Nursing (MN) program, followed by a one-year supervised clinical practice and licensure [97].

Despite its sophisticated healthcare system, Singapore continues to face challenges in healthcare access and delivery, particularly related to the growing demand for chronic disease management and the need to optimize healthcare workforce utilization [55]. Cultural factors, hierarchical professional norms, and resource limitations within certain sectors further complicate efforts to build a more person-centered and team-based model of care [47].

APN Role and Scope of Practice

The educational pathway for APNs in Singapore is rigorous. Candidates must be registered nurses with at least 5 years of continuous clinical practice and must be nominated and sponsored by their employing institutions to enroll in the MN program [97]. Following graduation, they must complete a supervised clinical practice before being eligible for full APN licensure [45]. More recently, APNs with additional training may also obtain Collaborative Prescribing rights, enabling them to prescribe medications under a structured governance framework. This framework refers to a formal system of oversight, accountability, and standardized procedures designed to ensure safe, effective, and legally compliant prescribing practices [98]. Under this prescribing model, APNs are authorized to prescribe medications within the parameters of a Collaborative Practice Agreement, developed jointly with their collaborating physicians and sanctioned by institutional credentialing committees [54].

In Singapore, the term *APN* is a legally protected title and the only recognized designation for nurses practicing at an advanced level. While the role encompasses functions commonly associated with both the NP and CNS titles in other countries, the titles "NP" and "CNS" are not used in the local context. Instead, the APN role in Singapore represents a hybrid model that integrates direct clinical care, advanced assessment and diagnostic functions, and system-level contributions such as education, leadership, and quality improvement [82]. In acute care hospitals, they manage patients requiring complex care, lead multidisciplinary teams, and contribute to quality improvement initiatives [45]. In primary healthcare, APNs play a key role in chronic disease management, providing continuity of care for patients with diabetes, hypertension, and other long-term conditions [95]. Increasingly, APNs are also engaged in community and specialist services, including oncology, cardiology, neurology, and mental health [95]. These roles are underpinned by specialized education and training aligned to their clinical focus, often involving advanced coursework, supervised clinical practice, and credentialing in their area of specialty.

The scope of APN practice is formally defined by the Singapore Nursing Board and is aligned with international competencies for Advanced Practice Nursing [82]. Advanced Practice Nurses (APNs) are authorized to perform comprehensive physical and psychosocial assessments, diagnose health conditions, order and interpret diagnostic tests, initiate and manage treatments, provide health education and counseling, and where appropriate, make specialist referrals or discharge patients from care.

Challenges to APN Clinical Autonomy

While the role of APNs in Singapore has expanded significantly, several challenges continue to constrain their clinical autonomy. At the policy and legal level, APNs have not yet been granted fully independent practice. Prescribing rights are limited to those with Collaborative Prescribing credentials, and even then, prescribing must occur within the scope of a jointly developed Collaborative Practice Agreement [54]. APNs without prescribing credentials must rely on physician collaborators to enact medication changes, which can delay care and affect professional autonomy.

Cultural and institutional barriers further complicate the practice environment [47]. Singapore's healthcare system remains strongly hierarchical, and traditional professional norms can inhibit APNs from fully exercising their advanced competencies. Both APNs and registered nurses have reported uncertainty about the APN role, overlap with nurse clinician functions, and occasional resistance from medical colleagues [94].

Workforce and interprofessional collaboration challenges also persist [45]. Inconsistent support from nursing leaders and institutional managers has further hindered efforts to grow and sustain the APN workforce. A recent national survey of registered nurses found that only 31% expressed interest in pursuing an APN role, citing concerns about workload, remuneration, and career progression [94].

Resource constraints also impact APN practice. Heavy clinical demands limit opportunities for APNs to engage in leadership, research, and professional development activities [95]. The role remains underrecognized in some settings, and career progression pathways are still evolving.

Finally, social and gendered perceptions of nursing may further influence APN workforce development [94, 96]. Woo et al. [96] found that gender stereotypes and limited role models contribute to a persistent gender gap in APN recruitment and retention, with men underrepresented and facing unique barriers to career advancement.

Strategies and Best Practices to Promote Clinical Autonomy

In recent years, Singapore's MoH has introduced targeted policies to promote greater clinical autonomy for APNs. Chief among these is the Collaborative Prescribing Framework, which authorizes selected APNs and pharmacists to prescribe medications independently, within the scope of carefully structured Collaborative Practice

Agreements [54]. By granting prescriptive authority and enabling APNs to manage a wider range of clinical decisions, this policy has significantly increased APN autonomy and their contribution to interprofessional and multidisciplinary care.

Formal training is a cornerstone of Singapore's approach to ensuring that APNs are equipped to practice at advanced levels. The foundational MN program prepares APNs with advanced clinical, diagnostic, and leadership competencies [57–59]. For those pursuing prescribing roles, the Collaborative Prescribing Program offers additional, competency-based training in pharmacology, clinical reasoning, interprofessional collaboration, and medication safety [57–59]. This structured pathway has not only enhanced clinical capabilities but also strengthened APN confidence in managing complex prescribing decisions, which is a critical enabler of autonomous practice.

A defining feature of Singapore's APN practice landscape is the emphasis on collaborative, team-based care. The Nurse-led Integrated Chronic Care E-enhanced Atrial Fibrillation (NICE-AF) Clinic offers a compelling example of this model in action [96]. In this community-based clinic, an APN leads the management of atrial fibrillation, supported by a family physician and a hospital-based cardiologist. Using evidence-based care pathways, electronic decision-support tools, and teleconsultation, the clinic exemplifies how interprofessional collaboration can expand APN roles while improving person-centered outcomes.

Singapore's APN-led innovations also demonstrate the power of technology to support clinical autonomy, especially in resource-constrained environments. In the NICE-AF Clinic, digital tools such as an APN-led online patient education platform and electronic decision-support flow sheets have enabled safe, guideline-based care at the community level [96]. Teleconsultation with hospital-based specialists ensures timely access to expert advice without requiring patients to travel to tertiary centers. Such digital solutions amplify the reach and impact of APNs, offering a scalable strategy for extending advanced nursing practice in settings where physician resources are limited and where APN contribution would provide safe and effective care.

The expansion of APN roles has yielded demonstrable benefits for patients. The NICE-AF Clinic has been associated with significant improvements in atrial fibrillation-specific quality of life, patient knowledge, medication adherence, and psychological well-being [96]. These outcomes illustrate that with appropriate support, APNs can lead high-quality, person-centered care that complements and enhances traditional models of care.

Impact and Lessons Learned

By enabling APNs to manage chronic conditions in community settings, these initiatives have improved access to care and reduced demand on specialized services. The NICE-AF Clinic, for example, allows stable atrial fibrillation patients to be managed closer to home, reducing unnecessary hospital visits and promoting continuity of care [96]. The Collaborative Prescribing Framework further enhances system efficiency by empowering APNs to initiate medications, adjust, and deprescribe independently, where appropriate, streamlining healthcare pathways and improving responsiveness [98].

Singapore's experience offers valuable lessons for increasing APN clinical autonomy that can be adapted to other settings. Structured governance frameworks, such as Collaborative Practice Agreements, provide a safe and pragmatic pathway for expanding APN roles. Importantly, Singapore's targeted, role-specific training builds the clinical expertise and professional credibility necessary for advanced practice. Delivered through the MN program, the curriculum is distinct from generalist postgraduate nursing education. It includes advanced diagnostics, pharmacology, and supervised clinical practice within a defined specialty, and is closely aligned with national regulatory requirements and service needs. This integrated approach, combining academic preparation with institutional sponsorship and clinical mentorship, differs from other systems that separate NP and CNS pathways.

The strategic use of digital tools, ranging from decision-support systems to teleconsultation, can extend APN impact in resource-limited environments. Fostering trust and collaboration within interprofessional teams is essential to embedding APN-led care in traditionally hierarchical systems. Most importantly, a strong person-centered ethos ensures that expanded APN roles not only improve system efficiency, but also deliver measurable gains in patient experience, empowerment, and outcomes. These lessons underscore that with thoughtful investment and cultural leadership, clinical autonomy for APNs can be a powerful driver of healthcare transformation, even in low-resource settings.

Country Case Study: Advanced Practice Nurses in Switzerland

Country Profile and Healthcare System

Switzerland is a high-income country located in the heart of Europe, with a population of approximately 8.9 million people with around 26% of people with migration background [23]. The life expectancy is high with women 85.8 years and men 82.2 years of age [24]. The country faces demographic challenges, such as an aging population, with over 20% of residents aged 65 and older [23]. The major diseases affecting the Swiss population reflect trends common in high-income countries. Non-communicable diseases (NCDs) are the leading causes of morbidity and mortality, particularly cardiovascular diseases, cancer, diabetes, and chronic respiratory conditions. Mental health issues, including depression and anxiety, are also increasingly recognized as public health priorities [24].

Switzerland is known for its decentralized political structure and healthcare system, which combines compulsory health insurance with a mix of public and private providers and high out-of-pocket costs [18]. Despite substantial investment and the goal of universal health coverage, structural fragmentation and strong cantonal autonomy contribute to regional and population-level disparities [56]. Vulnerable groups, including older adults with multimorbidity, migrants, and individuals with low health literacy and limited financial means, face barriers related to navigation, out-of-pocket costs, and uneven service availability, particularly in rural and mountainous regions [72]. The absence of a national health workforce monitoring and planning exacerbates these disparities, contributing to a general practitioner maldistribution, especially in rural areas, and nurse shortages in fields such as specialized cancer care [39]. These workforce challenges undermine retention efforts and hinder timely access to care. Moreover, care coordination across healthcare sectors remains fragmented, and access to supportive services such as palliative and psychosocial care varies widely between cantons due to limited reimbursement mechanisms for these services and interprofessional coordination interventions [70].

APN Role and Scope of Practice in Cancer Care

Nurse-led care provided by APNs is gaining recognition in Switzerland as a promising model to ensure timely, equitable, evidence-based and person-centered cancer care. Although the implementation of the APN and their roles, such as the CNS and NP, is still evolving, APN are increasingly involved across the entire cancer care continuum, from prevention and diagnosis to treatment, survivorship, palliative, and end-of-life care [27]. Most nurses working in an advanced practice role identify themselves as an APN, understood as a blended role combining role domains of the CNS and NP. Many other nurses identify themself as CNS and a few as NP. Nevertheless, the CNS and NP roles contribute in distinct yet complementary ways, depending on the healthcare setting, stakeholder support, and institutional regulatory policies. Clinical Nurse Specialist (CNS), most often implemented in secondary healthcare settings, coordinate interprofessional collaboration, manage cancer-related symptoms, and lead quality improvement initiatives. Whereas NP, often implemented in tertiary healthcare settings, such as designated cancer centers, frequently conduct comprehensive assessments, participate in tumor boards, and manage complex treatment pathways. In primary healthcare, NP are gradually becoming integrated into clinical teams, where they support cancer screening, manage treatment side-effects and late effects, and provide follow-up and palliative care coordination [27].

The development of Advanced Practice Nursing education in Switzerland began in 2000 with the introduction of the first master's programs [83]. Since then, educational models have continued to evolve and are informed by international frameworks such as Hamric's Advanced Practice Nursing core competencies [85], CanMEDS, developed by the Royal College of Physicians and Surgeons of Canada to define the roles and competencies of medical professionals [25], and PROFILES, the Principal Relevant Objectives and Framework for Integrative Learning and Education in Switzerland, which outlines core competencies for medical graduates [38].

However, master programs vary in structure, for example, with differences in credit load (90–120 European Credit Transfer System points) and the number of supervised clinical practice hours [7, 48]. A voluntary registration process for APN has been available for about 6 years through the national association called Advanced Practice Nursing—Switzerland (APN-CH), based on defined application criteria [1]. Although APN are not yet fully integrated into national legislation, such as the

Health Professions Act or the Health Insurance Law, they are being increasingly shaped and supported by practice-based and institutional efforts. Specialized cancer care in the primary healthcare setting remains limited but is gradually expanding as general practitioners and NP strengthen their collaboration [22, 27].

Challenges to APN Clinical Autonomy in Cancer Care

Several barriers hinder full clinical autonomy for APN in Swiss cancer care, particularly in resource-constrained environments such as rural areas or smaller regional hospitals. These barriers can be grouped into the following three key domains:

1. Policy and Legal Barriers: The absence of a national legal framework for APN and their roles limit role clarity and contributes to inconsistent implementation across cantons. Only a few cantons (e.g., Vaud, Neuchâtel, Valais) grant extended responsibilities such as advanced clinical decision-making and prescriptive authority [26], which are otherwise subject to local policies and institutional agreements. Further, in outpatient settings, APN face insufficient reimbursement for services such as patient education, psychosocial support, and care coordination, hindering role development and sustainability.

   The limited development of a coordinated national cancer care system continues to challenge progress in the expansion of the APN and their clinical autonomy. A national masterplan for cancer care has been developed, outlining actions to strengthen patient care, access to pharmaceutical treatment, medical research, and workforce retention. However, current discussions suggest that the focus on pharmaceutical treatment and medical research may overlook the importance of integrating other healthcare professions, such as APN and their clinical autonomy, to ensure a more holistic, evidence-based, person-centered and sustainable cancer care system [61].
2. Specialized Education and Health Workforce Gaps: While APN are required to complete a Master of Science in Nursing program [26], most receive generalist training with little exposure to cancer care. There is currently no standardized credentialing process in cancer care for APN. Existing cancer care credentials are limited to disease-specific areas (e.g., breast and cancer nursing) are not mandatory [20, 21] and do not effectively include professional development needs of APN [27]. Additionally, many oncologists, primary healthcare physicians, and nurse managers do not have a realistic understanding of APN competencies, which can lead to role conflict, restricted autonomy, and underutilization in the care of patients with cancer.
3. Institutional and Cultural Constraints: Many settings lack general administrative and managerial support necessary for autonomous Advanced Practice Nursing practice, that is reflected in specialized cancer care as well. This includes restricted access to electronic health records along the patients care pathway, absence of independent patient scheduling, and limited referral rights. In the

predominant oncologist- and general practitioner-led models of care, APNs often encounter skepticism regarding their clinical autonomy, particularly in diagnostic and treatment-related decisions [43].

Strategies and Best Practices to Promote Clinical Autonomy in Cancer Care

Despite the previously described barriers, several initiatives in Switzerland, led or facilitated by nursing and Advanced Practice Nursing associations, support greater APN implementation efforts, their recognition and therefore, the expansion of APN clinical autonomy in cancer care. At the policy level, the Swiss Federal Council's Action Plan for Health Professions promotes APN healthcare system integration and supports their legal recognition, with some cantons piloting prescriptive authority and reimbursement models for NP, offering scalable examples for broader implementation across regions and cantons. Targeted training programs, such as the European Oncology Nursing Society accredited Breast Cancer Nursing Framework [21] adapted for Switzerland, help build cancer care-specific competencies. However, a national credentialing pathway for APN, that recognizes their professional development needs in cancer care remains lacking and urgently needed [27]. Successful interprofessional models are emerging in certified cancer centers, where APN participates in tumor boards, symptom clinics, and survivorship care, such as services for patients with lung cancer [80]. These roles foster through their leadership skills clinical autonomy by participating in shared therapeutic decision-making and defined scopes of practice that provides more role clarity. Digital health tools, especially in low-resource settings, further enhance APN-led care. For example, electronic application-based symptom monitoring in post-stem cell-transplant care, facilitated by the SteM cell transplantatIon faciLitated by eHealth (SMILe) App, enables timely interventions without the need for direct physician involvement [88]. Similarly, APN-led initiatives using Patient-Reported Outcome Measures (PROMs) in sarcoma centers to help improve symptom control [28]. Another approach is laid in molecular and genomic profiling routed in the precision health approach, that empowers APN with structured data to guide independent clinical actions [16]. These strategies collectively demonstrate that supportive policy, targeted training, interprofessional collaboration, and digital tools can expand APN autonomy and improve cancer care delivery along the patients care pathway.

Impact and Lessons Learned

The implementation of APN in Swiss cancer care has led to perceived improved patient outcomes, particularly when APNs can practice to a fuller extent of their potential [27]. Reported benefits include better symptom control, especially in survivorship and palliative care, enhanced continuity and coordination, and increased patient satisfaction and perceived safety [27, 88]. At the system level, outcomes include reduced hospitalizations, improved treatment adherence, and more efficient use of physician and oncologist time. Fully integrated APN models of care also enhance interprofessional collaboration and staff satisfaction [5]. Key lessons for low-resource settings include starting with clear role definitions and stakeholder engagement, and leveraging digital tools (e.g., symptom-monitoring applications, PROMs) to support clinical decisions. It is also essential to embed APN in community-based follow-up or long-term care, where continuity is critical and access to medical care through general practitioners and oncologists is limited. Switzerland's experience shows that APN clinical autonomy depends not only on policy reform but also on institutional culture, interprofessional trust, and thoughtful healthcare system design.

Country Case Study: Primary Healthcare Nurse Practitioners in Québec, Canada

Country Profile and Primary Healthcare Organization in Québec, Canada

Canada is a high-income country with over 39 million people and a decentralized, publicly funded healthcare system known as Medicare [34]. Although private practices exist, the vast majority of healthcare services are delivered through the public system, and individuals covered by Medicare do not typically pay fees at the point of care. Governed by the Canada Health Act, healthcare is a shared responsibility: the federal government sets national standards and provides funding through the Canada Health Transfer, while provinces and territories manage service delivery [84].

In the province of Québec, the Ministry of Health and Social Services (MSSS) oversees the planning and funding of healthcare services, reflecting its distinct language, culture, and governance priorities [52]. Santé Québec, a public organization, is tasked with administering and operating these services [75]. In Québec, the predominant model for delivering primary healthcare is the Family Medicine Group (FMG). Some FMGs are affiliated with universities and serve as teaching sites for medical trainees. These are known as University-affiliated Family Medicine Groups (U-FMGs) and typically have more teaching resources than regular FMGs. FMGs and U-FMGs are typically privately owned clinics managed by physicians or private corporations, operating under the FMG framework established by the MSSS [53], which allows them to receive public funding and access to health network resources (e.g., registered nurses, nurse practitioners (NPs), physiotherapists, pharmacists, and social workers), to promote interprofessional collaboration and improving patient care [53]. Other models of primary care clinics also include Local Community Service Centers (CLSCs), publicly owned and managed FMGs, medical clinics, long-term care facilities, home care services, and more recently, NP-led clinics integrated into the public health network [51]. These services are covered under

Medicare. However, private clinics operating outside the public healthcare system are not, and patients must pay out-of-pocket for care received in those settings.

Despite its universal access to care, Canada continues to face persistent healthcare access challenges, particularly in rural, Indigenous, and northern communities [60, 81] and for people in vulnerable situations, such as refugee and asylum-seeker populations [37, 40]. Québec experiences similar challenges, including long wait times, healthcare workforce shortages, and gaps in primary care access [6].

In Canada, accepted refugees are covered under the same provincial health insurance as permanent residents and citizens [71]. In contrast, asylum seekers, also called refugee claimants, are covered by the Interim Federal Health Program (IFHP) [33], which is often unfamiliar to healthcare professionals and not universally accepted despite its intended purpose [44]. Despite having health insurance and theoretical universal access to care, these populations may still face significant barriers to access services [2]. These include language barriers, complex and specific health needs, limited understanding of how the healthcare system works, and practical challenges such as lack of accessible transportation, inability to miss work (due to wage loss), or limited access to childcare, all of which can impede their ability to attend medical appointments.

Primary Healthcare NP Role and Scope of Practice

While a pan-Canadian effort in 2006 called for the development of APN roles [13], each province proceeded independently and at its own pace. All healthcare professionals are regulated by professional orders, with Québec nurses regulated explicitly by the Ordre des infirmières et infirmiers du Québec (OIIQ), which also oversees Advanced Practice Nursing roles [64]. Québec currently recognizes and regulates two APN roles: specialized NP in five specialties (primary healthcare, adult care, pediatric care, neonatal care, and mental health) and clinical nurse specialist (CNS) in infection prevention and control [65].

In Québec, primary healthcare NPs are authorized to diagnose, prescribe medications, order and interpret diagnostic tests, and manage patient care within their area of specialization [64]. While they have significant clinical autonomy, they must refer to other healthcare professionals in certain situations, such as when an activity falls outside their scope of practice or expertise, when it is not needed based on the person's condition, or when it is not supported by evidence-based guidelines [64].

To become a primary healthcare NP in Québec, registered nurses with at least 2 years of recent clinical experience must complete a master's degree and a graduate diploma from an OIIQ-accredited university program, followed by passing the OIIQ licensure exam [64]. Continuing education is required to maintain certification and professional competence [63].

Primary healthcare NPs in Québec practice across a range of settings, including FMGs, U-FMGs, CLSCs, long-term care facilities, and home care services [64]. They play a pivotal role in delivering accessible, comprehensive care, particularly to underserved and marginalized populations [69, 77]. Many primary healthcare NPs work in rural, remote, and socioeconomically disadvantaged urban areas where access to healthcare is limited due to physician shortages, long wait times, and constrained health infrastructure. These challenges are especially pronounced in regions with significant economically vulnerable populations, where systemic inequities contribute to poor health outcomes. In this context, primary healthcare NPs address critical healthcare gaps and provide essential services in environments that align with a broader understanding of low-resource settings, even within a high-income province like Québec [42]. Additionally, a small number of primary healthcare NPs provide care to refugee and asylum-seeker populations. While not yet widespread, these initiatives represent innovative and responsive models of care that not only address urgent health needs but also offer opportunities to enhance clinical autonomy and optimize NP roles within an evolving healthcare system.

Challenges to Primary Healthcare NP Clinical Autonomy

Across Canada, primary healthcare NPs continue to face systemic and institutional barriers that limit their clinical autonomy despite consistently demonstrating their capacity to deliver high-quality, cost-effective care [41, 42]. Regulatory fragmentation between provinces and territories has created inconsistencies in the scope of practice, prescriptive authority, and clinical independence. In several jurisdictions, including Québec, progress toward full primary healthcare NP integration has been slowed by uneven policy support, physician-centric models of care, and institutional resistance to role expansion. Nevertheless, the scope of practice for NPs has undergone continuous expansion, and as of 2021, all jurisdictions in Canada permit independent NP practice without requiring collaborative agreements with physicians, as was previously the case [12, 64].

In Québec, there are now very few restrictions in the scope of practice of primary healthcare NPs. However, one current limitation that remains, relates to mental health care: primary healthcare NPs are not authorized to assess mental health disorders, which prevents them from diagnosing these conditions and developing treatment plans accordingly [64]. This restriction was implemented because of the high risk of stigma associated with mental health diagnosis and to avoid the scope of practice overlap between primary healthcare NPs and mental health NPs. In practice, this means that still, to this day, primary healthcare NPs who encounter patients with complex physical and mental health needs must refer these patients to other providers for mental health diagnosis and treatment. This situation causes a significant issue as access to physicians and mental health NPs to evaluate and follow patients for mental health disorders is very limited, thus threatening access and continuity of care. Recognizing this challenge, various stakeholders, including regulatory bodies, professional associations, and policymakers, have been actively collaborating in recent years to review and update the scope of practice for primary healthcare NPs and regulations for mental health disorder evaluation. New recommendations aimed at broadening the scope of primary healthcare NPs in mental health care are currently under development and are expected to be released in the near future, with the goal of improving access and continuity of care for patients.

Innovative Practice of Primary Healthcare NPs in Refugee and Asylum-Seeker Clinics

A recent descriptive multiple-case study conducted in Québec highlighted an innovative example of APN practice in low-resource settings, showcasing the added value of primary healthcare NPs in offering care to people in vulnerable situations, more specifically refugee and asylum-seeker populations [76]. The study examined two clinical settings, one non-urban and one urban, selected to reflect different structural contexts with similarly high levels of structural vulnerability and resource constraints. Both settings faced limited access to specialized services, fragmented infrastructures, and lacked on-site diagnostics, typifying low-resource conditions.

In both clinical settings, primary healthcare NPs worked in interdisciplinary teams spread across multiple locations. Despite challenges related to coordination and infrastructure, NPs demonstrated adaptability and clinical leadership, bridging gaps in care and navigating complexity within dispersed teams.

NPs cared for highly diverse patient populations with complex, intersecting needs. Operating at full scope, they conducted holistic assessments and managed care plans addressing biological, psychological, social, and cultural factors. Their responsibilities included preventive care, diagnostics, prescribing, treatment planning, and referrals, all performed with a high degree of autonomy, though in continuous collaboration with clinical team members.

A key constraint in both settings was the limited scope of primary healthcare NP practice in mental health care. Although initial assessments by nurses and social workers aimed to identify such needs early in the process, issues often emerged later as trust developed. When primary healthcare NPs identified mental health concerns, referral to physicians was required, which could disrupt care continuity and challenge the therapeutic relationship. This limitation highlights structural barriers in low-resource contexts, where workforce constraints and rigid scopes of practice can hinder responsive and continuous care.

Impact and Lessons Learned

The Québec case study presented revealed several important outcomes of NP-led care in refugee and asylum-seeker clinics. Outcomes observed and discussed by participants across both clinical settings included improved access to timely primary healthcare, high patient and family satisfaction, and improved patient health outcomes. Primary healthcare NPs also contributed to improving their clinical team dynamics and potentially reduced healthcare costs by providing timely preventive care [76].

From a patient care perspective, the presence of NPs led to significant improvements in continuity and quality of care. Patients reported feeling heard, respected, and well-supported in navigating complex health and social needs. The trusting relationships primary healthcare NPs were able to build, often across language and cultural barriers, were particularly impactful for individuals with histories of trauma or systemic marginalization. Holistic, person-centered assessments allowed NPs to identify physical, psychological, and social issues early on, preventing deterioration and reducing unnecessary emergency room visits [76].

Several key lessons from this experience are transferable to other low-resource settings globally. First, maximizing the full scope of NP practice, particularly when supported by interdisciplinary collaboration, can greatly enhance service delivery in underserved communities. Second, organizational flexibility and openness, which allow for the clarification of roles, enable each healthcare provider to practice within their full scope and implement a communication and documentation system compatible across sites, thereby enabling care delivery even in fragmented or non-integrated infrastructures. Third, a critical area for policy advancement is expanding the authority of primary healthcare NP in mental health care, where restrictive regulations currently hinder continuity and quality of care.

The Québec innovative practice of primary healthcare NPs in clinical settings serving refugee and asylum-seeker populations underscores that even within high-income countries, low-resource realities exist and can be mitigated by empowering NPs to lead innovative, responsive care models. These insights offer valuable guidance for other jurisdictions seeking to strengthen primary healthcare delivery in the face of limited resources and high patient complexity.

Country Case Study: Advanced Practice Nurses in Chile

Country Profile and Healthcare System

Chile is a developing country facing health challenges similar to those in developed nations, but with a more limited health budget [67]. The healthcare system in Chile is divided into public and private sectors. The Ministry of Health (MoH) is responsible for developing and managing healthcare policies and regulating healthcare services [32, 91].

The public system serves approximately 80% of the population and provides universal healthcare coverage focused on health promotion, prevention, and treatment. However, the public sector suffers from physician shortages, especially in economically disadvantaged and remote areas, requiring referrals for specialist care, and having long wait times, often exceeding a year [4, 32, 92]. Additionally, access to primary healthcare is primarily determined by the ability of individuals to pay for their care, leading to significant inequities.

In contrast, the private sector is profit-driven, risk-stratified, and emphasizes consumption of health services. It's characterized by greater availability of physicians, direct access to specialists, and minimal wait times [4, 30, 31]. These structural disparities result in a concentration of low-income individuals in the public sector and healthier, wealthier individuals in the private sector [4].

The healthcare system in Chile is under increasing pressure from major demographic and epidemiological shifts [36]. Non-communicable diseases (NCDs), particularly cardiovascular disease and cancer are the leading causes of death, and 56% of the population lives with multiple chronic conditions, a trend that has worsened since 2010 [50, 90]. Additionally, by 2050, an estimated 24% of the population will be over 65, increasing the demand for chronic and long-term care [66]. Moreover, obesity affects 67% of adults and 39% of children, especially among vulnerable populations, increasing the risk of NCDs and placing strain on the system [66].

Despite the fact that mental health problems affect 38% of the population, services provided mainly by psychologists in primary healthcare, remain inadequate and lack interdisciplinary support [29, 73]. Additionally, the migrant population from other LMICs has grown rapidly in recent decades, posing additional challenges related to cultural and structural barriers that hinder care [17].

These overlapping pressures exacerbate systemic barriers in the healthcare system and underscore the urgent need to expand professional roles, such as those of APNs, to improve access, equity, and responsiveness, especially in underserved communities.

APN Role and Scope of Practice

Although APNs are not yet formally integrated into Chile's healthcare system, significant progress has been made toward their inclusion over the past decade. Key developments include the creation of master's-level programs for APNs, the incorporation of Advanced Practice Nursing roles into the National Cancer Plan, and the deployment of APNs in oncology within public and private cancer centers [49].

Simultaneously, there is a growing debate on how to formally recognize nurses who, despite not holding a master's degree, are already practicing with expanded scopes in various settings, such as primary healthcare centers and specialty areas including intensive care, and emergency [14]. For example, rural nurses in southern Chile often demonstrate autonomous practice, leading public health initiatives and improving healthcare in underserved areas. While not formally recognized as APNs, these practices reflect nursing leadership and innovation in low-resource settings [74].

Advanced Practice Nursing education in Chile has developed gradually over the past decade, supported by a strong foundation in undergraduate nursing education, partnerships with international universities, faculty members training abroad, and physicians' involvement as clinical mentors. The first master's program was launched in 2011 by the Universidad de los Andes, focusing on the CNS role in a context where APN was unknown [10, 87]. In response to the Pan American Health Organization's [68] call to advance the introduction of APNs in Latin America, additional master's programs were established to address gaps in primary healthcare, oncology, and palliative care [49]. These two-year, clinically intensive programs, currently offered at four universities, include more than 800 hours of internship and cover seven core competencies aligned with international standards [10, 49]. Programs focused on mental health still need to be expanded, with adequate funding mechanisms [14].

Challenges to APN Clinical Autonomy

Despite collaborative efforts among universities and progress in Advanced Practice Nursing education, Chile still lacks coordinated national policies to ensure legal recognition and title protection for APNs. Additionally, nursing education leaders must advocate for the expansion of APN training beyond the capital and work to persuade the MoH to allocate funding for APN education and job creation [14, 49].

Although APNs are increasingly working in public and private oncology centers in Chile, with defined scopes of practice including patient follow-up, diagnosis, laboratory test ordering, and collaborative prescribing, significant challenges remain in achieving full clinical autonomy. These practices are not supported by national regulations, rather, depend on local agreements between physicians and APNs [49]. Broader integration is hindered by outdated legal frameworks, such as the Chilean Health Code, which restricts diagnostic, treatment, and prescribing authority to physicians only (Book V, Article 113).

Another challenge for the integration of APNs into the healthcare system is the limited awareness and understanding of their role and impact, particularly among patients and allied health workers [15]. While physicians and nurses may be familiar with Advanced Practice Nursing, many others remain unaware of the competencies, scope, and added value that APNs bring to patient care. This lack of recognition can hinder collaboration, reduce acceptance, lead role confusion, and delay role integration [8]. Raising public awareness and promoting interprofessional education are essential strategies to build trust, foster collaboration, and ensure the successful incorporation of APNs into multidisciplinary teams.

While there is consensus among health sector leaders on the transformative potential of APN roles, strong commitment from policymakers and decision-makers, along with systemic changes in the healthcare system, are required to formally incorporate APNs as autonomous providers [14]. One of the underlying reasons for the limited policy commitment to Advanced Practice Nursing in Chile is the historically hierarchical nature of the country's healthcare system, in which physicians occupy a central role. Policymaking processes have traditionally been physician-driven, with other stakeholders, including nursing associations, invited to participate but rarely positioned as equal decision-makers. Although a slow shift toward more inclusive governance is emerging, the influence of medical opinion leaders continues to shape healthcare policy priorities [15]. In this context, nursing associations have primarily assumed an advocacy role, working to raise awareness of the value of APNs and to promote the integration of their roles within the system. However, achieving full recognition and policy support for APNs will require stronger representation of nurses in decision-making tables and greater interprofessional collaboration to challenge entrenched hierarchies and drive systemic change ([3]; [15]; [49]).

Strategies and Best Practices to Promote Clinical Autonomy

One strategy to advance the clinical autonomy of APNs is to consolidate their role in oncology and expand it to regional public cancer centers, rural healthcare posts, and primary healthcare facilities. In areas with limited physician availability, many nurses already practice with an expanded scope of practice, though without formal recognition. Developing mechanisms to acknowledge and integrate these roles within the healthcare system would enhance their legitimacy and sustainability. Equally important is securing funding, such as research grants, to support implementation and generate measurable outcomes. These should capture the impact of APNs on patient health outcomes, team performance, organizational effectiveness, and the implementation process itself [9]. Evidence generated from such studies can support policy development, build the case for regulatory reform, and inform future strategies for scaling up APN roles in underserved healthcare contexts [79].

A second key strategy is for nursing educational leaders to establish an autonomous credentialing system for APNs and ensure the accreditation of master's-level programs based on agreed-upon standards. This would support the formal recognition of APNs, protect their title, and ensure consistency in role preparation across institutions [49]. These leaders should foster national university alliances to expand master programs beyond the capital, reducing geographic disparities in education access, and promoting equitable integration across the healthcare system [15].

Finally, another strategy is to advance broad, intersectoral policy advocacy to strengthen the clinical autonomy of APNs through regulatory and institutional change. This includes promoting national policies that clearly define and expand APNs' scope of practice, supported by clinical protocols that guide and legitimize their decision-making authority. Additionally, advocacy efforts should aim to formally recognize APNs as independent healthcare providers within the legal and institutional frameworks of the healthcare system. Achieving these changes will require sustained engagement with policymakers, medical associations, patient groups, and other stakeholders to build consensus and support for the role's full integration.

Impact and Lessons Learned

The implementation of Advanced Practice Nursing roles in Chile, particularly in oncology, has demonstrated their potential to improve access, continuity, and quality of care for populations with unmet health needs. Advanced Practice Nurses (APNs) have slowly but steadily integrated into oncology teams, contributing to the development of clinical protocols and taking on key responsibilities such as patient follow-up, and collaborative prescribing. These early successes illustrate the value of APNs in addressing health workforce shortages and enhancing care delivery, even within restrictive regulatory environments.

Progress has been driven by the leadership of nurse educators and professional associations, which have forged partnerships with policymakers, universities, and healthcare institutions. However, broader policy change requires stronger political advocacy and increased visibility of APN roles beyond the nursing profession. Nurses must strengthen their policy capacity, understand the legislative and regulatory landscape, and engage in intersectoral dialogue with key decision-makers. Institutionalizing APN roles will also require the creation of autonomous credentialing systems, regulatory reform, and sustainable financing. While policy windows like the National Cancer Plan have provided opportunities, critical needs remain in areas such as mental health, migrant care, and chronic disease management in primary healthcare. Sustaining momentum will require aligning the APN agenda with national priorities and generating local evidence to inform and influence policy.

Comparative Analysis and Key Takeaways

Advanced Practice Nurse (APN) roles are increasingly recognized as essential to strengthening healthcare systems, improving access, and enhancing care quality, particularly in low-resource settings. A critical factor in realizing their impact is the ability of APNs to practice autonomously and work to the full extent of their education and competencies. While the title and implementation of APN roles vary across countries, common themes, enablers, and challenges emerge from the case studies of Singapore, Switzerland, and Québec (Canada), Chile.

Common Themes Across Québec (Canada), Chile, Singapore, and Switzerland

Across all four countries, a strong policy impetus and recognition of APN contributions to healthcare quality and system efficiency underpin the expansion of advanced nursing roles. Although regulatory and structural differences exist, each setting demonstrates a trend toward expanding APN responsibilities in response to health workforce shortages, rising healthcare demands, and the need for more integrated, person-centered care. However, a persistent gap remains in health workforce planning that adequately accounts for expanded roles such as APNs. In low-resource settings, shortages of specialized personnel and systemic constraints are prevalent. Therefore, strategically aligning patient needs with the capabilities of healthcare professionals, including APNs, is not only critical for delivering quality and efficient care, but also fundamental to the long-term sustainability of health systems [62].

Another shared theme is the hybridization of APN roles In Singapore, the APN represents a hybrid of both NP and CNS function [95]. This approach is comparable to Switzerland in the early years of Advanced Practice Nursing role development and implementation. As understanding and experience with the APN role increased, particularly regarding its contributions and requirements in Switzerland, the canton of Vaud facilitated the differentiation between the CNS and NP roles. It opted to implement the NP role in primary care to better address the rising care demands and the declining number of general practitioners in rural areas. Nevertheless, many nurses in cancer care in Switzerland continue to identify with the broader APN role, with only a few aligning themselves specifically with the CNS or NP titles [27]. In contrast, Québec maintains distinct NP and CNS roles that are deployed collaboratively [65].

Chile also reflects a blended model, often shaped more by practical need than by regulatory clarity [14]. Across all settings, APNs are embedded in a wide range of clinical areas, including primary healthcare, cancer care, mental health, and acute care, with a shared emphasis on holistic, longitudinal care for populations with complex or unmet needs.

Structured education and credentialing frameworks are another consistent feature. Each country has developed master's-level programs with supervised clinical practice to ensure APNs are equipped with advanced competencies. These educational pathways often align with international standards while reflecting national healthcare system priorities. In parallel, credentialing frameworks, such as licensure, certification, and registration processes, serve to formally recognize an APN's qualifications and scope of practice. While education focuses on preparing APNs with the necessary knowledge, skills, and competencies, credentialing ensures accountability, role clarity, and public trust by validating their readiness to practice. The formality and rigor of these credentialing mechanisms vary across countries, often influenced by the degree of professional regulation and integration of APN and their roles within national workforce planning.

Factors Enabling APN Autonomy in Low-Resource Settings

Several enabling factors are evident in supporting APN autonomy, particularly in low-resource or underserved settings:

1. *Structured governance mechanisms:* Collaborative Practice Agreements in Singapore and regulatory guidelines in Québec provide legal and procedural clarity, enabling APNs to practice safely and independently within defined scopes. These frameworks and guidelines offer replicable models for settings where full independent practice may not yet be feasible.
2. *Role-specific, competency-based education:* Master-level programs in Québec, Chile, Singapore and Switzerland incorporate clinical internships, ensuring APNs are equipped to practice autonomously and safely.
3. *Innovative care models:* Advanced Practice Nurse (APN)-led clinics for atrial fibrillation in Singapore and refugee care in Québec show how targeted innovations can address healthcare gaps and build APN credibility. These models

improve outcomes, reduce pressure on the healthcare system, and demonstrate APN leadership in addressing complex patient needs.

4. *Technology integration:* Digital tools, including electronic decision-support systems, teleconsultation, and PROMs, enhance APN decision-making and care coordination, particularly in low-resource contexts such as rural Switzerland or community settings in Singapore.
5. *Community and patient trust:* Across all case studies, APNs demonstrated the ability to build trusted relationships with patients, especially among vulnerable or marginalized populations. This trust enables early issue identification, continuity of care along the care pathway, and improved adherence to treatment plans.

Challenges Impeding APN Autonomy in Low-Resource Settings

Despite significant progress, key barriers to APN autonomy persist:

1. *Legal and regulatory fragmentation:* In Chile and Switzerland, the lack of national legislation protecting APN roles creates inconsistency, limits role clarity, and impedes title protection. In Québec, while regulation is well-established, restrictive mental health scopes still limit comprehensive practice in some clinical specialties.
2. *Hierarchical healthcare culture:* In Singapore and Chile, embedded physician-dominant care models constrain APN decision-making authority. Cultural resistance among physicians and institutional leaders delays role integration and limits trust.
3. *Inadequate role awareness:* Across countries, limited understanding of the APN and their roles among the public, other healthcare professionals, and even within nursing hierarchies results in underutilization of the APN and role confusion.
4. *Workforce and resource constraints:* Heavy workloads, limited clinical support, and restricted access to infrastructure (e.g., diagnostics, referral systems) particularly affect APNs in rural or underserved settings, as seen in refugee clinics in Québec and primary healthcare settings in Chile.

Recommendations for Policymakers, Educators, and APN Leaders

Based on the lessons from these case studies, several recommendations can guide future efforts to advance APN autonomy globally:

1. *Develop enabling legislation and regulation:* Governments should prioritize legal recognition, title protection, and clearly defined scopes of practice for the APN and their roles. Where full independence is not yet feasible, structured models like Collaborative Practice Agreements can serve as transitional mechanisms.

2. *Strengthen APN education and credentialing:* National nursing councils and academic institutions should ensure access to accredited, role-specific APN programs that include clinical specialization and supervised clinical practice. Credentialing processes should be transparent and aligned with both international standards and local service in needs.
3. *Promote interprofessional education and collaboration:* Building mutual understanding and trust between nurses, physicians, and allied healthcare professionals is crucial. Joint training, shared clinical placements, and co-leadership models, where APNs, nurses, physicians, and other healthcare professionals jointly oversee care delivery, program development, or clinical teams, can foster a culture of collaboration and shared accountability. These approaches help dismantle professional silos and promote more integrated, interprofessional team-based healthcare.
4. *Support APN-led innovation in underserved settings:* Ministry of Health (MoH) and healthcare organizations should invest in APN-led clinics and pilot projects targeting populations with limited access to healthcare. These initiatives should be rigorously evaluated and scaled where successful.
5. *Invest in digital tools to support APN practice:* Governments and healthcare systems should integrate digital decision-support tools, PROMs, and telehealth platforms to extend APN capabilities, especially in low-resource and remote areas.
6. *Address gender and cultural barriers:* Efforts should be made to promote diversity in APN recruitment and leadership, address gender stereotypes, and foster inclusive career pathways. Public education campaigns can improve the visibility of the APN and support access to APN-led care models.
7. *Embed APNs in healthcare system planning:* Advanced Practice Nurses (APNs) should be actively involved in policy development, workforce planning, and healthcare reform efforts. Their frontline experience offers critical insight into service design, patient needs, and system inefficiencies.

By adopting these strategies, countries can advance the autonomy and effectiveness of APNs, ultimately improve health outcomes and strengthen healthcare systems in both high- and low-resource contexts.

Conclusion

The case studies of Singapore, Switzerland, Québec, and Chile reveal a diverse yet convergent landscape in the global development of Advanced Practice Nursing. Each setting reflects different stages of APN integration, ranging from formalized national credentialing frameworks to innovative but locally negotiated roles. Despite contextual variations, common threads emerge: a commitment to addressing workforce shortages, improving access to healthcare, and advancing person-centered, holistic models of care delivery.

In all four countries, APNs have demonstrated their capacity to operate effectively in resource-constrained environments, whether through community-based care for atrial fibrillation in Singapore, refugee and asylum-seeker health clinics in Québec, oncology services in Chile, or integrated cancer care in Switzerland. Their contributions include improved patient outcomes, stronger interprofessional collaboration, and enhanced system efficiency. Crucially, these roles are most successful when supported by enabling policies, targeted education, interdisciplinary trust, and digital infrastructure.

Looking ahead, advancing APN autonomy in low-resource settings will require sustained investment in legislation, role-specific training, and institutional readiness. Ensuring equitable access to education and credentialing, and embedding APNs in underserved settings must be prioritized. Furthermore, digital tools offer an opportunity to extend APN reach and support autonomous decision-making, especially in geographically dispersed or infrastructure-limited environments.

Global collaboration and advocacy are essential to accelerating this momentum. Policymakers, educators, nursing leaders, and professional associations must work together to exchange best practices, harmonize standards, and champion regulatory reform. Cross-country learning initiatives, joint capacity-building programs, and international research networks can support the global advancement of the APN and their roles.

Ultimately, empowering APNs to practice to the full extent of their training and expertise is not only a professional imperative but also a public health necessity. As healthcare systems worldwide face increasing pressures from ageing populations, chronic disease, and health inequities, APNs offer a scalable, evidence-based solution to deliver high-quality, equitable access to care. Strengthening APNs' clinical autonomy, particularly in low-resource settings, is both a strategic investment and a moral obligation to ensure better health outcomes and healthcare access for all.

References

1. APN-Switzerland (APN-CH). Registration to become an advanced practice nurse. 2019. https://apn-ch.ch/home/downloads/
2. Barbo G. Resilience of refugees and asylum seekers in Canada. Int J Migr Health Soc Care. 2023;19(3/4):417–34. https://doi.org/10.1108/IJMHSC-11-2022-0113.
3. Barzegar Safari M, Bahadori M, Alimohammadzadeh K. The related factors of nurses' participation and perceived benefits and barriers in health policy making. J Nurs Res. 2020;28(4):1–8. https://doi.org/10.1097/jnr.0000000000000385.
4. Bernales-Baksai P. Tackling segmentation to advance universal health coverage: analysis of policy architectures of health care in Chile and Uruguay. Int J Equity Health. 2020;19:106. https://doi.org/10.1186/s12939-020-01176-6.
5. Bologna F, Kaufmann S, Staudacher S, Spichiger E. Betreuung durch eine advanced practice nurse: Erfahrungen von patient:innen mit Sarkom und Angehörigen [Care provided by an advanced practice nurse: experiences of patients with sarcoma and family members. A qualitative study]. Pflege. 2023;36(1):2–10. https://doi.org/10.1024/1012-5302/a000917.
6. Breton M, Deslauriers V, Lamoureux-Lamarche C, Smithman MA, Sauvé C, Beauséjour M, Laberge M, Motulsky A, Pomey M-P. Organizational innovations related to primary care access points (GAP) for unattached patients in Quebec: a multi-case qualitative study. BMC Prim Care. 2024;25(1):363. https://doi.org/10.1186/s12875-024-02614-y.

7. Brügger U. Bildungsabschlüsse, Kompetenzen und Tätigkeitsfelder der Gesundheitsberufe in der Schweiz: Ein Fokus auf advanced practice nurses [Educational qualifications, competencies and fields of activity of healthcare professions in Switzerland: a focus on advanced practice nurses]. Bern: Schweizerische Akademie der Medizinischen Wissenschaften (SAMW); 2025.
8. Bryant-Lukosius D, Wong FKY. International development of advanced practice nursing. In: Tracy MF, O'Grady ET, Phillips SJ, editors. Hamric and Hanson's advanced practice nursing: an integrative approach. 7th ed. Amsterdam: Elsevier; 2023. p. 137–66.
9. Bryant-Lukosius D, Spichiger E, Martin J, Stoll H, Kellerhals SD, Fliedner M, Grossmann F, Henry M, Herrmann L, Koller A, Schwendimann R, Ulrich A, Weibel L, Callens B, De Geest S. Framework for evaluating the impact of advanced practice nursing roles. J Nurs Scholarsh. 2016;48(2):201–9. https://doi.org/10.1111/jnu.12199.
10. Bryant-Lukosius D, Martin-Misener R, Donald F, Peña LM, Brousseau L. Advanced practice nursing: a strategy for achieving universal health coverage and universal access to health. Rev Lat Am Enfermagem. 2017;25:e2826. https://doi.org/10.1590/1518-8345.1677.2826.
11. Busca E, Savatteri A, Calafato TL, Mazzoleni B, Barisone M, Dal Molin A. Barriers and facilitators to the implementation of nurse's role in primary care settings: an integrative review. BMC Nurs. 2021;20:1–12.
12. Canadian Institute for Health Information. Nurse practitioners. 2024, July 25. https://www.cihi.ca/en/nurse-practitioners
13. Canadian Nurses Association. The Canadian nurse practitioner initiative: a 10-year retrospective. 2016. https://ia903103.us.archive.org/30/items/5762376-Canadian-Nurse-Practitioner-Initiative-a-10-Year/5762376-Canadian-Nurse-Practitioner-Initiative-a-10-Year.pdf
14. Cerón C, Bryant-Lukosius D. Reporte del Foro de Discusión: "Optimizando la contribución de la enfermería y la enfermería de práctica avanzada a la atención primaria de salud en Chile en el contexto de la reforma de salud" [Report]. Universidad de los Andes; 2024. https://www.uandes.cl/wp-content/uploads/2024/07/Reporte-Foro-final-version-Espanol_-002.pdf
15. Cerón Mackay MC, Marquez Doren F, Dias BM. Expansion of the scope of practice for nurses in Chile. Acta Paulista de Enfermagem. 2025;38(spe1), eSPE01i. https://doi.org/10.37689/acta-ape/2025SPE01i
16. Colomer-Lahiguera S, Gentizon J, Christofis M, Darnac C, Serena A, Eicher M. Achieving comprehensive, patient-centered cancer services: optimizing the role of advanced practice nurses at the core of precision health. Semin Oncol Nurs. 2024;40(3):151629. https://doi.org/10.1016/j.soncn.2024.151629.
17. Cruz-Riveros C, Portilla-Saavedra D, Lay-Lisboa SL, Mardones-Macaya C, Macaya-Sanzana C, Vidal-Saavedra L. Primary healthcare accessibility from the perspective of migrants and health professionals in Antofagasta, Chile. Ciencia y Enfermería. 2023;29:Article e60032. https://doi.org/10.29393/CE29-32AACL60032.
18. De Pietro C, Camenzind P, Sturny I, Crivelli I, Edwards-Garavoglia S, Spranger A, Wittenbecher F, Quentin W. Switzerland: health system review. Health Syst Transit. 2015;17(4):1–288. xix
19. Department of Statistics, Singapore. Population and population structure. 2024. Retrieved June 6 from https://www.singstat.gov.sg/find-data/search-by-theme/population/population-and-population-structure/latest-data
20. Eicher MR, Marquard S, Aebi S. A nurse is a nurse? A systematic review of the effectiveness of specialised nursing in breast cancer. Eur J Cancer. 2006;42(18):3117–26. https://doi.org/10.1016/j.ejca.2006.07.007.
21. Eicher M, Kadmon I, Claassen S, Marquard S, Pennery E, Wengstrom Y, Fenlon D. Training breast care nurses throughout Europe: the EONS post-basic curriculum for breast cancer nursing. Eur J Cancer. 2012;48(9):1257–62. https://doi.org/10.1016/j.ejca.2011.07.011.
22. Eisner D, Zoller M, Rosemann T, Huber CA, Badertscher N, Tandjung R. Screening and prevention in Swiss primary care: a systematic review. Int J Gen Med. 2011;4:853–70. https://doi.org/10.2147/ijgm.s26562.
23. Federal Statistics Office Switzerland. Switzerland's population in 2022. 2023. https://www.bfs.admin.ch/bfs/de/home/statistiken/kataloge-datenbanken.assetdetail.28425364.html

24. Federal Statistics Office Switzerland. Taschenstatistik 2025. 2025. https://www.bfs.admin.ch/bfs/en/home/statistics/health.assetdetail.34027817.html
25. Frank JR, Snell L, Sherbino J, editors. CanMEDS 2015 physician competency framework. Royal College of Physicians and Surgeons of Canada; 2015. https://canmeds.royalcollege.ca/uploads/en/framework/CanMEDS%202015%20Framework_EN_Reduced.pdf
26. Gaylord J, Ribaut J, Gentizon J, Colomer-Lahiguera S, Robatto L, Mabire C, Zúñiga F, Eicher M. Establishing educational entry to practice requirements for advanced practice nursing in Switzerland: current debate and nursing perspective. Swiss Med Wkly. 2025;155:4301. https://doi.org/10.57187/s.4301.
27. Geese F, Bryant-Lukosius D, Zwakhalen S, Hahn S. Advanced practice nurses and their roles in Swiss cancer care: a cross-sectional study. Semin Oncol Nurs. 2024a;40(3):151626. https://doi.org/10.1016/j.soncn.2024.151626.
28. Geese F, Kaufmann S, Sivanathan M, Sairanen K, Klenke F, Krieg AH, Müller D, Schmitt KU. Exploring the potential of electronic patient-reported outcome measures to inform and assess care in sarcoma centers: a longitudinal multicenter pilot study. Cancer Nurs. 2024b;47(6):E395–403. https://doi.org/10.1097/NCC.0000000000001248.
29. Goldstein E. Carga mundial de los trastornos de salud mental: Evolución pre-pandemia y efectos de la aparición de COVID-19. Biblioteca del Congreso Nacional de Chile, Santiago, Chile; 2022. https://obtienearchivo.bcn.cl/obtienearchivo?id=repositorio/10221/33592/2/BCN__Carga_mundial_de_Salud_Mental__FINAL_repos.pdf
30. Goldstein E, Paredes LC. El recurso humano en el sector de la Salud. Biblioteca del Congreso Nacional de Chile, Santiago, Chile; 2021.
31. Gómez L, Núñez A. Vigilancia del acceso a la salud en Chile: Un sistema de indicadores para monitoreo multidimensional. Rev Med Chile. 2021;149(1):62–75. https://doi.org/10.4067/S0034-98872021000100062.
32. González C, Castillo-Laborde C, Matute I. Estructura y funcionamiento del sistema de salud chileno. CEPS, Facultad de Medicina, Clínica Alemana Universidad del Desarrollo, Santiago, Chile; 2019.
33. Government of Canada. Interim Federal Health Program Policy. 2023a. https://www.canada.ca/en/immigration-refugees-citizenship/corporate/mandate/policies-operational-instructions-agreements/interim-federal-health-program-policy.html
34. Government of Canada. About Canada's health care system. 2023b, October 10. https://www.canada.ca/en/health-canada/services/canada-health-care-system.html
35. Horton M, Dixon J, Turi E, Balusu C, Paikoff R, Maier CB, Poghosyan L. Advanced practice nurses in primary care and their impact on health service utilisation, costs and access globally: a scoping review. J Clin Nurs. 2025;34(5):1592–601. https://doi.org/10.1111/jocn.17614.
36. Instituto Nacional de Estadística. Cifras de población y censos demográficos [Data page]. INEbase; 2024. Retrieved July 21, 2025, from https://www.ine.es/dyngs/INEbase/en/operacion.htm?c=Estadistica_C&cid=1254736176992&idp=1254735572981
37. Iqbal MP, Walpola R, Harris-Roxas B, Li J, Mears S, Hall J, Harrison R. Improving primary health care quality for refugees and asylum seekers: a systematic review of interventional approaches. Health Expect. 2022;25(5):2065–94. https://doi.org/10.1111/hex.13365.
38. Joint Commission of the Swiss Medical Schools. Principal relevant objectives and framework for integrative learning and education in Switzerland (PROFILES). 2017. https://www.profilesmed.ch
39. Jolidon V, Jubin J, Zuercher E, Roth L, Carron T, Oulevey Bachmann A, Gilles I, Peytremann-Bridevaux I. Health workforce challenges: Key findings from the Swiss Cohort of Healthcare Professionals and Informal Caregivers (SCOHPICA). International Journal of Public Health. 2024;69, Article 1607419. https://doi.org/10.3389/ijph.2024.1607419
40. Kamran H, Hassan H, Ali MUN, Ali D, Taj M, Mir Z, Pandya M, Steinberg SR, Jamal A, Zaidi M. Scoping review: barriers to primary care access experienced by immigrants and refugees in English-speaking countries. Qual Res J. 2022;22(3):401–14. https://doi.org/10.1108/QRJ-02-2022-0028.

41. Kilpatrick K, Tchouaket E, Savard I, Chouinard M-C, Bouabdillah N, Provost-Bazinet B, Costanzo G, Houle J, St-Louis G, Jabbour M, Atallah R. Identifying indicators sensitive to primary healthcare nurse practitioner practice: a review of systematic reviews. PLoS One. 2023;18(9):e0290977. https://doi.org/10.1371/journal.pone.0290977.
42. Kilpatrick K, Savard I, Audet L-A, Costanzo G, Khan M, Atallah R, Jabbour M, Zhou W, Wheeler K, Ladd E. A global perspective of advanced practice nursing research: a review of systematic reviews. PLoS One. 2024;19(7):e0305008.
43. Koller M, Zúñiga F, De Geest S, Simon M. Institutional readiness and barriers for advanced nursing practice: a cross-sectional study in Swiss hospitals. J Nurs Scholarsh. 2019;51(5):544–53. https://doi.org/10.1111/jnu.12480.
44. Leps C, Monteiro J, Barozzino T, Bowry A, Rashid M, Sgro M, Suleman S. Interim Federal Health Program: survey of access and utilization by paediatric health care providers. Paediatr Child Health. 2022;27(1):19–24. https://doi.org/10.1093/pch/pxab045.
45. Lin XLS, Tan SW, Wang HYS, Ang KHM, Maniya S, Woo BFY. Healthcare professionals' perspectives towards the role of ward-based advanced practice nurses: a cross-sectional study. J Adv Nurs. 2025;81(6):3083–95. https://doi.org/10.1111/jan.16401.
46. Lockwood EB, Lehwaldt D, Sweeney MR, Matthews A. An exploration of the levels of clinical autonomy of advanced nurse practitioners: a narrative literature review. Int J Nurs Pract. 2022;28(1):e12978. https://doi.org/10.1111/ijn.12978.
47. Lyu Y, Xu Q, Liu J. Exploring the medical decision-making patterns and influencing factors among the general Chinese public: a binary logistic regression analysis. BMC Public Health. 2024;24(1):887. https://doi.org/10.1186/s12889-024-18338-8.
48. Mahrer-Imhof R, Altherr J, Eissler C, Petrig M, Piattini S, Ullmann-Bremi A, Weibel L, Spichiger E. Minimal standards for certificates and specializations of advanced practice nurses (MiS-APN). 2024. https://apn-ch.ch/assets/MiS-APN/240712_MiS-APN-paper.pdf
49. Márquez-Doren F, Palma-Rivadeneira S, Soto-Fuentes P, Lucchini-Raies C, Peña-Durán J, Nervi-Nattero B, Suárez-Pierart P, González-Rodríguez R, Rojas-Silva N, Bustamante-Troncoso C, Alcayaga-Rojas C, Catoni-Salamanca MI, Arechabala-Mantuliz MC. Una propuesta para mejorar el acceso y cobertura en oncología para Latinoamérica: enfermería de práctica avanzada. Rev Med Chile. 2021;149(4):591–7. https://doi.org/10.4067/s0034-98872021000400591.
50. Martínez-Sanguinetti MA, Leiva-Ordoñez AM, Petermann-Rocha F, Celis-Morales C. ¿Cómo ha cambiado el perfil epidemiológico en Chile en los últimos 10 años? Rev Med Chile. 2021;149(2):149–52. https://doi.org/10.4067/S0034-98872021000100149.
51. Ministry of Health and Social Services (MSSS). Clinique d'infirmières praticiennes spécialisées (IPS): Cadre de référence pour les établissements de santé et de services sociaux. 2024a. https://publications.msss.gouv.qc.ca/msss/document-003651/?&date=DESC
52. Ministry of Health and Social Services (MSSS). Gouvernance et organisation des services. 2024b, February 19. https://www.msss.gouv.qc.ca/reseau/systeme-de-sante-et-de-services-sociaux-en-bref/gouvernance-et-organisation-des-services/
53. Ministry of Health and Social Services (MSSS). Programme de financement et de soutien professionnel pour les groupes de médecine de famille (GMF). Direction des communications du Ministère de la Santé et des Services Sociaux; 2025. https://publications.msss.gouv.qc.ca/msss/document-001527/?&date=DESC&sujet=gmf&critere=sujet
54. Ministry of Health, Singapore. Guidelines for implementation of collaborative prescribing services. MOH Singapore; 2018. https://www.moh.gov.sg/docs/librariesprovider4/guidelines/guidelines-for-implementation-of-collaborative-prescribing-services.pdf
55. Ministry of Health, Singapore. Expanding healthcare capacity and transforming the healthcare workforce. 2025. https://www.moh.gov.sg/newsroom/expanding-healthcare-capacity-and-transforming-the-healthcare-workforce
56. Muili A, Tangmi A, Shariff S, Awad F, Oseili T. Exploring strategies for building a sustainable healthcare system in Africa: lessons from Japan and Switzerland. Ann Med Surg. 2024;86(3):1563–9. https://doi.org/10.1097/MS9.0000000000001767.

57. National University of Singapore. Collaborative Practitioners Prescribing Programme (CP3). n.d.-a. Retrieved 6 June from https://medicine.nus.edu.sg/dgms/continuing-ed-training-programmes/national-collaborative-prescribing-programme/
58. National University of Singapore. Master of Nursing. n.d.-b. Retrieved 6 June from https://medicine.nus.edu.sg/nursing/education-programmes/postgraduate/masters/master-of-nursing/
59. National University of Singapore. National Collaborative Prescribing Programme. n.d.-c. Retrieved 14 April from https://pharmacy.nus.edu.sg/national-collaborative-prescribing/
60. Nguyen NH, Subhan FB, Williams K, Chan CB. Barriers and mitigating strategies to healthcare access in indigenous communities of Canada: A narrative review. Healthcare. 2020;8(2). https://doi.org/10.3390/healthcare8020112.
61. OncoSuisse. Newsletter July 2025—Update National Cancer Plan. 2025, July. https://oncosuisse.ch/nationaler-krebsplan/
62. Ono T, Lafortune G, Schoenstein M. Health workforce planning in OECD countries: a review of 26 projection models from 18 countries (OECD Health Working Papers No. 62). OECD Publishing; 2013. https://doi.org/10.1787/5k44t787zcwb-en.
63. Ordre des infirmières et infirmiers du Québec (OIIQ). IPS: Tout savoir sur la norme de formation continue. 2019. https://www.oiiq.org/ips-tout-savoir-sur-la-norme-de-formation-continue
64. Ordre des infirmières et infirmiers du Québec (OIIQ). Specialized nurse practitioners and their practice: Guidelines 2021. https://www.oiiq.org/documents/20147/2943833/2530-np-guidelines-web.pdf
65. Ordre des infirmières et infirmiers du Québec (OIIQ). Pratique avancée. Pratique Professionnelle. 2025. https://www.oiiq.org/pratique-professionnelle/pratique-avancee
66. Organization for Economic Co-operation and Development (OECD). Estudios de la OCDE sobre salud pública: Chile hacia un futuro más sano, evaluación y recomendaciones. 2019. https://www.oecd.org/health/health-systems/Revisión-OCDE-de-Salud-Pública-Chile-Evaluación-y-recomendaciones.pdf
67. Organization for Economic Co-operation and Development (OECD). Health at a glance 2021: OECD indicators. 2021. doi:https://doi.org/10.1787/ae3016b9-en.
68. Pan American Health Organization. Report: universal access to health and universal health coverage: advanced practice nursing summit. 2015. https://www.observatoriorh.org/es/report-universal-access-health-and-universal-health-coverage-advanced-practice-nursing-summit
69. Pelletier J, Vermette S, Lauzier S, Bujold M, Bujold L, Martin É, Guillaumie L. Challenges faced by Canadian primary health care nurse practitioners in chronic disease management: a qualitative study among key informants. J Am Assoc Nurse Pract. 2019;31(5):300–8. https://doi.org/10.1097/JXX.0000000000000141.
70. Reeves E, Schweighoffer R, Liebig B. An investigation of the challenges to coordination at the interface of primary and specialized palliative care services in Switzerland: a qualitative interview study. J Interprof Care. 2021;35(1):21–7. https://doi.org/10.1080/13561820.2020.1724085.
71. Régie de l'assurance maladie (RAMQ). Connaître les conditions d'admissibilité à l'assurance maladie. 2020. https://www.ramq.gouv.qc.ca/fr/citoyens/assurance-maladie/connaitre-conditions-admissibilite
72. Remund A, Cullati S, Sieber S, et al. Longer and healthier lives for all? Successes and failures of a universal consumer-driven healthcare system, Switzerland, 1990–2014. Int J Public Health. 2019;64:1173–81. https://doi.org/10.1007/s00038-019-01290-5.
73. Rojas G, Martínez V, Martínez P, Franco P. Improving mental health care in developing countries through digital technologies: a mini narrative review of the Chilean case. Front Public Health. 2019;7:Article 391. https://doi.org/10.3389/fpubh.2019.00391.
74. Sandoval Arias F, Rivas Riveros E, Catalán Melinao Y, Painecura Rayman P, Urra Valenzuela C. Profesionalización de enfermería rural, circulación de saberes y políticas estatales de salud en La Araucanía-Chile, años 1970–1990 [Rural nursing professionalization, knowledge circulation and state health policies in the Araucania Region-Chile, 1970–1990]. Cultura de los Cuidados. 2021;25(60):97–112. https://doi.org/10.14198/cuid.2021.60.08.
75. Santé Québec. Une approche humaine. 2025. https://sante.quebec/

76. Savard I. Understanding the added value of primary healthcare nurse practitioners for people in vulnerable situations: a descriptive multiple case study. Doctoral thesis. McGill University; 2025.
77. Savard I, Jabbour M, Tchouaket E, Gauthier N, Kilpatrick K. Evaluating the influence of primary healthcare nurse practitioners' interventions in home care on hospitalizations and emergency department transfers. J Eval Clin Pract. 2024;30:440–52. https://doi.org/10.1111/jep.13960.
78. Schirle L, Norful AA, Rudner N, Poghosyan L. Organizational facilitators and barriers to optimal APRN practice: an integrative review. Health Care Manag Rev. 2020;45(4):311–20. https://doi.org/10.1097/hmr.0000000000000229.
79. Schober MM, Gerrish K, Mcdonnell A. Development of a conceptual policy framework for advanced practice nursing: an ethnographic study. J Adv Nurs. 2016;72(6):1313–24. https://doi.org/10.1111/jan.12915.
80. Serena A, Dwyer AA, Peters S, Eicher M. Acceptance of the advanced practice nurse in lung cancer role by healthcare professionals and patients: a qualitative exploration. J Nurs Scholarsh. 2018;50(5):540–8. https://doi.org/10.1111/jnu.12411.
81. Shah TI, Clark AF, Seabrook JA, Sibbald S, Gilliland JA. Geographic accessibility to primary care providers: comparing rural and urban areas in southwestern Ontario. Can Geogr. 2020;64(1):65–78. https://doi.org/10.1111/cag.12557. Academic Search Complete.
82. Singapore Nursing Board. Core competencies of advanced practice nurse. 2023. Retrieved 6 June from https://isomer-user-content.by.gov.sg/78/164d803e-ce80-45ef-82d9-f8154ef89759/core-competencies-of-apn_2023.pdf
83. Spirig R. 10 Jahre advanced nursing practice in der Schweiz: Rückblick und Ausblick [10 years advanced nursing practice in Switzerland: retrospect and prospects]. Pflege. 2010;23(6):363–6. https://doi.org/10.1024/1012-5302/a000075.
84. Tiedemann, M.. The Canada Health Act: An overview. Canada Health Act. 2019, December 17. https://lop.parl.ca/staticfiles/PublicWebsite/Home/ResearchPublications/BackgroundPapers/PDF/2019-54-e.pdf
85. Tracy MF, O'Grady ET. Hamric and Hanson's advanced practice nursing: an integrative approach. 7th ed. Amsterdam: Elsevier; 2023.
86. Unsworth J, Greene K, Ali P, Lillebø G, Mazilu DC. Advanced practice nurse roles in Europe: implementation challenges, progress and lessons learnt. Int Nurs Rev. 2024;71(2):299–308. https://doi.org/10.1111/inr.12800.
87. Urrutia-Egaña MJ, Perucca-Gallegos D. Enfermera de práctica avanzada en Chile: Identificando barreras y oportunidades para el ejercicio del rol. Enfermería Universitaria. 2021;18(2):130–7. https://doi.org/10.22201/eneo.23958421e.2021.2.952.
88. Valenta S, Ribaut J, Leppla L, Mielke J, Teynor A, Koehly K, Gerull S, Grossmann F, Witzig-Brändli V, De Geest S, SMILe Study Team. Context-specific adaptation of an eHealth-facilitated, integrated care model and tailoring its implementation strategies: a mixed-methods study as a part of the SMILe implementation science project. Front Health Serv. 2023;2:977564. https://doi.org/10.3389/frhs.2022.977564.
89. van Zyl C, Badenhorst M, Hanekom S, Heine M. Unravelling 'low-resource settings': a systematic scoping review with qualitative content analysis. BMJ Glob Health. 2021;6(6):e005190. https://doi.org/10.1136/bmjgh-2021-005190.
90. Vargas I, Barros X, Fernández MJ, Mayol M. Rediseño en el abordaje de personas con multimorbilidad crónica: Desde la fragmentación al cuidado integral centrado en las personas. Rev Med Clin Condes. 2021;32(4):400–13. https://doi.org/10.1016/j.rmclc.2021.05.003.
91. Vergara M. Conceptualización y método para revisitar la gestión de la salud pública y la provisión de servicios de salud en los municipios de la Región Metropolitana. Rev Med Chile. 2020;148(8):1195–201. https://doi.org/10.4067/S0034-98872020000801195.
92. Vergara M. La falta de perspectiva sanitaria en el sistema de salud chileno. Rev Med Chile. 2021;149(9):1347–51. https://doi.org/10.4067/S0034-98872021000901347.

93. Wheeler KJ, Miller M, Pulcini J, Gray D, Ladd E, Rayens MK. Advanced practice nursing roles, regulation, education, and practice: a global study. Ann Glob Health. 2022;88(1):42. https://doi.org/10.5334/aogh.3698.
94. Woo B, Koh K, Zhou W, Wei Lim T, Lopez V, Tam W. Understanding the role of an advanced practice nurse through the perspectives of patients with cardiovascular disease: a qualitative study. J Clin Nurs. 2020;29(9–10):1623–34. https://doi.org/10.1111/jocn.15224.
95. Woo BFY, Zhou W, Lim TW, Tam WW S. Practice patterns and role perception of advanced practice nurses: A nationwide cross-sectional study. Journal of nursing management. 2019;27(5):992–1004. https://doi.org/10.1111/jonm.12759.
96. Woo BFY, Goh YS, Zhou W. Understanding the gender gap in advanced practice nursing: a qualitative study. J Nurs Manag. 2022;30(8):4480–90. https://doi.org/10.1111/jonm.13886.
97. Woo BFY, Ng WM, Tan IF, Zhou W. Practice patterns, role and impact of advanced practice nurses in stroke care: a mixed-methods systematic review. J Clin Nurs. 2024;33(4):1306–19. https://doi.org/10.1111/jocn.16970.
98. Woo BFY, Cashin A, Higgins A, Casey M, Buckley T, Zhou W. Prescribing practices and behaviours of advanced practice nurses and pharmacists: a nationwide cross-sectional survey. J Adv Nurs. 2025. https://doi.org/10.1111/jan.70111.

Global Nurse–Midwifery Clinical Autonomy: Contextual Differences, Similarities, and Challenges Across Three Economically and Culturally Divergent Countries Comparing Urban and Rural Settings (Uganda, Indonesia, and the United States)

Michelle Telfer, Rachel Zaslow, Qorinah Estiningtyas Sakilah Adnani, and Scovia Nalugo Mbalinda

Introduction and Context

The World Bank annually designates countries by their economies based on their per capita gross national income (G7410NI). There are five country classifications; "not classified" (currently only Venezuela is in this category); low-income countries (LICs), lower–middle income countries (LMICs), upper–middle-income countries (UMICs), and high-income countries (HICs) [1]. Table 1 details the per capita income ranges for these designations. Countries move up or down based on economic progress or faltering, though progress tends to be linear in an upwards trend.

M. Telfer (✉)
Midwifery Specialty, Yale School of Nursing, Orange, CT, USA
e-mail: michelle.telfer@yale.edu

R. Zaslow
Mother Health International, Atiak, Uganda

Mother Health International, Richmond, VA, USA
e-mail: Rachel@motherhealth.org

Q. E. S. Adnani
Department of Public Health, Faculty of Medicine, Universitas Padjadjaran, Bandung, Indonesia
e-mail: qorinah.adnani@unpad.ac.id

S. N. Mbalinda
Department of Health Sciences, Midwifery, Makerere University, Kampala, Uganda
e-mail: Scovia.mblalinda@mak.ac.ug

A. Kapu et al. (eds.), *A Global View on Clinical Autonomy for Advanced Practice Nurses*, Advanced Practice in Nursing,
https://doi.org/10.1007/978-3-032-21458-4_19

Table 1 Definitions for World Bank classifications of world economies income groups

World Bank Classifications of World Economies Income Groups [1] (based on gross national income per capita)	
Low-income countries (LICs)	</= $1135
Lower–middle income countries (LMICs)	$1136–$4495
Upper–middle income countries (UMICs)	$4496–$13,935
High-income countries (HICs)	>$13,935

Table 2 Definitions for urban, rural and maternity deserts

Urban, rural and maternity deserts	
Urban Areas	There is no set definition of urban areas as countries define it differently. For this chapter, urban refers to regions characterized by high population density, well-developed healthcare infrastructure, and access to specialist providers.
Rural areas	There is no set definition for rural areas; often they are simply defined as not urban. Rural areas defined here are sparsely populated, rely on agricultural farming, often marked by limited healthcare facilities, greater distances to tertiary care healthcare facilities, workforce shortages, and greater reliance on APNs or nurse–midwives as sole providers.
Maternity care deserts	Geographic areas, such as counties in the US, that do not have maternity services, including facilities such as a hospital or birth center, or clinicians such as obstetricians, family physicians who attend birth, certified nurse–midwives, and certified midwives [2].

A country may falter through economic and political upheaval caused by war, natural disasters such as famine or drought, or a pandemic such as COVID-19. Shifting economic realities impact not only healthcare but also health practitioners' scope of practice and their ability to practice autonomously. This was demonstrated in the United States (US) during the COVID-19 pandemic. Many states extended the scope of practice for nurse–midwives due to the increased demand for out of hospital birth related to fears of exposure to COVID-19 in hospitals.

Uganda, Indonesia, and the US, sit in three of the seven World Health Organization (WHO) regions: Sub-Saharan Africa, Western Pacific, and North America. The authors, representing each of these regions and a fourth with expertise in two of them, explore the differences, similarities, and challenges between urban and rural healthcare settings as well as nurse–midwives' clinical autonomy in their respective countries. Table 2 provides definitions of urban, rural, and "maternity deserts" used throughout the chapter. The experiences of one fictional nurse–midwife, Sara, and her client, Lina, are woven through the discussions of the different countries and settings to demonstrate the realities that both nurse–midwife and patient face, and how the state of clinical autonomy can negatively or positively impact both. Despite significant differences across economies and culture, both challenges and solutions to nurse–midwives' clinical autonomy are remarkably similar.

The focus only on nurse–midwives rather than APNs is intentional. Neither Uganda nor Indonesia recognize APNs, yet they do recognize nurse–midwives as APNs who work autonomously with defined scopes of practice. All four authors are nurse–midwives or midwives and are well-positioned to discuss the status and challenges of clinical autonomy in the countries where they practice. It is the hope that future editions of this book will forward the discussion of APN clinical autonomy as APNs become recognized across the global south.

Background and Conceptual Framework

The history of midwives and midwifery predates education programs, licensure, and regulation. Over the course of the last 300 years, the professionalization of midwifery developed differently in different contexts. In most of the world before professionalization, traditional midwives were selected and trained by elders in their communities for centuries. They were healers as well as birth attendants and well-versed in their specific cultural and community setting.

The British Empire introduced nurse–midwives to Uganda in the 1800s during colonization. Their training was based in the Western medical patriarchal model and centered on memorization. Over time, different levels or cadres of midwives came into being. Following on heels of the Safe Motherhood Conference to reduce maternal mortality in 1987, Uganda expanded the role of nurses and midwives with increased training and new competencies in 1994 [3]. The Nurses and Midwives Act of 1996 enshrined the different cadres and their scope of practice. In 2010, Uganda outlawed traditional midwives as birth attendants to move birth into facilities in an effort to decrease mortality rates [4]. Though meant to improve care, this law precluded implementation of the midwifery model of care, which requires knowledge of cultural context and significant community understanding. Despite being illegal, many women today still seek care from traditional midwives, women they know and trust who treat them with culturally appropriate care.

In Indonesia, "Dukun," or traditional midwives, customarily accompanied women in childbirth and assisted with fertility, contraception, and abortion. Beginning in the 1800s, Dutch colonizers moved to replace Dukun and began to train Indonesian women to practice European-style midwifery starting in 1809 and opening a school for midwives in 1850 [5]. However, Indonesian women did not trust the European-trained midwives and the school closed in 1875. When Indonesia gained independence in 1945, midwifery schools once again opened but they too closed by the 1980s.

In response to the International Safe Motherhood Conference in Nairobi in 1987, Indonesia launched a three-year, post-secondary diploma program in 1993 [5]. Recognizing that women trusted Dukun more than they did midwives, the Indonesian government implemented several policies in attempt to bridge the trust gap. Unfortunately, these policies have largely failed. Policymakers failed to both fully support collaboration between midwives and Dukun, and to address competition between midwives and Dukun. Additionally, policymakers continue to blame Dukun for poor outcomes despite the absence of evidence [6].

American midwifery has taken a different route than that of Europe or colonized countries, where traditional midwifery was respected and integrated into the medical model. Indigenous midwives on the unceded land now known as the US served indigenous communities long before colonization and continue to practice traditional midwifery in some communities today. In the colonial period, midwives were respected, sought after, and salaried. Enslaved African midwives attended births of the enslaved and frequently those who enslaved them. The first American midwifery school, Boston Female Medical College, was founded in 1848 to educate women in the care of women. It closed in 1873 due to opposition from the overwhelmingly male physician community [7]. The mid-1800s saw the rise of physicians and medical obstetricians. Physicians viewed midwives as competition. Fearing losing income to midwives, they falsely claimed that midwives were "unsanitary" or unskilled, though the physicians themselves that had higher mortality rates. Despite the spread of misinformation, less than 5% of births were attended by obstetricians in 1900. The 1910, Flexner Report declared obstetric training as "the worst in medical education" producing ill-trained, underskilled graduates. With this report recommending the abolition of midwifery and encouraging hospital deliveries, physicians succeeded in diminishing midwifery in the US. From 1910 to 1935, US obstetricians waged a war on midwives in obstetric journals, claiming that birth was inherently pathologic and required interventions [7].

At the same time, European countries were granting midwives national licensure, and public health officials evaluated the midwifery model in Europe demonstrated that it was associated with better outcomes than the medical model. Not long after, the Sheppard–Towner Maternity and Infant Protection Act of 1921 (US) gave state governments more power and funds to design programs to improve maternal and newborn care. Midwifery schools were opened in New York, New Jersey, and Pennsylvania, however opposition from the American Medical Association persuaded Congress to let the Shepard Towner Act to expire and midwifery schools to close. New laws stripped apprentice-trained midwives from practicing overnight. Most of these midwives were Black and had served rural communities throughout the Southern US. In the state of Alabama alone, over 150 Black grand or "granny" midwives as they were commonly known, were blocked from practicing with no pathway to licensure.

United States nursing programs grew into hospital-based programs and nursing leaders abandoned support for midwifery. Nursing education developed the role of maternity nursing wherein nurses with expertise in maternity care follow physicians' orders and call a physician to attend births. In the early twentieth century, the first formal school for nurse–midwives was opened in Kentucky, The Frontier Nursing Service. With outstanding health outcomes, nurse–midwife programs were opened again in New York [7]. This shift to licensure and nurse–midwifery effectively ended apprenticeship midwifery in the US at the time, as well as eliminated midwives of color who were disenfranchised and not admitted to nurse–midwifery programs until the late 1930s–40s and still are a small proportion of the nurse–midwives in the US at less than 8% [7]. The growth continued to what is now primarily graduate-level education with most located within nursing schools and colleges.

Conceptual Framework

Clinical autonomy among nurse–midwives is influenced by several interconnected factors; individual competence informed by education and training, regulatory bodies, health system infrastructure, and sociocultural context.

Individual Competence and Education

Individual competence covers formal education, training, and licensure which encompasses clinical skills, specialized and local expertise, critical decision-making, access to ongoing continuing professional development, and ethical and professional judgment. In all settings discussed here, national certifying bodies issue requirements for licensure and continuing professional development. It is important to note that the level of education for nurse–midwives varies widely across geographic settings.

Regulatory Environment

The regulatory environment encompasses the interplay between national laws and professional regulations, defined scopes of practice, and established codes of conduct that are specific and responsive to the needs of a community. In Uganda, where it may be impossible to call a physician in a rural setting that is far from a hospital, nurse–midwives are authorized to perform advanced procedures such as vacuum-assisted birth autonomously. In Indonesia, nurse–midwives are restricted from such a procedure. Only physicians may perform vacuum-assisted birth. In the US, nurse–midwives can be trained in vacuum-assisted birth as an additional skill to basic core competencies, but individual hospitals may approve or restrict nurse–midwives from performing this procedure regardless of training and experience. As the global healthcare environment continues to limit access to maternity care, this life-saving skill may soon need to be permitted as an autonomous skill for all nurse–midwives.

Health System Infrastructure

Health system infrastructure varies greatly across geographic settings, with large discrepancies in access and quality of care between urban and rural areas. Infrastructure as it is defined here includes the structure of healthcare at the national and local levels, whether it is non-profit or for profit, governmental privatized, or a hybrid of the two. Infrastructure also includes the structures, staffing, supply chain, protocols, hierarchies, and policies within institutions. Access to potable water, sanitation, electricity, transportation, safe roads, and internet and cell service are a part of the health system infrastructure often taken for granted in HICs.

Sociocultural Context

A single country may contain multiple languages, religions, cultures, ethnicity, and races. These factors create complex, context-specific meanings surrounding community trust, gender norms, cultural expectations, and individuals' perspectives on and involvement in their care that collectively determine what care looks like. A care provider must adjust dietary recommendations, for example, for a client whose religion and access to resources impact what she eats during pregnancy. The provider must be willing to work with a client on a nutrition plan that works for her. Community trust and collaboration is especially vital in rural areas where nurse–midwives may be the only accessible healthcare providers.

Sara and Lina

Behind every clinical case is a story centering on the lived experiences, specific needs, beliefs, and desires of a person seeking care. To understand the unique experiences of nurse–midwives' clinical autonomy across contexts and the impact on the people they serve, the authors created a "universal" midwife, Sara and her client, Lina. These fictional characters are based on real stories from the archives and experiences of the authors in their countries and contexts. Sara and Lina's stories will provide a view into to how policy and regulation impact and influence clinical practice and experiences beginning in Uganda, then to Indonesia before arriving in the US (Fig. 1).

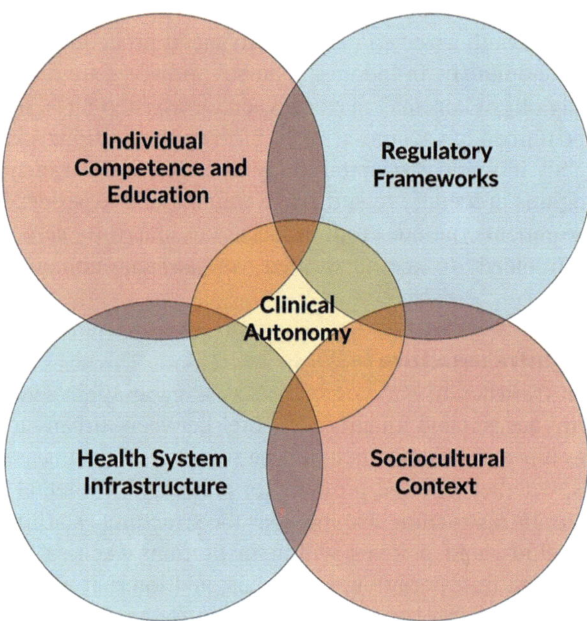

Fig. 1 Clinical autonomy arises from the dynamic intersection of individual competence and education, regulatory frameworks, health system infrastructure, and sociocultural context shaping nurse–midwifery practice

Uganda

Uganda, a LIC in East Africa, shares borders with other LICs such as Congo DRC and South Sudan as well as LMICs including Kenya and Tanzania. Uganda's maternal mortality ratio stands at 189 per 100,000 live births [8]. Though far below the World Health Organization (WHO) Sustainable Development Goals of less than 70 deaths per 100,000, it continues to improve [9]. The neonatal mortality has also decreased significantly to 22 per 1000 live births in 2024 but is still nearly double the WHO target of 12 per 1000 live births [10]. Though the WHO recommends a minimum of 6 midwives per 1000 people, the ratio in Uganda 2.3, with few trained to International Confederation of Midwives (ICM) or International Confederation of Nurses (ICN) APN standards [11]. About 74% of births in Uganda are attended by a skilled attendant, the majority of whom are nurse–midwives whose training is suboptimal [12].

Current Landscape

In Uganda, nurse–midwives practice autonomously and across four distinct cadres—certificate, diploma, bachelors, and masters—with each cadre having a defined scope of practice that is meant to build off of the other. "Certificate"-level midwives are trained in nursing before specializing in basic maternity care and becoming licensed nurse–midwives. With limited training, nurse–midwives at this level comprise 90% of nurse–midwives in Uganda and have the narrowest scope of autonomous practice [13]. As a result, Uganda is facing a massive nurse–midwife shortage.

Certificate-level nurse–midwives may take an additional 2 years of midwifery specialized training for a "diploma" and attain higher pay. Though more comprehensive "bachelors" and "masters" degrees are available, access is limited by high entry requirements and significant school fees. As a result, far too few nurse–midwives have advanced to the higher cadres leaving many health centers staffed with entry-level nurse–midwives and otherwise understaffed. Certificate-level nurse–midwives are often hired to work in rural health centers without a doctor or higher-level nurse–midwife, thus find themselves practicing beyond their scope. Additionally, infrastructure challenges such as poor roads and long distances between rural health centers and hospitals place undue burden on rural nurse–midwives. This leads to the "Three Delays" which contribute to the majority of unnecessary death in childbirth [14–17]: A delay in:

1. the decision to seek care if a condition seems minor,
2. reaching care, compounded by limited access to transportation and money, and,
3. the hospital due to overcrowding, lack of clinicians, and lack of essential medicine.

Most rural health centers in Uganda are between 30 and 50 miles from the closest hospital with a physician on duty. There is no central emergency ambulance system, and private ambulances can be prohibitively expensive. Few rural people own cars or have money to hire a car. Unpaved and rutted roads mean that a 50-mile emergency transport can take 4–5 h. Cell phone service is spotty and costly, limiting who and when calls for help can be made. These factors mean that nurse–midwives must be not only adept at assessing risk factors and knowing when to transfer, but also at being the sole practitioner working with women from even more remote areas with no time or resources for an arduous transfer. The scope of practice for nurse–midwives in these contexts are thus fluid; they must attend to women who would be considered too high risk for nurse–midwifery care as the only option.

Urban hospitals are staffed with physicians who care for the most high-risk cases including referrals from lower level and rural centers but are often overcrowded. At Kawempe, the national referral hospital in Kampala is one of the world's busiest maternity hospitals with an average of 100 births every 24 hours. In a 12-hour shift, a nurse–midwife might support care for women with twins, breech presentation, preeclampsia, placenta previa, obstructions, and more [18]. Due to the general shortage of nurses and doctors, nurse–midwives in urban settings must "be prepared for anything." They describe working entire shifts without sitting down, eating, or even going to the bathroom. To handle the astronomically high volume of people needing care despite a relatively small number of nurse midwives, Kawempe Hospital sorts patients by condition or risk into "pods" of 10 beds. Each pod is managed by one nurse–midwife. Every morning, obstetricians make rounds, identify risks and write orders for medications. Nurse–midwives carry out those orders for her pod, attend each woman through birth, and see her off to the postpartum ward shortly after birth, so the next woman can take the bed. While nurse–midwives practice in collaboration with obstetricians, they oversee each woman at the time of birth and must make real-time decisions regarding care. As labor progresses and different care needs arise, nurse–midwives make changes to the orders in the chart autonomously. Despite this level of responsibility, a nurse–midwife in this setting is not permitted to order a simple blood test without a physician's order, even though it is within her scope of practice. Though these nurse–midwives attend to the highest risk patients in the country, most have only achieved the certificate level of education which does not include high-risk training.

Lina" is a 16-year-old in her first-term pregnancy. Lina labored for several days at the rural health center but was referred to the main hospital to failure to progress in labor after remaining at 6 cm for 12 h with membranes ruptured. Tired, dehydrated, and scared to come to the big hospital, she traveled 30 km by motorcycle in active labor. Upon arrival, an obstetrician wrote orders for oxytocin to augment her labor. Sara, a certificate-level nurse–midwife who was in charge of the high-risk pod for the day, greeted her and pointed to a delivery bed. Though Sara is not supposed to manage high-risk clients without supervision under the certificate-level scope of practice, the hospital is short staffed. Lina presented with several high-risk factors: her young age and small pelvis size were initial factors, overlain by risk of infection from prolonged ruptured membranes. Sara took Lina's vital signs, placed an intravenous line, and administered the oxytocin. As Sara shared one fetoscope for monitoring fetal heart tones with multiple nurse–midwives overseeing their own pods, she was unable to adequately monitor how the fetus was responding to the oxytocin. Lina's pain increased with the rate of her contractions. Sara attends the births of two other high-risk clients while monitoring the 10 women in her pod. After several hours, Lina birthed a 2.5 kg baby girl into Sara's hands. Sara assessed both Lina and her baby, determining that the baby likely suffered from an infection due to prolonged rupture of membranes. She pointed them to the postpartum ward and wrote a note for the baby to be assessed by a pediatrician and given antibiotics. Sara then went back to greet the new laboring person admitted to Lina's bed. Beyond the initial writing of orders for oxytocin, the obstetrician did not see Lina again.

Sara technically practices in collaboration with a team of obstetricians, although she largely works alone, managing high-risk conditions and autonomously makes care decisions. The high volume of clients relative to the number of clinicians and high-risk needs of many of the people makes collaborative care as defined in Sara's scope of practice almost impossible. This extreme example illustrates the conditions faced by Ugandan nurse–midwives working in an urban setting, illustrating the real systemic challenges that must be addressed for nurse–midwives to practice both autonomously and with support when needed.

Challenges and Barriers to Clinical Autonomy

Scope of Practice: Clinical autonomy for nurse–midwives is essential for delivering high-quality person-centered care and improving maternal health outcomes. The WHO called for healthcare infrastructures to "Transition to midwifery models of care" [19]. To do that, nurse–midwives must be able to practice autonomously and effectively with collaborative support. Though the Uganda Nurses and Midwives Council (UNMC) provides guidelines for nursing roles, formal scopes of practice covering nurse midwives' rights to assess, diagnose, prescribe, and treat remain underdeveloped and inconsistently applied [20, 21]. The following story highlights these challenges.

Sara works in Uganda as a trained and licensed nurse–midwife at the certificate level. As she is not trained to independently manage a client who has severe pre-eclampsia, she is required to consult a colleague with more advanced training to ensure such a client has adequate medicine and monitoring. However, Sara is working alone at a rural clinic that is 75 km from a referral hospital. At 3 am, Lina comes through the doors in active labor with a blood pressure of 180/120, lower extremity edema, and a severe headache. Sara diagnoses preeclampsia but there is no ambulance or public transportation at this time of night to transfer Lina. If she sends her to the next clinic, it is several hours away, Lina could have a seizure and die en route. Instead, Sara starts an intravenous line to deliver essential medications and manages the birth safely. Lina and the baby do well.

These very real barriers and infrastructure challenges force nurse–midwives to operate in legal grey zones, balancing necessary extended practice often with fear of liability or professional sanctions [18]. A less experienced nurse–midwife than Sara may not have known what to do, leading to grave consequences for both Lina and her baby. Advanced training such as appropriate dosing and timing of medications are skills that midwives across all levels must be trained for even if it is not technically within their scope of practice due to workforce shortages of physicians and specialists in rural settings. A rural nurse–midwife might act as the sole clinician for large populations, handling everything from maternal healthcare, infectious disease, and primary care with limited backup.

On a Monday morning shift, Sara is responsible for managing clients in labor and birth as well as people needing antenatal care in a small village clinic. She spends her time moving between the long line for antenatal care and the two women in labor. Lina has come to the clinic for both antenatal and wound care as she has a deep laceration on her foot from working on her farm. Though the laceration technically is considered primary care, Sara sutures the laceration as that skill is within her training and scope of practice.

Nurse–midwives must frequently provide complex care while lacking higher-level support, sufficient supplies, diagnostic tools, referral options, and for entry-level midwives, training. This broad level of responsibility increases practical autonomy but also causes role overload, burnout, and moral conflict. Shortages of essential drugs and equipment, limiting the ability of rural nurse-midwives to practice safely despite the requirement to manage wider clinical roles [22]. Taking time to suture the foot of a patient might seem simple, but it also means that the women in labor while Sara was suturing, are not being adequately monitored or supported.

Infrastructure and Technology Constraints

Successful clinical autonomy relies on robust health system infrastructures that enable information access, communication, diagnostics, and collaboration. In urban centers like Kampala, nurse–midwives have access to multidisciplinary teams, electronic health records systems (EHRs), and telehealth initiatives that support clinical decision-making within defined practice limits. Hospitals like the main referral hospital have piloted EHRs and telemedicine platforms to support clinical decision-making and improve interdisciplinary collaboration [23]. By contrast, clinics in rural areas of Uganda often lack electricity and have limited internet, and nurse–midwives must rely on paper-based records. Ugandans carry a Ministry of Health-designed booklet to share health records across facilities and clinicians without the need for technology. Nurse–midwives in rural areas lack access to a consulting physician and the ability to safely transfer a person making paper records critical for understanding health histories and increasing the need for autonomous decision-making.

It is late at night and Sara is the only nurse–midwife on duty at a small rural clinic that is two hours from the nearest hospital. Lina arrives reporting vaginal bleeding in a term pregnancy. Sara assesses the bleeding using 'point of care ultrasound' and determines Lina has a placenta previa, a dangerous condition and requires an urgent cesarean birth.

In a city like Kampala, Sara would likely have access to Lina's EHR, collaborating physicians who can perform a cesarean birth, and a sonographer for diagnostic confirmation. At the same time, urban hospitals are often overcrowded and understaffed with frequent stock outs of medicine. If Lina had presented in the same scenario at the main referral hospital, she likewise may have had to wait to be diagnosed until the morning, when she would have been placed into a queue that could mean a several hour delay for her cesarean birth. Despite being in the main referral hospital, this delay could still have resulted in Lina's death.

The outcomes are connected to the "Three-delays" and the absence of infrastructure to reduce those delays. Clinical autonomy in resource-scarce settings can become meaningless if the nurse–midwife lacks access to higher level or emergency care, staffing, or supplies. Nurse–midwives working across settings must weigh these barriers when making clinical decisions [24].

Accountability

As described above, inadequate infrastructure and unclear accountability frameworks force nurse–midwives to work in legal grey zones. Fear of reprimand or legal consequences may provoke defensive clinical behaviors or avoidance of autonomous decision-making, sometimes to the detriment of the patient [25].

Sara is once again the sole nurse–midwife on duty at her rural clinic. According to the law, she must refer grand multiparas (women who have given birth to more than six babies) to a higher-level facility because of the increased risk of hemorrhage after birth. Lina, however, does not see the need to travel to the higher-level facility. She is sure, based on her previous births, that she will give birth quickly and easily. Her family are subsistence farmers. Without income, they must weigh expense of paying for transportation to a hospital against the high likelihood that she will give birth before she reaches a distant hospital. The Ministry of Health is performing its monthly case file audit on Sara's clinic, so she must take extra care to ensure she remains within her scope of practice. Both because Sara fears that Lina will come to the clinic too far into labor to be transferred and she fears disciplinary action, she refuses to see Lina for prenatal care. When Lina arrives, Sara tells her she does not qualify for care, and she must go to see a high-risk specialist. This puts Lina in a difficult position. As Lina is unable to pay for transportation and has an otherwise healthy pregnancy, Sara's defensive act results in her skipping prenatal care altogether. When it is time to give birth, Lina calls a local traditional healer to help her instead of going to the health center.

Both Sara and Lina have made difficult decisions that neither of them should have had to make, but all too often in rural settings, such decisions are being made from lack of support, regulations that don't mirror the realities of the environment, and lack of infrastructure. If the Ministry of Health guidelines supported nurse–midwives to make autonomous decisions around parity and risk, knowing that many people like Lina would otherwise have to give birth with unlicensed healers as they cannot afford transportation for care at the health facility, then Sara could have offered Lina care without worry over sanctions. Alternatively, if Sara's facility had an ambulance, she could have easily transferred Lina in labor without putting that financial burden onto Lina's family.

Sociocultural Factors

The midwifery model of care is evidence-based and rooted in clinical autonomy [19, 26]. The model is bolstered by strong community ties, trust that is built on cultural understanding, and longstanding relationships: across decades and across multiple pregnancies. Nurse–Midwives understand individual's religious beliefs, food accessibility, home responsibilities, and even more intimately, how they feel about their pregnancies including specific desires and needs. With clinical autonomy, nurse–midwives can participate in shared decision-making with their clients which improves trust, satisfaction, and outcomes.

In Uganda, implementing this evidence-based ideal is often compromised. Nurse–midwives themselves are typically transferred from facility to facility. Working outside of their communities or religions may limit the development of community trust and cultural understanding. Language barriers and cultural bias between tribes can strain communication between communities and nurse–midwives who have been transferred to their region. In these scenarios, people may be reluctant to use midwifery care. Skepticism about the ability of nurse–midwives to execute advanced procedures may lead them to seek physician-led care if it is available. Resolving these tensions requires establishing trust by educating people and engaging communities on nurse–midwives' roles and competence. National policies that support longitudinal placements for nurse–midwives within their own communities may strengthen community acceptance and provide higher job satisfaction (Table 3).

Table 3 Comparison of Factors Affecting Nurse–Midwife Autonomy in Urban and Rural in Uganda

Factor	Urban	Rural
Workforce density	Multidisciplinary teams, specialist access, though staffing can be tight with high patient volume	Frequently are sole clinical decision-makers
Technology	Electronic health record pilots, telemedicine emerging	Paper-based documentation, basic communication tools
Regulatory environment	More adherence to protocols, moderate supervision	Ambiguity, autonomy by necessity, ad hoc referrals, intermittent supervision
Infrastructure	Fairly well-equipped, better supply chains, cell service, internet, electricity, running water	Frequent stock-outs, unreliable transport, poor roads, intermittent electricity, poor cell reception, usually running water
Continuing professional development opportunities	Regular workshops, digital continuing education, mentorship	Infrequent, reliant on mobile learning, irregular training
Community trust	Varied, often dependent on hospital leadership	Strong, with nurse midwives as trusted frontline providers

Strategies, Innovations, and Best Practices

The experiences of Sara and Lina have illustrated some of the challenges limiting clinical autonomy of nurse–midwives in Uganda. The UNMC, educational institutions, and the Ministry of Health are working to develop solutions that address the barriers and reinforce evidence-based care to ensure these barriers get addressed [3]. The goal is to formalize and expand nurse–midwifery scope of practice, improve access to continuing education, enhance infrastructure and technology, and promote collaborative professional cultures supporting safe and effective autonomous practice. As Uganda's economy continues to develop, the country will mitigate structural barriers such as poor roads, transportation, and internet access which will significantly impact provider clinical autonomy, community access to care, and health outcomes.

Formalizing Scopes of Practice and Regulatory Reforms

Because Uganda nurse–midwives practice is in so many legal grey zones by necessity of infrastructure and economic realities, the UNMC must clarify and codify the legal scope of practice in ways that are realistic to the landscape. The scope of practice must simultaneously reduce ambiguity and protect professional autonomy [27]. The UNMC has been actively finalizing comprehensive scopes of practice that reflect the realities of rural and urban settings, task-shifting policies, and expanded prescribing rights for nurse–midwives [28]. These reforms align with WHO recommendations on task shifting, supporting the delegation of specific services from physicians to nurses and midwives to address workforce shortages.

Expanding Access to Continuing Professional Development

Access to ongoing Continuing Professional Development (CPD) is a cornerstone for establishing and maintaining competencies necessary for clinical autonomy. Many LICs are now leveraging digital technologies to overcome geographic and resource barriers to CPD participation. Uganda's Ministry of Health has adopted mHealth platforms and group text chat peer learning groups to facilitate ongoing clinical education and case consultations [29].

Sara is part of several peer discussion group chats that allow her to share clinical cases with colleagues in her region and receive expert guidance in real time. These chats allow nurse–midwives to access critical information and support decision-making, reducing professional isolation, even when the internet is limited. Sara and peers from her point of care ultrasound training are in a group chat with a sonographer from the US who helps to review cases that they encounter. When Sara diagnoses a placenta previa, she sends the image via *a group chat to her sonography mentor who confirms the diagnosis and helps Sara make a management plan. These groups require very little data and allow nurse–midwives to access critical information and support, even when the internet is limited.*

Best Practice Example: Midwife-Led Clinics

In parts of Uganda, the Ministry of Health has piloted policies that enable nurse–midwives to own or manage maternal health clinics, allowing nurse–midwives to utilize fully their autonomous clinical skills and scope. These initiatives improve service accessibility and continuity of care. Nurse–midwife-led clinics demonstrate improved maternal outcomes and client satisfaction, correlating with expanded clinical responsibilities and autonomy [30].

After several years at a government clinic, Sara chooses to open a private clinic close to her family home. The convenience of working close to home means she doesn't have to choose between time spent with her patients and her children. She can set the standards of how many patients she can see in a month, has more control over her protocols and guidelines, does not fear being transferred to a new location, and can deeply embed her practice in the needs of her community. She goes to the market and sees her patient, Lina. Lina is also buying fish, and they compare recipes. Sara sees other patients when she picks up her kids at school, and they discuss the challenges of parenting, working, and staying healthy. Sara is fully integrated into the community and intimately understands the unique stressors her patients are experiencing.

Future Considerations and Directions

The evidence for midwifery-led care—the backbone of clinical autonomy for nurse–midwives—is rooted in community connection and cultural fluency that allows for true continuity of care [31]. Nurse–midwives are vital to strengthening health systems, particularly in low-income countries like Uganda where shortages of healthcare workers and infrastructural challenges are endemic and complex [32]. This section highlights how levels of clinical autonomy in Uganda are built on a web of clinical skills, regulatory frameworks, infrastructure, and sociocultural factors that influence trust. Urban nurse–midwives work within structured environments that provide relatively clear scopes of practice and offer technological support and collaborative multidisciplinary teams. Though this environment provides safer and more consistent autonomous practice, it is plagued by overcrowding, understaffing and much higher rates of burnout [33]. Conversely, rural nurse–midwives have high levels of practical autonomy driven by necessity in the face of limited resources, regulatory uncertainties, and infrastructure challenges.

It is critical to design care that is highly responsive to the barriers, delays, and needs of the Ugandan community. Nurse–midwives' autonomy is a crucial response to gaps within the health system, underscoring the importance of supportive policies and investments in networks of care. Innovative strategies such as task shifting, mobile digital platforms for ongoing professional development, telehealth initiatives, and inclusion of community health worker practice models have demonstrated promising methods to enhance nurse–midwives' autonomy safely and effectively. These innovations, alongside ongoing regulatory reforms and interprofessional collaboration, are essential to formalizing and expanding autonomous nurse–midwifery roles that improve access to quality care and lead to better outcomes. Uganda has made significant strides in lowering perinatal mortality in the last decade and the majority of care given to pregnant women in Uganda is midwife-led.

Indonesia

Background

Indonesia has the fourth most populous nation and is the world's largest archipelago with over 17,000 islands. It was the largest economy in Southeast Asia until May 2025 when it was officially moved from the WHO Southeast Asia Region to the Western Pacific Region. Indonesia has made significant economic and health gains in the past 20 years and is now an UMIC. The 2022 Indonesia Health Survey reported the maternal mortality ratio at 189 per 100,000 live births, which is significantly higher than the Sustainable Development Goal target of 70 per 100,000 live births by 2030 [34]. High rates of maternal mortality are linked to geographic obstacles that come with being on small islands, inequitable distribution of health facilities, poor referral infrastructures, and other intersecting sociocultural factors [35]. The neonatal mortality rate has significantly reduced at 11 per 1000 live births in 2023 [36]. The ratio of nurses and midwives is also improving with an average of 4.2 nurses and midwives per 1000 population [11]. There are more than 850 midwifery schools and over 750,000 registered midwives in Indonesia who attend the births of nearly 70% of women; physicians attend less than 20% of births [37]. The stories of Sara and Lina, now in Indonesia, demonstrate the way these challenges arise in regions with a variety of different influences on midwifery autonomy.

In a mountainous district of South Sulawesi, Sara, a midwife, frequently functions as the sole healthcare provider responsible for high-risk births. Travelling to referral hospitals during periods of heavy rainfall necessitates hours of additional travel time due to the winding and slippery roadways. To prevent this issue, she refers women to a maternity waiting home to ensure that those individuals with high-risk pregnancies receive care at the onset of labor. Lina has come to Sara for prenatal care with a twin pregnancy. She lives in a village far from the referral hospital. Lina has two other children at home, ages 3 and 5 years. Sara recommends Lina move to the maternity waiting home at 36 weeks for safety. At first, Lina was very reluctant to do this as she would need to leave her two other children behind. Because Sara knew her family well, she was able to meet with her family and discuss the risks and benefits for Lina and the family. The family agreed upon a plan to support Lina's children in her absence and her husband agreed to support her staying at the maternity home.

This local midwifery care is culturally responsive and has the infrastructure to support necessary care, contributing to better perinatal outcomes [38]. Sara is autonomous in the care she provides and works directly with the family, addressing both the barriers to care and their concerns. If Sara was working in an urban environment like Bekasi, West Java, hundreds of miles to the west, she would be in a hospital that is equipped with sophisticated technologies and substantial medical staff [39]. With a team of collaborative obstetricians, she must call for support during a normal birth and steps aside while a physician attends the birth. Of course, even in the most well-staffed hospitals, there are situations such as a maternal hemorrhage prior to the arrival of a physician, when a midwife must utilize her advanced practice skills to execute lifesaving care in accordance with established protocols, maneuvering between hospital standard operating procedures and professional hierarchy pressures [40]. Midwives must have the clinical skills to practice autonomously, regardless of the context they work in.

Urban areas are characterized by high population density, relatively complete health infrastructure, and rapid access to referral facilities with specialist healthcare providers. In such settings, midwives often work within multidisciplinary teams where their clinical autonomy is shaped by institutional protocols and professional hierarchies. Rural areas of Indonesia conversely have low population density, limited infrastructure, unequal distribution of clinicians, and as a result, a reliance on midwives as primary healthcare providers, particularly during emergencies. In many rural regions of Indonesia, like in Uganda, midwives serve as the frontline health professionals managing both normal births and complications until a referral can be made. Because Indonesia has over 17,000 islands, reaching a higher-level service frequently requires a boat trip, weather permitting, in addition to overland travel creating significant barriers and potential delays to life-saving care [41]. Thinking back to the "Three Delays" discussed in Uganda, the need for a boat ride that is also dependent on the tide, poses significant delay-based threats to perinatal outcomes that are well beyond the control of even the most prepared midwives but make clear the need for midwives to be "ready for anything" [42].

The degree of autonomy that can be exercised by midwives across rural and urban settings varies significantly in Indonesia. It is shaped by the concentration of healthcare providers, service infrastructure, cultural norms, and legislative frameworks. This can lead to confusion among midwives about their role and underscores the need for measures that incorporate augmented clinical autonomy for midwives, fortified referral mechanisms, thorough care of comorbidities, and customization of services to local contexts.

Individual Competence and Education

In Indonesia, midwifery is its own profession, distinct from nursing. A midwife has successfully finished an accredited midwifery education program, either nationally or internationally and fulfills the criteria to practice midwifery [5]. Midwives are skilled health professionals with the expertise, autonomy, and authority to deliver holistic care for women, babies, families, and communities [43] In this section, we will refer to midwives and not nurse midwives as they are distinct in Indonesia but exemplify the role of an APN.

According to WHO midwifery competence at its best is a weaving of scientific knowledge and evidence that informs mastery of clinical skills [44]. Midwives offer support that is person-centered and culturally relevant. Midwives skilled at critical decision-making serve their community with a clear understanding and respect for their scopes of practice. These competencies are critical but be confusing when there is not one standard educational pathway for midwifery licensure.

In Indonesia, like Uganda, there are multiple cadres of midwives. Midwives enter training with either a Diploma III or via a Professional Midwives Program. Midwives can upgrade their education and scope of practice with an Advanced Diploma of Midwifery (D4), Bachelor of Midwifery and Professional Program, and then a Masters in Midwifery, which allows for the most clinical autonomy. Graduates at all levels are equipped with basic nursing and midwifery knowledge that is generally correlated with improved outcomes [45]. Like the certificate in midwifery in Uganda, the majority of midwives in Indonesia hold the Diploma III degree which is a three-year entry-level vocational education program [46]. Beyond formal education, additional certifications and continuing professional development are crucial to maintaining high-level clinical competency for the duration of a midwife's career [37].

Regulatory Environment

Indonesia has worked hard over the last two decades to promote "skilled birth attendance" and create a network in which every mother can be attended by a licensed midwife. To achieve this goal, regulations, frameworks, and policies have had to develop alongside the rural women that might rather deliver at home with a trusted traditional healer and in the cities where overregulation and lack of clinical autonomy push a lot of licensed midwives out of the system. Midwives are caught in a confusing liminal space where they are both regulated with an ever-looming risk of litigation and malpractice, alongside the reality of how unpredictable childbirth is, a complex infrastructure with many geographic limitations, and the need to "be prepared for anything" to save a life. In 2023, Indonesia passed "Law no. 17," a regulation aimed to improve the quality of health services by simplifying licensing procedures for low-risk services, offering stronger legal protection, and integrating health technology into practice [47]. The policy has explicit protections written into law that increase the authority of midwives, but also created challenges in terms of regulatory adaptation, licensing costs, and the need for additional training [48]. The reality is that regulating and licensing midwifery requires systems level change that is in direct relationship with the barriers that clinicians face when carrying out their duties.

Health System Infrastructure

The organizational system within healthcare facilities directly shapes the scope of midwives' autonomy and in Indonesia there are large differences across settings [49]. In secondary and tertiary referral hospitals, service delivery of clinical care is hierarchical, with specialist doctors serving as the leads. In such settings, midwives' clinical decisions often must follow written protocols and require physician approval even if it's within their normal scope per national guidelines. This means that even highly competent midwives may have limited opportunities for autonomous decision-making [50].

In a busy urban hospital in Java, Sara, our midwife is caring for a laboring person, Lina. The fetal heart for Lina's baby is a little high. Sara wants to give intravenous fluids, which is well within her scope of practice, however, in this hospital she must first consult the obstetrician before implementing any management changes. She consults with the doctor and then provides a fluid bolus and helps Lina with position changes. The fetal heart improves and Lina is now ready to push and progresses quickly. Sara calls in the obstetrician who will be attending the birth, even though Sara has cared for Lina throughout her pregnancy and now in labor. This is the standard in an urban hospital. Sara feels demoralized as she formerly worked in a rural hospital where she managed births on her own every day. Not only is she clinically competent in attending this birth, but it is within her clinical scope. She has a relationship with Lina and wants to offer continuity of care, but because of her position within an urban hospital, her clinical autonomy is undermined. For Lina, having an unknown obstetrician attend her most intimate moment is confusing and uncomfortable. She had come to trust Sara through her pregnancy.

In community health centers and hospitals, midwives have a broader role, especially in areas with limited medical staff [51]. In urban settings, midwives may practice below their scope while in rural settings, they may be forced to practice outside of their scope because there are no other providers. Clinical autonomy supports midwives decision-making freedom, though it comes with greater legal responsibilities and risks that may not always be supported [48]. When autonomy is supported by regulations, professional competence, and strong referral networks with hospitals and other healthcare providers, we see the best possible outcomes [52].

We understand from the experiences of Sara and Lina that geographical context and infrastructure conditions directly impact midwives' roles, responsibilities, and critically, their levels of autonomy. In urban areas of Indonesia, healthcare facilities are generally well-equipped, medical personnel are relatively abundant, and referral systems are efficient. While these conditions should serve to enhance midwives' autonomy, the irony is that autonomy is more restricted due to strict hierarchical structures and standardized protocols. Conversely, in rural areas, midwives practice almost exclusively without physician support. Shortages of other healthcare providers, long distances to referral hospitals, poor transportation infrastructure, and weather constraints present major challenges. A midwife on a small island with no major hospital will often serve as the sole, trained health provider, requiring her to take on broader clinical roles. Emergency situations may exceed her normal scope of practice, driven by the urgent need to save lives [53].

Sociocultural Context

There are many factors that influence the acceptance and effectiveness of midwives' roles in any setting. Community trust is critical to and must be embedded into the midwifery model of care. It is not a coincidence that in communities with strong midwifery systems where midwives practice with clinical autonomy, women report higher satisfaction with care and better outcomes [54]. Positive collaborative relationships between midwives, physicians, nurses, and other health workers ultimately strengthen midwives' positions within healthcare teams. Unfortunately, regulatory dynamics are often driven by institutional hierarchies and limit midwives' ability to do what they do best: care for women in ways that are responsive to their lived experiences. For example, in Indonesia, strong religious beliefs and a

Table 4 Comparison of Midwives' autonomy in urban and rural Indonesia

Factor	Urban areas	Rural areas
Number of healthcare providers	Work within multidisciplinary teams with immediate access to medical specialists	Midwives act as the main decision-makers; physicians are not always available
Technology	Use of electronic health records (EHR), digital referral systems, and limited telemedicine	Manual documentation, basic communication through phone calls or texting
Regulatory context	Must comply with standard operating procedures (SOPs); clinical decisions follow institutional protocols	Greater autonomy driven by field demands, safeguarded by emergency provisions
Infrastructure	Comprehensive medical equipment with a reliable supply chain	Limited equipment, irregular medicine stock, and challenging transportation access
Continuing professional development opportunities	Frequent training, online courses, and seminars	Rare training opportunities; dependent on online learning when internet connection is available
Community trust	Varies and is often shaped by physician decisions	Experienced midwives are viewed as the primary healthcare providers in the community

culture of shyness and privacy around reproduction often keep pregnant women from seeking care in hospitals, preferring instead a trusted midwife. If a midwife is blocked from providing care because of hospital hierarchies, trust may be broken, leading to people seeking the care of unlicensed "traditional birth attendants." These cultural barriers lead to a lower uptake of licensed midwifery care and unfortunately lead to higher mortality. When considered alongside the reality of geographical barriers and the expense of complex transportation and cost of a health center, midwives need to work extra hard to gain trust and provide continuity of care. While midwives are working through these complex systems, gender norms simultaneously shape how communities perceive midwives' authority. In some regions, beliefs that place women in subordinate positions may hinder recognition of midwives as primary decision-makers, regardless of their competence, experience, and legal clinical autonomy. Conversely, in communities where midwives are esteemed figures, social support for their clinical decisions is likely to be stronger (Humaedi et al., 2025) (Table 4).

Current Landscape

"The Midwifery Act" gave legal autonomy to midwives in 2019 in Indonesia. This Act enables midwives to govern their own practices and work autonomously across the vast network of islands throughout the country. The aims of the act are to: increase the quality of midwifery education and practice, provide legal protection for midwives and clients, improve perinatal outcomes via midwifery care [5].

Challenges still exist for midwives to provide high-level care including confusing differences in autonomy based on settings. There are several innovations across districts in Indonesia that are clear evidence of the concerted effort to improve midwifery care. Providing midwifery service in maternity waiting homes and offering mobile midwifery care in the most rural of areas are examples of creative thinking that gets midwives into even the hardest to reach areas [55]. Because needs are so different depending on geography, the majority of districts in Indonesia set their own protocols for health service delivery that are based on the real needs and challenges of the families in those communities. This includes a written protocol for licensed midwives to work alongside community health workers or traditional midwives who support rural women as keepers of local custom and knowledge. This reflects an understanding that improving outcomes requires community participation and targeted placement of clinicians to strengthen health service delivery. Indonesia has significantly reduced perinatal mortality over the past decade by responding to the "Three delays" and implementing programs that reduce barriers that are intrinsic to a country made up of many islands. The geographical constraints to midwifery service in Indonesia vary so widely that midwifery autonomy needs to be designed and implemented at the most local of levels. Currently, family-based surveillance for neonatal danger signs using an app, monitoring for pregnant women and infants with midwives via chat groups, and ambulance systems for referrals to healthcare facilities in larger districts are innovations that greatly improve midwives' abilities to serve the needs of the community [56].

Challenges and Barriers to Clinical Autonomy

Scope of Practice

While laws and regulations within the Midwifery Act define the scope of practice for midwives, the interpretations and implementation vary greatly by setting. Local regulations, hospital internal policies, or institutional practices frequently narrow the professional space midwives practice in. As described in Lina's story, some hospitals require many routine procedures like giving intravenous fluids, and must await a doctor's instruction, even though national regulations permit midwives to make these clinical decisions autonomously. This creates uncertainty, leaving many midwives hesitant to make autonomous decisions even when rapid action is necessary.

Infrastructure and Technology Constraints

Transportation challenges with long distances to referral facilities often across several islands, pose a huge barrier to midwives practicing safely. Best practices for clinical autonomy for midwives must include a functional and swift referral system [56].

Sara is working a night shift on a remote island in the south of Indonesia. Lina, a client, experienced a severe hemorrhage after birth and needs a blood transfusion. The boat that would take them off the island will not be available until seven in the morning. While waiting, Sara must keep Lina stable, so calls the hospital on the bigger island, prepare them for a transfer to hopefully expedite matching blood products once they reach the hospital.

As we can see from this story, limited transportation via boat often causes delays in referrals in remote areas. In such circumstances, midwives must manage complicated cases longer than intended, thereby exercising "forced" autonomy [57]. The challenge is that without adequate equipment and medicines, this expanded autonomy becomes a heavy and risky responsibility that can lead to secondary trauma and emotional exhaustion for midwives [58].

Accountability (Legal Safety, Ethics, Clinical Pressure)

Midwives often hesitate to make autonomous decisions in critical situations due to fear of legal repercussions, complaints, or institutional sanctions including threats to job security [59]. Medical decisions made by midwives are subject to litigation if the midwife does not practice in accordance with regulations. This can be confusing when interpretation of the regulations vary by district. This fear is reinforced by colleagues' experiences with being sued or losing a job as a result of a bad outcome. Such psychological pressure may lead midwives to choose the administratively safest course of action, even if it is not the most clinically appropriate choice for the person receiving care at the time.

Sara is practicing in a small hospital in Southern Indonesia. Lina has arrived in active labor with her second baby. Her first baby was an emergency cesarean birth after a prolonged second stage. This labor, however, is moving swiftly and things seem to be progressing normally. Sara knows she could likely safely support the birth of Lina's baby and that the risk of uterine rupture is small, but she is scared. She has a midwifery colleague who was recently sued after she did not transfer a person in labor with a previous cesarean birth. She tells Lina she must take a cab to a larger hospital where she can be assessed by a doctor and will likely have a cesarean birth. This added transfer comes at a huge financial and emotional cost for Lina, not to mention the physical toll of a second cesarean birth. Sara feels terrible for days afterwards, as she knows given different circumstances, she could have provided comprehensive care for her client.

Sociocultural Factors

In some regions, medical decisions are highly influenced by local leaders, traditional birth attendants, or extended families. Strong trust in traditional practices can make it challenging for licensed midwives to gain trust for clinical decisions despite clear medical indications [60]. In certain areas, home birth is perceived as safer, more comfortable or "more natural" than facility-based birth, leading to refusals or delays in referrals recommended by midwives. Midwives who recognize and respect cultural norms, often gain the trust of the community and work with their patients through shared decision-making to ensure smooth transitions when needed and safety for all [61].

Strategies, Innovations, and Best Practices

Clear and Standardized Guidelines

Enhancing midwives' autonomy and independence in Indonesia requires strengthening protocols for practice, both within healthcare facilities and in administration. The first step is to ensure that every facility, whether a community health center, maternity clinic, or hospital, has clear and standardized guidelines that align with national practice authority. These should outline the clinical scope midwives can perform autonomously, proper documentation procedures, and structured consultation and referral pathways. Such guidelines provide legal protection for midwives and prevent delays in critical care, ultimately saving the lives of mothers and newborns.

At the policy level, strategic measures are needed both nationally and regionally to ensure that midwives' clinical autonomy is optimized and consistent. Midwifery practice regulations must make sense for the contexts they are in. They must clearly define the scope of practice, including legal protection for midwives who act autonomously during emergencies, eliminating interpretative differences or restrictive barriers in the field. Optimally, midwives would be integrated with collaborating healthcare professionals so that everyone understands the roles and responsibilities of colleagues and offer care within a supportive system that does not abandon midwives or people needing essential care [62].

Education and Continuing Professional Development

Streamlining the midwifery educational cadres and ensuring all levels meet ICM standards is essential. At present, there are 856 midwifery schools in Indonesia. The most recent national data recorded that midwifery schools have produced 749,866 registered midwives [5]. Inconsistent entry to midwifery practice leads to varying knowledge and confusion for collaborating healthcare providers as well as the public as to scope of practice. Continuing professional training is essential for a clinically competent workforce in an ever-evolving field and must be standardized so that midwives in remote and rural areas have the same learning and advancement opportunities as those in urban areas.

Teleconsultation and Digital Referral Networks

The implementation of telehealth and digital referral networks should be expanded to connect midwives in primary care facilities with specialist doctors. There is evidence that telemidwifery in Indonesia significantly increases midwives' ability to offer continuity of care across wide geographical areas especially remote islands that depend on boats for transfer. With technological support, midwives can access real-time clinical guidance without waiting for physical referral processes, enabling quicker and more targeted interventions and saving people time and arduous travel at great expense [40, 63].

Incentives for Midwife Placement in Remote Areas

To address the unequal distribution of healthcare workers, retention policies for midwives in remote areas should include financial incentives, career development pathways, and scholarships for continuing professional development. These policies must be accompanied by adequate facility and infrastructure support, ensuring that midwives are not only willing to work in hard-to-reach areas but are also able to deliver quality services. Alternatively, recruiting potential midwifery students early in the education process from rural areas can provide opportunities to women who might not otherwise have access to higher education and who will likely want to return to their home region to support their community once they enter the workforce [64].

Future Considerations

Future considerations for the autonomy of midwives in Indonesia is complex: there is no one size fits all solution to offering care in a country composed of so many rural islands. As the country works to improve maternal and child health outcomes, uplifting and supporting the role of midwives is the evidence-based solution. Increasing entry to practice levels that are aligned with ICM standards and that focus on organization of care and clearly defined scopes of practice, including partnerships between local leaders and midwives in rural areas, will foster ease of practice in areas where midwives are also asked to be primary healthcare providers. Revising institutional frameworks to support midwives in making clinical decisions autonomously is crucial. Collaboration is needed to integrate midwives into multidisciplinary teams and vital to ensuring that midwives can fully exercise their autonomy while providing essential care across all settings.

United States

Background

The history of nurse–midwives in the US is complex, and the profession lags most other countries in recognizing and integrating midwives into the healthcare system. Currently, nurse–midwives attend around 12 percent of births nationally [65]. The US has only four midwives per 1000 live births, below the WHO recommended minimum of six per 1000 live births and far lower than most other HIC ratios of 12 per 1000 live births [11]. High-income countries (HIC) with higher midwife to patient ratios have significantly lower perinatal mortality rates than the US [66]. The maternal mortality ratio in the US has been rising over the past three decades from 10 per 100,000 live births in 1990 to 14.5 in 2000 and a peak of 33 in 2021 and now at 18.7 in 2023 [67]. This is far higher for Black women with nearly 50 per 100,000 live births [67]. The US is the only HIC with an increasing maternal mortality rate, all while outspending all other HIC countries per capita by up to two to four times. This is especially true for Black, Brown, Indigenous, and Alaskan Native populations where mortality rates are up to eight times those of their White counterparts, regardless of education level and income [68]. Further aggravating the US maternal health crisis, more than 2.3 million women of childbearing age currently live in maternity care deserts. More than 150,000 babies are born each year in counties with limited access to maternity care. Currently, there is a shortage of 8200 nurse–midwives in the US, which would still only meet minimum requirements for a ratio of 6 midwives per 1000 live births [69].

Individual Competence and Education

Individual competence in the US for nurse–midwives is high and meets ICM standards for autonomy with a master's level degree required for entry to practice. Many degree programs are moving to a Doctor of Nursing requirement as entry to practice. This is not supported by the American College of Nurse Midwives (ACNM), the national professional organization, or by the evidence on clinical care outcomes [70]. Nurse–midwifery clinical education in the US has always been competency based. A student will not matriculate unless they have had a "Declaration of Safety" signed off deeming them competent as a safe beginning nurse–midwife. All nurse–midwives must pass the national certifying exam through the American Midwifery Certification Board and recertification is maintained every 5 years through continuing professional education and completion of three required modules on key midwifery content areas in intrapartum, ambulatory gynecologic care, and primary care. There are non-nursing pathways for midwifery in the US which are discussed in depth in another chapter.

Regulatory Environment

American College of Nurse Midwives (ACNMs) defines "full practice authority" as the ability of certified nurse–midwives to autonomously practice to the full extent of their education, clinical training, and certification [71]. The nurse–midwife credential is recognized in all 50 states; however, each state sets its own regulations. Currently 31 states and the District of Columbia license and regulate nurse–midwives autonomously. Seventeen states require a signed collaborative practice agreement with a supervising physician as a condition for licensure and two states still require physician supervision. These state regulations prohibit nurse–midwives from working to their full scope of practice, often restricting ability to write prescriptions and practice autonomously. Additional restrictions on practice include failure to reimburse nurse–midwives at the same rate as their physician counterparts for the same procedures and restricting nurse–midwives' ability to directly admit people to hospitals. Individual state regulations for nurse–midwife run birthing centers often restrict autonomy through prohibitive requirements such as required written physician collaborative agreements, proximity to collaborating hospitals, or unnecessary facility standards imposed by state medical associations [71]. This effectively ensures control of where women give birth. The result is a restriction of a woman's autonomy as well as nurse–midwives' clinical autonomy. Additionally, it has devastating health consequences for many rural women when maternity wards or hospitals close and physicians move to urban centers and nurse–midwives can no longer practice, increasing difficulty in access to care [72].

The utilization of nurse–midwives and the US maternity care system compared to other HIC countries demonstrates five key areas that could lead to improved perinatal outcomes: affordable/accessible healthcare, a maternity workforce that emphasized midwifery care and interprofessional collaboration, respectful care, evidence-based guidelines, and national data collection [73]. While critical in all settings, clinical autonomy becomes imperative in rural settings. The ACNM position statement on "Rural Midwifery Practice" outlines the challenges and potential solutions to increasing, empowering, and supporting nurse–midwives in rural settings [74]. These recommendations are similar to nurse–midwives in HMIC and LICs such as ensuring the skills and training of rural nurse–midwives are supported to ensure access to high-level critical thinking and management skills, regulatory support for practicing to their full-scope, and facilitating peer support and interprofessional collaboration. This includes skills in managing emergencies and the ability to access and transfer to higher-level care and providers during emergencies.

Nurse–midwives often struggle to gain admitting privileges at nearby hospitals where administrators and physicians do not agree with a woman's choice to give birth when, where, and with whom they choose. This barrier has a detrimental effect on nurse–midwifery autonomy, patient safety, collaborative relationships, and perinatal outcomes [71].

In a small town in the state of Connecticut, Sara is practicing as a community nurse–midwife and attending births in homes. She recently moved her practice from Vermont as her husband's job moved to Connecticut. She sees women throughout their pregnancy usually for hour-long visits. She gets to know them well and they develop strong relationships and trust over time. Lina is a first-time mother who has had an uncomplicated pregnancy and is now in active labor. Sara arrived at her home an hour ago and after listening to the fetal heart and taking vitals, is quietly supporting Lina as she labors. As the hours go by, Lina begins to tire, and progress is slow. She is well-supported but she has not slept and the pain is increasing. Together, they make the decision to go to their nearby hospital for better pain management and augmentation of labor. Lina is worried her choices for birthing positions at the hospital won't be respected. Sara reassures her that she will accompany her at the hospital. Sara calls ahead and speaks to the physician on call to let them know they were en route. Sara sent Lina's prenatal and labor records ahead. Upon arrival, they are greeted harshly and Lina is asked why she would be selfish and try to have a home birth when the hospital is safer. Sara is not allowed into triage and not allowed to speak with the physician to give a report. Sara never had this issue when she worked in Vermont where there is a well-integrated health system between hospitals and community providers. There, transfers were seamless, with strong guidelines, protocols, and admitting privileges in place. Interprofessional respect was the norm and even in emergency situations, she was treated as an autonomous provider, and her clients were welcomed into the facility. Sara worries about Lina and feels that not only has she disappointed Lina, but also Lina's care is potentially compromised due to lack of communication with the new provider.

Such scenes play out all over the US where only two states mandate admitting privileges for nurse–midwives and very few have invested in creating seamless transfers of care from community settings to hospitals. Nurse–midwives, fearing the treatment they and their clients may receive, may delay transfers out of fear and a desire to protect the trust of their client. Delays can cost lives and result in further eroding of trust with interprofessional colleagues when the transfer occurs too late [66].

Health System Infrastructure

Urban health centers and tertiary hospitals care for large diverse populations and are staffed with multidisciplinary teams with ready access to emergency services. Overcrowding and long wait times may occur, but usually staffing is adequate and supplies are readily available in the US. It is rare for essential drugs or supplies to be out of stock, however, this has become more common since the COVID-19 pandemic. Natural disasters that impact medication and supply production are often overly reliant on one or two production centers leaving the supply chain fragile and vulnerable to disruptions.

While urban settings in the US. provide access to skilled maternal fetal medicine physicians and multidisciplinary care teams, often a medicalized version of pregnancy care is provided, even for a healthy, uncomplicated pregnant person [75]. This translates to overuse of interventions that lead to complications leading to additional interventions: commonly referred to as the "cascade of interventions."

Reports of overmedicalization and unnecessary interventions are high across the US [75]. The unnecessarily high cesarean birth rate, at 34%, is one example of how the medical model as well as the legal repercussions of a highly litigious society have occupied the birthing space and limited women's choices [76, 77].

One of Sara's longtime clients, Lina, birthed her first two children at the small community hospital in an urban city. Now she is in labor with her third child. When Lina arrives at the community hospital, she is told the labor unit closed three months ago, she must instead go to the large hospital across town where Sara now practices. She remembers that Sara did tell her this, but when the labor contractions started, she just went into auto pilot and began the same walk through her neighborhood to the hospital she had done with her previous two babies. Now, Lina must find a friend to drive her as she does not have a car. When she arrives an hour later at the large hospital, it feels very different: chaotic, with lots of hallways, unfamiliar faces, and bright lights. She is feeling anxious. Lina is seen in triage by a resident doctor whom she does not know as Sara was busy with another birth. After she is evaluated, she is to be moved to a labor room, but there is a two-hour wait. She labors on her own in triage. When she arrives to the labor room, she is told she needs to have continuous electronic fetal monitoring as they do not have enough nurses to support intermittent auscultation. The continuous monitoring makes it difficult for Sara to move freely about in labor, and she finds it more difficult to cope with contractions lying in bed attached to the monitors. Sara arrives as Lina is pushing because she has been attending other laboring people. She apologizes to Lina, but the fact remains that she labored without her midwife.

Sara then explains she will need to call in her consulting physician for the birth, though they would only be standing in the back of the room. The physician would ultimately bill for the birth at the higher-reimbursed insurance rate which pays physicians more than nurse–midwives for the same procedure. Sara is embarrassed explaining this to Lina, but she wants her to know why the physician would be present. She also knows Lina's history of past sexual trauma makes additional people in the room more stressful, but she is helpless to do anything about this if she wants to keep her job as billing and revenue is calculated closely for each provider.

Both Lina and Sara suffer loss of autonomy and unnecessary barriers to the kind of care they each have come to expect despite being in a well-resourced facility. Healthcare costs, nursing shortages, liability concerns, and a for-profit healthcare system are the drivers for loss of nurse–midwife clinical autonomy and person-centered care. Large hospital systems continue to consolidate small hospitals and private practices into their ever-growing corporate system. With this comes depersonalized care that is often not designed to support clinical autonomy. Maternity units in the US almost universally lose more money than they generate due to the high staffing needs and fluctuating admission volume [72, 78, 79]. Healthy birthing women and their babies do not generate enough income to keep labor and delivery floors open. High intervention rates, cesarean births, and neonatal intensive care units contribute to larger profit margins, putting both people who need care and nurse–midwives at odds with a system that does not necessarily value low-cost, low intervention care.

Over the past decade, privatized healthcare corporations have been consolidating health facilities and closing maternity units that don't make enough money, creating larger and larger "maternity care deserts" and leaving expectant mothers to travel sometimes hundreds of miles and spend hours to access basic prenatal and birthing care [80]. Nearly six million women in the US now live in maternity care deserts and while nurse–midwives currently attend less than 10% of births nationally, they attend over 30% of births in rural hospitals [66, 80–82]. Between 2016–2019, the maternal mortality rate increased significantly, but women in rural areas experienced significantly higher rates of ICU admissions and maternal mortality than urban areas as a direct result of these gaps in care [83].

Lina lives in rural Neshoba County in Mississippi, an hour drive away from the nearest hospital or birth center that is staffed by a maternity care provider. The local hospital closed its maternity unit three years ago to cut costs. She did not have 'proof' of pregnancy from the Public Health Department to qualify for Medicaid at her first prenatal visit, so the office turned her away. This was after taking the day off from work. She did not receive care, and she also had a lost day of wages and the cost of gas round trip. When she was able to reschedule and take another day off from work, she was already 18-weeks pregnant. She saw Sara, a nurse–midwife, at the clinic whom she liked and who completed her initial prenatal visit. Due to the distance and cost of keeping prenatal appointments, Lina skipped her next two appointments and planned to return at 30 weeks. A week before her next appointment, she started having headaches and felt swollen, especially in her hands and face. She didn't call Sara as she had only seen her once, she did not have a direct number, and she knew that pregnant women often get swelling. Two days before her appointment, the headache became worse, and she was seeing spots. Her husband urged her to call Sara who then urged her to go to the nearest hospital emergency room, even though they do not have a maternity provider on staff. Sara called ahead so the staff would be ready for her and would know what tests to order as Sara suspected Lina may have preeclampsia. Her husband drove Lina but she had a seizure in the car. By the time they reached the emergency department 15 minutes later, she had stopped seizing but was not responding. She was taken in immediately for evaluation and found to have severe range blood pressures which were treated, but her fetus was in distress. She was prepared for an emergency cesarean birth. Lina spent three days in the ICU, and her baby was transferred to a hospital an hour away for neonatal intensive care. Lina was eventually also transferred, and Sara and her collaborating physician were able to resume care for Lina.

In this scenario, we see how "The Three Delays" plays out even in a HIC. Barriers to care that include distance and financial considerations, lack of continuity of care, and ultimately access to midwifery care, create a combination of events that can result in poor health outcomes.

Sociocultural Context

It is difficult to write about nurse–midwives and maternal health in the US without contextualizing the conversation within the history of obstetric racism in the US and poor birth outcomes. Disparities in mortality rates, particularly among Black and Indigenous populations are extreme. Black women die at up to eight times the rate as White women while giving birth in the US. This systemic issue manifests through implicit bias from care providers, lack of access to culturally sensitive care, and inadequate social support for the diversity of family needs.

For example, a standard prenatal visit lasts 35–40 min and covers not only clinical care but also time for the nurse–midwife to learn about the needs of the pregnant person and for the person to ask questions. In this way, a trusting relationship is beginning to be built, and the person's unique needs are known and addressed. This trusting relationship is an essential element of the midwifery model of care. In hospitals with a high number of individuals with Medicaid (public insurance), only 15 min may be allocated based on patient volume and the revenue billing and collection strategies in the practice (Medicaid reimburses less per patient than private insurance). Cutting the time short for prenatal care means the focus is limited to lab results and clinical signs, eliminating the human connection element of nurse–midwifery care. The midwifery model of care is grounded in values of person-centered care and is thus the antidote to implicit bias; building relationships of trust and understanding are at the forefront of the model [84, 85]. Especially in urban areas with diverse populations and languages, there is evidence that having nurse–midwifery care at scale is critical to improving disparities in outcomes [26]. Nurse–midwives provide personalized, respectful, and culturally sensitive care that is rooted in addressing the complexities each family faces throughout their pregnancies. Nurse–midwives, when empowered to work autonomously, build trusting relationships, advocate for their clients, and strive to ensure their needs are met. In this way, nurse–midwives, practicing with autonomy, are instrumental in dismantling barriers to equitable care. An increased focus on anti-racist training and collaboration with healthcare organizations are needed to ensure policies reflect an understanding of and responsiveness to the unique challenges faced by marginalized communities, ultimately leading to improved birth outcomes for all (Table 5).

Table 5 Comparison of Nurse–Midwife autonomy in urban and rural United States

Factor	Urban areas	Rural areas
Number of healthcare providers	Work within multidisciplinary teams with immediate access to specialist doctors	Act as the main decision-makers; doctors are not always available
Technology	Use of electronic health records (EHR), digital referral systems, and telemedicine	Varies, can have EHR or paper records,
Regulatory context	Must comply with standard operating procedures (SOPs); clinical decisions follow institutional protocols	Greater autonomy driven by field demands, less oversight
Infrastructure	Comprehensive medical equipment with a reliable supply chain	Limited equipment and increasingly challenging transportation access
Continuing professional development opportunities	Frequent training, online courses, and seminars	Fewer training opportunities; dependent on online learning or travel to conferences which can be prohibitively expensive
Community trust	Varies and is often shaped by hospital protocols	Often viewed as the primary healthcare provider in the community

Current Landscape: Where We Are Now

Nurse–midwives attend births in varying numbers by state from 1% in Alabama to 32 percent in Vermont. Only 11 states out of 50 meet the WHO-recommended adequate midwifery workforce of 6 midwives per 1000 live births. Distribution of midwives is incongruous with the majority concentrated in urban counties. Licensure and regulation vary by state. Some states have independent midwifery boards while in other states midwifery is regulated by nursing boards. American College of Nurse Midwives (ACNM) and state affiliates are key drivers in shaping legislation and regulations that restrict or infringe upon nurse–midwifery autonomy. In many states ACNM and APN organizations work together to advance autonomy for all APNs. Despite the barriers to clinical autonomy, demand for nurse–midwives continues to grow as families seek person-centered and culturally appropriate care with fewer interventions. Past experiences with the healthcare system have left many women with lasting trauma around pregnancy and birth [86]. It is estimated that up to 40% of women experience some form of traumatic birth experience and this number is likely undercounted. Women want their voices heard and their individual needs and choices to be respected. Nurse–midwives could be a solution to many of these issues, however, clinical autonomy, state regulations, integration into the healthcare system, and seamless transfer protocols must be systematically addressed [86, 87].

Challenges and Barriers to Clinical Autonomy

Scope of Practice

Current challenges to clinical autonomy in the US stretch across legislative bodies. Urban settings offer collaborative teams, ready technology, and consultative services which bolster clinical autonomy within a supportive framework. However, at times these frameworks can lead to overreach of institutional and physician restrictions on autonomous practice. For example, because many urban hospitals are also teaching hospitals that train resident physicians which means there may be no clinical learning opportunities for student midwives. Expanded skills such as vacuum-assisted birth, point of care ultrasound, and first assist at cesarean births are all within the expanded clinical scope of nurse–midwives yet training in them or ability to apply those skills can be difficult.

Sara is working at a hospital in Philadelphia. As a nurse–midwife, she completed point of care ultrasound training last year and has received certification. She is working in the labor and delivery unit when Lina comes into triage in early labor. Lina's baby had been breech, but she thinks the baby has turned. Sara agrees based on a manual assessment. Sara has been unsuccessful in gaining the ability at her hospital to perform and bill for ultrasound. Instead of performing a quick ultrasound to quickly confirm the position of Lina's baby and then help her get comfortable in a labor room, she must call and wait for the collaborating physician to perform (and bill for) the ultrasound.

In a previous example, Sara needed to call in the consulting obstetrician for a normal birth so the physician can bill at the higher reimbursement rate. This continues to be a reality in many institutions. It undermines autonomy and infringes on patient– provider relationships. Addressing insurance and Medicaid reimbursement rates across the country must be seen as a priority that supports clinical autonomy for all APNs and nurse–midwives.

Much like in Uganda and Indonesia, rurally placed nurse–midwives may work outside their scope or to stretch it to uncomfortable limits based on availability of collaborating physicians and distance to higher-level hospitals. This creates an unsafe working environment where fear of managing emergencies outside their scope may lead midwives to work in a legally ambiguous area and worry about loss of licensure if emergency care is provided [88]. Ensuring nurse–midwives in rural areas have access to frequent emergency training and legislation that expands their scope of practice can create a safer environment for both nurse–midwives and their patients. Working in unsupported rural environments leads to high turnover which further erodes community trust [89, 90].

Infrastructure and Technology Constraints

Nurse–midwives working in rural US face infrastructure and technology constraints that sometimes mirror those of their colleagues in Uganda and Indonesia, limiting their ability to provide consistent, high-quality care. Many rural communities rely on satellite internet access, which restricts the use of telehealth services, electronic medical records, and remote consultations with specialists. Limited cell service can also make emergency communication difficult during urgent maternal or neonatal complications. Long distances from hospitals and ambulances can delay access to advanced care when complications arise. Furthermore, rural clinics and birth centers may not have up-to-date medical equipment or even at times, reliable power sources, creating gaps in monitoring and treatment capabilities. These systemic limitations increase the risks for mothers and newborns and place additional stress on nurse–midwives who must often rely on resourcefulness and community networks to bridge critical gaps in care [82, 88, 91].

Accountability

Nurse–midwives working in large, urban hospitals have clinical autonomy if the institution and individual practice support them. In one city in the Northeast of the US, one nurse–midwife-owned practice co-manages nearly all high-risk pregnant people collaboratively with maternal–fetal medicine consultations. This practice rarely risk-out clients, thus the practice has developed a dedicated patient following. In the same town and same facility, another nurse–midwife-led practice has much stricter risk-out guidelines thus limiting patient acuity and risk. It is important that both clinicians and clients understand the full scope of nurse–midwifery clinical autonomy and what conditions risk-out patients whether it is for necessary care or preference versus state or institutional regulations.

Sociocultural Factors

The long and complicated history of nurse–midwifery in the US has also complicated what the sociocultural make-up of the midwifery workforce looks like in the US beyond the eradication of traditional midwifery in the 1800s and 1900s that excluded Indigenous and Black midwives along with European midwives by physicians. When nurse–midwives reorganized themselves in the 1950s, they systematically excluded any non-White nurse–midwives from their national association. Nursing and midwifery in the US mirrored the larger national milieu and created a deeply segregated profession that actively kept out midwives of color [92]. It has only been in the last decade that distinct strides have been made to make the profession not only more inclusive, but also supportive and welcoming toward nurse–midwives from diverse backgrounds. American College of Nurse Midwives (ACNMs) came out with a Truth and Reconciliation Resolution to address the historical and current inequities [92]. Because of this, the current nurse–midwifery workforce is 98% White and therefore severely lacking in sociocultural representation of those they care for [93].

Strategies, Innovations, and Best Practices

National and State Consistency and Full Practice Authority

National and State legislation that seeks to codify and expand nurse–midwife clinical autonomy and scope is a priority [71]. A recent legislative win in Illinois demonstrates this advocacy with a new law that strengthens clinical autonomy while expanding access to families in maternity deserts. House Bill 2688 was signed into law on August 15, 2025; nurse–midwives can now provide out-of-hospital birth services in licensed birth centers without a written collaborative agreement if they hold clinical privileges from the center's clinical director [90]. Additionally, nurse–midwives may offer out-of-hospital birth services with a written collaborative agreement with another APN or nurse–midwife who has full practice authority if they are in a federally designated primary healthcare Health Professional Shortage Areas or in recognized maternity deserts [90].

Out of Hospital Birthing Options

Expanding state legislation and regulations for licensing of birth centers that do not require "certificates of need" (CON) and physician oversight or physician directors is another priority area for rural and urban areas. The COVID-19 Pandemic demonstrated the need for birthing options outside of healthcare facilities in both rural and urban areas as fear of infection led many to question the need for hospital birth for normal pregnancies [94]. States with CON requirements which increase start-up costs have far fewer birth centers than states that do not have CON requirements. A recent example is in Connecticut which had one of the most restrictive regulatory environments for birth centers. New regulations have passed allowing a waiver for a CON as well as establishing clear guidelines for birth centers that can be directed by APNs, nurse–midwives, or physicians [95]. The hope is that the newer, more flexible regulations will foster growth in birth centers in the state and provide nurse–midwives and patients alternatives to hospital births. Making birth centers easier to open and maintain will also help to close the gaps in care in the ever-growing maternity care deserts [96].

Integrating Midwifery Care at All Levels and Interprofessional Integration

As maternity deserts grow and as more women seek out of hospital birth, nurse–midwives must be well-integrated into community birth care. One example of how this can strengthen clinical autonomy comes from a collaborative in Vermont, New Hampshire, and Maine. These three states created a strong interprofessional organization that addresses these critical gaps, the Northern New England Perinatal Quality Improvement Network [97]. They created an interprofessional referral network with clear transfer guidelines from community to facility birth that respects not only nurse–midwifery autonomy but supports the patient's transition in a patient-centered manner. This impacts outcomes as it eliminates a barrier to care that both nurse–midwives and their patients may perceive when deciding if and when to transfer. If they know the transfer will be smooth and they will be welcomed into the system in a non-threatening way, it reduces unnecessary delays based on fear and allows decisions based on clinical and personal indications.

A new quality-improvement program, Step Up Together from Primary Maternity Care, is seeking to train healthcare professionals to implement seamless transfers from community settings to facilities across the US [98]. They offer a Drill Kit, which contains everything needed to plan, run, and debrief a drill for clinical emergencies involving transfers from the community setting to a hospital. It includes the community team, the emergency responder team, and the hospital team who all work together to improve client transfers for the goal of improved care and health outcomes. Such programs not only serve to improve the transfer process but also strengthen interdisciplinary communication, understanding, and relationships which are critical to clinical autonomy.

Education and Continuing Professional Development

Currently, there is no nationally funded support or mandate for nurse–midwifery education as there is for physicians with Graduate Medical Education that is funded largely through different US Government programs with the aim to grow the physician workforce. Such programs are managed through agencies within the Department of Health and Human Services, Department of Veteran Affairs, and Department of Defense. Currently, the biggest barrier to expanding nurse–midwifery education is finding preceptors and clinical sites [99]. A government program that would support and guarantee training sites in hospitals akin to those that resident physicians receive would allow nurse–midwifery education programs to increase their enrollment and graduate more nurse–midwives. The "Midwives for MOMS Act of 2025" is one such piece of legislation introduced to rectify this disparity through grants for midwifery education programs and students to support education costs and training costs including preceptors. It would also give priority to students who plan to practice in a health-professional shortage area which are mostly rural areas [100].

Mobile Health Units

Mobile Health Units are an innovative model that has the potential to support APN and nurse–midwifery clinical autonomy while addressing health provider shortage areas especially maternity deserts, though they are also used in urban environments where access to care also has barriers. Mobile Health Units are a type of van or bus that is equipped to treat and examine people wherever it is parked. The units can travel long distances to bring healthcare to individuals or small communities that otherwise would have to travel hours to reach care each way. This increases care opportunities and decreases the burden of costs. Advanced Practice Nurses (APNs) and nurse–midwives are cost-effective and essential to staffing mobile units if clinical autonomy is supported in the areas in which they are working [78, 101].

Maternity Waiting Homes

While maternity waiting homes are common in low-resource settings outside the US, rural areas in the US are beginning to use this model. Alaska, a state with a small population spread across a vast terrain that is challenging to navigate, often requiring flights to reach the nearest healthcare facility. One such home is in Bethel with a population under 7000 and more than 350 miles from any other town in any direction but serves a region the size of Oregon. Women are encouraged to arrive at the home for the last 30 days of pregnancy. Benefits of staying at waiting homes include access to prenatal and birth care as well as reported benefits of living with other pregnant women going through similar conditions. However, women also report feeling isolated and missing their children during this time [102].

Future Considerations and Directions

Expanding legal and regulatory full practice authority for nurse–midwives is critical to expand care and reduce perinatal mortality in childbirth. In many states, nurse–midwives are still required to operate under supervisory or collaborative agreements with physicians, which limits their ability to practice to the full scope of their training. Strengthening state legislation and licensing regulations to remove unnecessary barriers, such as supervision mandates, constrained prescriptive authority, and limited privileges, will ensure nurse-midwives can deliver care more efficiently.

Increasing reimbursement for nurse–midwives and payment equity with other maternal care providers is also critical to achieve the ratio of nurse–midwives to childbearing women recommended by the WHO. Without equitable compensation, autonomy has limited value, as financial considerations strongly influence where and how midwifery services are available. Federal recognition, clearer Medicaid policies, and policies that influence insurance coverage all need implementation. Building a strong evidence base through research and adopting global best practices will further aid policy decisions aimed at optimizing nurse–midwives' autonomy.

Ensuring regulations in maternity deserts support the introduction and functioning of birth centers, mobile health units and community birth that is integrated into the greater healthcare system will help to ensure safe and timely care as well as transfers when needed. Improving autonomy isn't just about policy; it's about real day-to-day ability to support the communities in which nurse–midwives are called to serve.

Conclusion

The comparative exploration of nurse–midwifery autonomy in Uganda, Indonesia, and the US reveals striking differences shaped by economic resources, cultural norms, health system structures and surprising similarities in the challenges nurse–midwives face across diverse contexts. In rural Uganda and Indonesia, infrastructure limitations, uneven regulatory frameworks, and reliance on community trust underscore how autonomy is both constrained and creatively redefined in resource-limited settings. In the US, despite advanced infrastructure and greater access to technology, nurse–midwives encounter legal and institutional barriers that curtail full practice authority, especially in rural communities where their skills are most urgently needed. What emerges across these contexts is the universal tension between nurse-midwives' capacity to provide comprehensive, evidence-based care, and the external constraints. Structural, cultural, and political influences shape how care is delivered. Recognizing parallels across multiple settings invites a reframing of autonomy not simply as a legal or professional designation, but as a dynamic interplay between nurse–midwives, the communities they serve, and the systems within which they operate. It is said that nurse–midwifery is more than just a profession, it's a calling. This can be seen clearly from the many scenarios that our nurse–midwife, Sara, found herself in as she attempts to care for her community across many intersecting barriers. They can be understood through another lens, our exemplar Lina, whose experiences navigating the complexities of various health systems highlight the real need for person-centered care everywhere in the world. Future global efforts should prioritize strengthening regulatory systems, equitable resource distribution, and interprofessional collaboration, while honoring local cultural contexts, so that nurse–midwives everywhere can practice to the full extent of their training. This is slow and measured change that may, in many instances, require infrastructure overhaul. In doing so, however, the shared vision of advancing safe, respectful, and accessible maternity care across urban and rural divides becomes a truly global endeavor.

References

1. Metreau E, Young K, Eapen S. World Bank Data Blog. 2025 [cited 2025 Oct 7]. Understanding country income: World Bank Group income classifications for FY 26 (July 1, 2025–June, 2026). Available from: https://blogs.worldbank.org/en/opendata/understanding-country-income%2D%2Dworld-bank-group-income-classifica
2. March of Dimes. Nowhere to Go: Maternity Care Deserts Across the US, 2024 Report [Internet] 2024. Available from: https://www.marchofdimes.org/
3. Munabi-Babigumira S, Nabudere H, Asiimwe D, Fretheim A, Sandberg K. Implementing the skilled birth attendance strategy in Uganda: a policy analysis. BMC Health Serv Res. 2019;19(1):655.
4. Graham S, Davis-Floyd R. Indigenous midwives and the biomedical system among the Karamojong of Uganda: introducing the partnership paradigm. Front Sociol. 2021;6
5. Adnani QES, Gilkison A, McAra-Couper J. A historical narrative of the development of midwifery education in Indonesia. Women Birth. 2023;36(1):e175–8.
6. Wallace LJ, Macdonald ME, Storeng KT. Anthropologies of global maternal and reproductive health from policy spaces to sites of practice [Internet]. Wallace L, MacDonald M, Storeng K, editors. Cham: Springer; 2022. Available from: http://www.springer.com/series/15852
7. Capitulo K. The RISE, FALL, and RISE of nurse–Midwifery in America. MCN, Am J Matern Child Nurs. 1998;23(6):314–21.
8. Maternal mortality rates and statistics - UNICEF DATA [Internet]. [cited 2022 Apr 16]. Available from: https://data.unicef.org/topic/maternal-health/maternal-mortality/
9. United Nations. Global indicator framework for the Sustainable Development Goals and targets of the 2030 Agenda for Sustainable Development. Work of the Statistical Commission pertaining to the 2030 Agenda for Sustainable Development [Internet]. 2020;1–21. Available from: https://unstats.un.org/sdgs/indicators/GlobalIndicatorFrameworkafter2019refinement_Eng.pdf, https://unstats.un.org/sdgs/indicators/GlobalIndicatorFramework_A.RES.71.313Annex.pdf.
10. United Nations Iner-agency Group for Child Mortality Estimation. Levels and Trends in Child Mortality: Report 2024. 2025.
11. World Bank Data. World Bank Data: Nurses and Midwives (per 1,000 people). 2022.
12. Telfer M, Zaslow R, Chalo Nabirye R, Nalugo Mbalinda S. Review of midwifery education in Uganda: toward a framework for integrated learning and midwifery model of care. Midwifery [Internet]. 2021;103(August):103145. https://doi.org/10.1016/j.midw.2021.103145.
13. Telfer M, Zaslow R, Chalo Nabirye R, Nalugo Mbalinda S. Review of midwifery education in Uganda: toward a framework for integrated learning and midwifery model of care. Midwifery Churchill Livingstone. 2021;103
14. Thaddeus S, Maine D. Too far to walk: maternal mortality in context. Soc Sci Med. 1994;38(8):1091–110.
15. Mohammed MM, El Gelany S, Eladwy AR, Ali EI, Gadelrab MT, Ibrahim EM, et al. A ten year analysis of maternal deaths in a tertiary hospital using the three delays model. BMC Pregnancy Childbirth. 2020;20(1):585.

16. Wilmot E, Yotebieng M, Norris A, Ngabo F. Missed opportunities in neonatal deaths in Rwanda: applying the three delays model in a cross-sectional analysis of neonatal death. Matern Child Health J. 2017;21(5):1121–9.
17. Alobo G, Ochola E, Bayo P, Muhereza A, Nahurira V, Byamugisha J. Why women die after reaching the hospital: A qualitative critical incident analysis of the € third delay' in postconflict northern Uganda. BMJ Open. 2021;11(3):e042909.
18. LoPoni CT, Rujumba J, Ssekatawa W, Adupet M, Kashesya JB, Sule I, et al. 'They just told me to go to theatre': women's experiences and support needs following emergency caesarean section in Kawempe national referral hospital, Uganda. BMC Pregnancy Childbirth. 2025;25(1)
19. World Health Organization. Transitioning to midwifery models of care: Global Position Paper. 2024 Oct.
20. Maier C, Aiken L, Busse R. Nurses in advanced roles in primary care [Internet]. Berlin; 2017 Nov. (OECD Health Working Papers; vol. 98). Available from: https://www.oecd.org/en/publications/nurses-in-advanced-roles-in-primary-care_a8756593-en.html
21. Uganda Nurses and Midwives Council. Scope of professional practice for nurses and midwives. Uganda Nurses and Midwives Act, Chapter 274 Uganda: https://ulii.org/akn/ug/act/1996/2/eng@2000-12-31; 1996.
22. Namutebi M, Nalwadda GK, Kasasa S, Muwanguzi PA, Ndikuno CK, Kaye DK. Readiness of rural health facilities to provide immediate postpartum care in Uganda. BMC Health Serv Res. 2023;23(1):22.
23. Sturrock S, Davies H, Rukundo G, Komugisha C, Kipyeko S, Nakabembe E, et al. Sociodemographic factors associated with established and novel antenatal vaccination uptake in a cohort of pregnant women in Uganda. Pediatr Infect Dis J. 2025;44(2):S92–6.
24. Sserwanja Q, Mukunya D, Musaba MW, Kawuki J, Kitutu FE. Factors associated with health facility utilization during childbirth among 15 to 49-year-old women in Uganda: evidence from the Uganda demographic health survey 2016. BMC Health Serv Res. 2021;21(1):1160.
25. Ackers L, Webster H, Mugahi R, Namiiro R. What price a welcome? Understanding structure agency in the delivery of respectful midwifery care in Uganda. Int J Health Govern. 2018;23(1):46–59.
26. Renfrew MJ, McFadden A, Helena Bastos M, Campbell J, Amos Channon A, Fen Cheung N, et al. Midwifery 1 Midwifery and quality care: findings from a new evidence-informed framework for maternal and newborn care. Lancet [Internet]. 2014;384:1129–45.
27. Kemp J, Bannon EM, Mwanja MM, Tebuseeke D. Developing a national standard for midwifery mentorship in Uganda. Int J Health Govern. 2018;23(1):81–94.
28. Ugandan Legislature. The nurses and midwives act. Uganda; 1996.
29. Meyer AJ, Armstrong-Hough M, Babirye D, Mark D, Turimumahoro P, Ayakaka I, et al. Implementing mHealth interventions in a resource-constrained setting: case study from Uganda. JMIR Mhealth Uhealth [Internet]. 2020;8(7):e19552. Available from: http://mhealth.jmir.org/2020/7/e19552/
30. Waiswa P, Akuze J, Peterson S, Kerber K, Tetui M, Forsberg BC, et al. Differences in essential newborn care at birth between private and public health facilities in eastern Uganda. Glob Health Action. 2015;8(1):24251.
31. Bazirete O, Hughes K, Lopes SC, Turkmani S, Abdullah AS, Ayaz T, et al. Midwife-led birthing centres in four countries: a case study. BMC Health Serv Res. 2023;23(1):1105.
32. Turigye B, Mulogo EM, Kajjimu J, Ngonzi J. Quality of maternal and newborn care services in Uganda: a scoping review. J Med Surg Public Health [Internet]. 2025;7:100210. Available from: https://linkinghub.elsevier.com/retrieve/pii/S2949916X25000349
33. Namutebi M, Nalwadda GK, Kasasa S, Muwanguzi PA, Kaye DK. Midwives' perceptions towards the ministry of health guidelines for the provision of immediate postpartum care in rural health facilities in Uganda. BMC Pregnancy Childbirth. 2023;23(1):261.
34. Republic Indonesai. PROFIL KESEHATAN INDONESIA, 2021 [Internet]. Jakarta; 2022 [cited 2025 Oct 7]. Available from: Website: http://www.kemkes/go.id

35. Misnaniarti, Sariunita N, Idris H. Regional perinatal mortality differences in Indonesia: evidence from Indonesian demographic health survey. Public Health in Practice. 2024:7.
36. World Bank Group. World Bank Data: Neonatal Mortality Rate Indonesia. 2023.
37. Adnani QES, Chairiyah R, Argaheni NB, Khuzaiyah S, Widyasih H, Telfer M. Decoding newly graduated midwives: a value-based philosophy of vocational and professional Midwifery program in Indonesia. Midwifery [Internet]. 2025;141:104239. Available from: https://linkinghub.elsevier.com/retrieve/pii/S026661382400322X
38. Dewi A, Sugiyo D, Sundari S, Puspitosari WA, Supriyatiningsih, Dewi TS. Research implementation and evaluation of the maternity waiting home program for enhancing maternal health in remote area of Indonesia. Clin Epidemiol Glob Health. 2023 Sep 1:23.
39. Adnani QES, Okinarum GY, Muchlis M, Susanti AI, Gumilang L, Adepoju VA, et al. Scope, significance and sustaining the midwifery profession in Indonesia: commentary. Midwifery. 2025;142:104286.
40. Susanti AI, Ali M, Hernawan AH, Rinawan FR, Purnama WG, Puspitasari IW, et al. Midwifery continuity of care in Indonesia: initiation of Mobile health development integrating midwives' competency and service needs. Int J Environ Res Public Health. 2022;19(21)
41. Mutiar A, Abbas KA. Narra J Challenges in maritime evacuation during pre-hospital emergency anesthesia on a remote island in Indonesia: a case report. https://doi.org/10.52225/narra.v5i2.1643
42. Muliyati M, Jaya R. Customer satisfaction as a mediator of service quality and perceived value in building customer trust. J Ilmiah Manajemen Kesatuan. 2025;13(3):1871–80.
43. Profil-Kesehatan-Indonesia-2019.
44. World Health Organization. Transitioning to midwifery models of care [Internet]. Geneva; 2024. [cited 2025 Feb 1]. Available from: https://www.who.int/publications/i/item/9789240098268
45. ICM Essential Competencies for Midwifery Practice 2024. 2024.
46. Bogren M, Alesö A, Teklemariam M, Sjöblom H, Hammarbäck L, Erlandsson K. Facilitators of and barriers to providing high-quality midwifery education in South-East Asia—an integrative review, vol. 35. Women Birth; 2022. p. e199–210.
47. Prayuti Y. Transformation of Midwives' Independent Practice in The Era of Law No. 17 of 2023: Between regulations, Challenges and Opportunities.
48. Vitrianingsih Y, Suhartono S, Arie Mangesti Y. Doctors' legal protection of midwives and nurses professionals in medical actions in hospitals. 2023;
49. Humairaa Haji Zolkefli Z, Brunei Darussalam Khadizah Haji Abdul Mumin U, Rudita Idris D. Literature review autonomy and its impact on midwifery practice. Br J Midwifery. 2020;28
50. Alsaqqa HH. Healthcare organizations management: analyzing characteristics, features and factors, to identify gaps "scoping review". Health Services Insights. SAGE Publications Ltd. 2023;16
51. Indrayani FH, Sarbini A, Andriyani A, Sari D, Bachtar M, Bebasari M, et al. The Midwifery practice challenges in the rural populations of Indonesia. Res J Med Sci. 2017;(11)
52. Hasanbasri M, Maula AW, Wiratama BS, Espressivo A, Marthias T. Analyzing primary healthcare governance in Indonesia: perspectives of community health workers. Cureus. 2024;16:e56099.
53. Homer CSE, Turkmani S, Rumsey M. The state of midwifery in small Island Pacific nations. Women Birth. 2017;30(3):193–9.
54. Lambung U, Banjarmasin M. The power of social norms: exploring the influence of cultural factors on economic decision-making Eny Fahrati. West Sci Interdiscipl Stud. 2023;01
55. Muharram FR, Sulistya H, Swannjo J, Firmansyah F, Rizal M, Izza A, et al. Adequacy and distribution of the health workforce in Indonesia. WHO South-East Asia J Public Health. 2025;13(2):45.
56. Halimah, Sutanto E, Suparmi, Baskoro A, Maulana N, Adani N, et al. Exploration of district-level innovations to address maternal and neonatal mortality in Indonesia. Indonesian J Health Admin. 2022;10(2):206–18.

57. Diba F, Ichsan I, Muhsin M, Marthoenis M, Sofyan H, Andalas M, et al. Healthcare providers' perception of the referral system in maternal care facilities in Aceh, Indonesia: a cross-sectional study. BMJ Open. 2019;9(12):e031484.
58. Naughton SL, Harvey C, Baldwin A. Providing woman-centred care in complex pregnancy situations. Midwifery Churchill Livingstone. 2021;102
59. Kebidanan Tahirah Al Baeti Bulukumba A, Zakariya H, Maulana Zanuar K. Aspects of legal protection against midwife profession in Indonesia. J Midwifery Nurs Stud. 2022;4(1)
60. Aynalem BY, Melesse MF, Bitewa YB. Cultural beliefs and traditional practices during pregnancy, child birth, and the postpartum period in east Gojjam zone, Northwest Ethiopia: a qualitative study. Women's Health Rep. 2023;4(1):415–22.
61. Puskesmas K, Kabupaten P, Selatan BK, Kasus S, Sungkai P, Palimbo A, et al. Pelaksanaan Sistem Rujukan Kasus Ibu Hamil Risiko Tinggi oleh Bidan Desa implementation on the referral system of high risk pregnant women from villages midwives to primary healthcare center with basic obstetric and neonatal emergency Care in Banjar District, South Kalimantan (a case study in Sungkai primary healthcare center). 2015.
62. Silvia E, Asmawati D, Syaptiani W. Barriers and facilitators to optimal midwife competence in Normal delivery care: perspectives from community health centers in Padang Pariaman, Indonesia. Sriwijaya J Obstetr Gynecol. 2024;2(2):103–15.
63. Algifinita A, Prasetyo B, Wittiarika I. View of perceptions, attitudes, And practices of midwives towards the use of telehealth. Indonesian J Health Adm. 2017;
64. Indriani D, Damayanti NA, Teguh D, Ardian M, Suhargono H, Urbaya S, et al. The maternal referral mobile application system for minimizing the risk of childbirth. J Public Health Res. 2020;9
65. Speer K, Fouladi F. Workforce Supports: Improving Maternal Health Outcomes. 2024.
66. Vedam S, Stoll K, MacDorman M, Declercq E, Cramer R, Cheyney M, et al. Mapping integration of midwives across the United States: impact on access, equity, and outcomes. PLoS One. 2018;13(2):e0192523.
67. Centers for Disease Control. Data from the Pregnancy Mortality Surveillance System. 2025.
68. Fishman SH, Hummer RA, Sierra G, Hargrove T, Powers DA, Rogers RG. Race/ethnicity, maternal educational attainment, and infant mortality in the United States. Biodemography Soc Biol. 2020;66(1):1–26.
69. Sakala C, Hernández-Cancio S, Mackay E, Wei R. Improving our maternity care now through Midwifery. J Perinatal Educ. 2022;31(4):181–3.
70. American College of Nurse Midwives. Position statement: Midwifery education and doctoral preparation. ACNM Position Statement. Silver Spring: ACNM; 2019.
71. POSITION STATEMENT Statutory and Regulatory Language Differentiating Scope of Practice/Practice Authority by Practice Setting [Internet]. Available from: https://www.midwife.org/acnm/files/acnmlibrarydata/uploadfilename/000000000266/Definitio
72. Fontenot J, Brigance C, Lucas R, Stoneburner A. Navigating geographical disparities: access to obstetric hospitals in maternity care deserts and across the United States. BMC Pregnancy Childbirth [Internet]. 2024. [cited 2025 Sep 30];24 https://doi.org/10.1186/s12884-024-06535-7.
73. Kennedy HP, Balaam MC, Dahlen H, Declercq E, de Jonge A, Downe S, et al. The role of midwifery and other international insights for maternity care in the United States: an analysis of four countries. Birth. 2020;47(4):332–45.
74. American College of Nurse Midwives Rural Midwifery Task Force. POSITION STATEMENT Rural Midwifery Practice [Internet]. Washington, DC: American College of Nurse Midwives; 2023 [Cited 2025 Dec 7]. https://doi.org/10.1111/birt.12516.
75. Clesse C, Lighezzolo-Alnot J, de Lavergne S, Hamlin S, Scheffler M. The evolution of birth medicalisation: a systematic review. Midwifery [Internet]. 2018;66:161–7. Available from: https://www.sciencedirect.com/science/article/abs/pii/S0266613818302377
76. Main EK. Leading change on labor and delivery: reducing nulliparous term singleton vertex (NTSV) cesarean rates. The Joint Commission Journal on Quality and Patient Safety [Internet]. 2017;43(2):51–2. https://doi.org/10.1016/j.jcjq.2016.11.009.

77. Antoine C, Young BK. Cesarean section one hundred years 1920-2020: the good, the bad and the ugly. J Perinat Med. 2020;49(1):5–16.
78. Brigance C, Lucas R., Jones E, Davis A, Oinuma M, Mishkin K, et al. Nowhere to go: maternity care deserts across the U.S. (Report No. 3) March of Dimes [Internet]. 2022 [cited 2025 Oct 7]. Available from: https://www.marchofdimes.org/research/maternity-care-deserts-report.aspx
79. Nearly six million women in the US live in maternity care deserts. Vol. 382, BMJ (Clinical research ed.). NLM (Medline); 2023. p. p1919.
80. Adashi EY, O'Mahony DP, Cohen IG. Maternity care deserts: key drivers of the national maternal health crisis. J Am Board Fam Med Am Board Fam Med. 2025;38:165–7.
81. Atwani R, Robbins L, Saade G, Kawakita T. Association of maternity care deserts with maternal and pregnancy-related mortality. Obstet Gynecol. 2025;146(2):181–8.
82. Access to Maternity Providers: Midwives and Birth Centers.
83. Harrington KA, Cameron NA, Culler K, Grobman WA, Khan SS. Rural–urban disparities in adverse maternal outcomes in the United States, 2016–2019. Am J Public Health. 2023;113(2):224–7.
84. Njoku A, Evans M, Nimo-Sefah L, Bailey J. Listen to the whispers before they become screams: addressing black maternal morbidity and mortality in the United States. Healthcare (Switzerland). 2023;11(3)
85. Post W, Thomas A, Sutton KM. "Black women should not die giving life": The lived experiences of black women diagnosed with severe maternal morbidity in the United States. Birth. 2025;52(1):36–45.
86. Watson K, White C, Hall H, Hewitt A. Women's experiences of birth trauma: a scoping review. Women and Birth. 2021;34:417–24.
87. McKelvin G, Thomson G, Downe S. The childbirth experience: a systematic review of predictors and outcomes. Women and Birth. 2021;34(5):407–16. Available from: https://www.sciencedirect.com/science/article/abs/pii/S1871519220303395
88. Sheffield EC, Fritz AH, Interrante JD, Kozhimannil KB. The availability of Midwifery care in rural United States communities. J Midwifery Womens Health. 2024;69(6):929–36.
89. Thumm EB, Smith DC, Squires AP, Breedlove G, Meek PM. Burnout of the US midwifery workforce and the role of practice environment. Health Serv Res. 2022;57(2):351–63.
90. Morris Y, et al. Public Act 104-0244 (formerly House Bill 2688). Chicago: House; 2025.
91. Friesen M, Josewski V, Sanders C. Barriers to rural Midwifery: an integrative review. J AdvNurs. 2025;
92. ACNM. Truth and reconciliation resolution from the American College of Nurse Midwives. Silver Springs; 2021.
93. Mehra R, Alspaugh A, Joseph J, Golden B, Lanshaw N, McLemore MR, et al. Racism is a motivator and a barrier for people of color aspiring to become midwives in the United States. Health Serv Res. 2023;58(1):40–50.
94. Quattrocchi P. Policies and practices on out-of-hospital birth: a review of qualitative studies in the time of coronavirus. Curr Sexual Health Rep. 2023;15:36–48.
95. Porter R, et al. An act protecting maternal health. [Internet]. Hartford: CT State Legislature; 2023. Available from: https://portal.ct.gov/governor/news/press-releases/2023/07-2023/governor-lamont-signs-legislation-licensing-free-standing-birth-centers?language=en_US
96. Jolles D, Stapleton S, Wright J, Alliman J, Bauer K, Townsend C, et al. Rural resilience: the role of birth centers in the United States. Birth. 2020;47(4):430–7.
97. NNEPQIN. Northern New England Perinatal Quality Improvement Network, A Dartmouth Health Program. 2025.
98. Step Up Together. Stepping up safety and teamwork for perinatal care, starting in communities. 2025.
99. ACNM. Executive summary final (1) [Internet]. Silver Spring; 2023 [cited 2025 Oct 8]. Available from: https://midwife.org/midwifery-workforce-study/

100. Lujan, Murkowski, Merkeley, Klobuchar, Kelly. To address maternity care shortages and promote optimal maternity outcomes by expanding educational opportunities for midwives, and for other purposes. 19TH CONGRESS 1ST SESSION [Internet]. D.C.; 2025 [Cited 2025 Oct 2]. Available from: https://www.congress.gov/bill/119th-congress/senate-bill/1599/text.
101. McGuinness C, Mottl-Santiago J, Nass M, Siegel L, Onyekwu OC, Cruikshank A, et al. Dyadic care Mobile units: a collaborative Midwifery and pediatric response to the COVID-19 pandemic. J Midwifery Womens Health. 2022;67(6):714–9.
102. Johnson K. Pregnant and far from home, a sisterhood of the expecting. New York Times 2017 Aug 24;

Global Demographic and Epidemiologic Trends in Advanced Practice Nursing

Kelly A. Goudreau

Introduction

Advanced practice nursing has been part of the nursing profession for a relatively short period of time with the first role being defined and specifically educated in 1956 [34]. The International Council of Nurses (ICN) define an Advanced Practice Nurse (APN) as a "registered nurse who has acquired the expert knowledge base, complex decision-making skills and clinical competencies for expanded practice, the characteristics of which are shaped by the context and/or country in which they are credentialed to practice" [20]. A master's degree is most often recommended for entry level [14, 20, 50].

The focus of this chapter will be a global perspective on the two primary advanced practice nursing roles (CNS and NP), in relation specifically to trends in demographics of the roles, populations served, and epidemiologic factors that enhance or inhibit the full development of the roles. These will be discussed within the framework of legislation and policy, the universal healthcare focus of the sustainable development goals, and the impact of technology, telehealth, and digital health tools on advanced practice. This exploration will focus on how these elements vary by country and advanced practice role. Additionally, dialogue will be presented that identifies what needs to occur into the future for the betterment of the health and welfare of the global community.

K. A. Goudreau (✉)
School of Nursing, University of Victoria, Victoria, BC, Canada
e-mail: kgoudreau@uvic.ca

A. Kapu et al. (eds.), *A Global View on Clinical Autonomy for Advanced Practice Nurses*, Advanced Practice in Nursing,
https://doi.org/10.1007/978-3-032-21458-4_20

The Global Demographics of Advanced Practice Nursing

The primary driver of the addition of advanced practice roles to the healthcare team is the current and worsening global shortage of healthcare workers—in particular—physicians. In most instances the shortage of physicians is focused on the rural environment in each country with most physicians choosing the urban areas for their practice. It is noted that nurses, especially advanced practice nurses, can best address local and rural healthcare needs since they know the population and geography of the areas where they practice and have the skillset needed to provide basic care, develop policies, educate the population, and bring a focus to wellness. The APN that is allowed to function to the full scope of their education and training work to introduce efficiencies into health systems that improve the reach and outcomes of care [27].

The roles of Clinical Nurse Specialist (CNS) and Nurse Practitioner (NP) are the most commonly found designations of advanced practice nurses on a global level [20, 25]. The United States has two additional roles that are considered advanced practice: Nurse Midwife and Nurse Anesthetist. Although the role of Certified Nurse Midwife (CNM) is not solely in the United States and does exist on a global level in some form (lay midwives as well as nurse–midwives), the Certified Nurse Anesthetist (CNA) is unique to the United States at this time. Although these roles exist, they are not the primary roles identified by the ICN as advanced practice. As such, these additional roles are not a focus of this discussion.

The global distribution of APNs (both NP and CNS) is interesting to note. A survey conducted by the World Health Organization (WHO) in 2022 received responses from 167 countries with 62% of the responding countries reporting having APN roles in place [65]. Of note is that the lower income countries reported the highest numbers of APN practitioners with 74% indicating they had the APN roles in place [65]. This was primarily found in countries that had a lower density of physicians to care for the population. The thought is that this potentially reflects a prioritization of the APN role where physicians are not readily available [65].

It is interesting that globally only 67% of the responding countries identified that professional regulations that provide structure and expectations for the APN roles were in place [65]. This means that the countries that have either partially or have no defined regulation of APN roles may have many individuals who are claiming to be APNs but have not had the education, training, or validation of competency that could potentially harm the public. In spite of the potential for harm, there is far greater potential for positive outcomes of care.

The demographics of the APN roles on a global level are hard to specifically quantify. The primary reason is that, as noted previously, only 67% of countries identified that they had regulatory boundaries outlined for the APN role, which in turn, would provide title protection for the role [65]. Title protection and specific regulation of the role would allow an accurate count of the number of APN providers. Since this is not the case in 33% of the reporting countries globally, the true number of APNs cannot be validated [65].

When looking at the Sustainable Development Goals (SDGs) outlined by the United Nations (UN) in 2022, there are many that can be enacted, enhanced, or enabled through the work of nursing in general and APNs in particular [49]. The WHO identified that in particular, "advanced practice nursing represents a powerful strategy for addressing global health challenges and achieving UHC [Universal Health Care]" [65].

Clinical Nurse Specialist

The first designation of an advanced practice role was the Clinical Nurse Specialist (CNS), when Frances Reiter gave a speech to the American Nurses Association (ANA) discussing the "nurse clinician" in 1943 [33]. However, little was done of a substantive nature at that time to specifically acknowledge or prepare these nurses. It was not until a need was identified by Hildegard Peplau that specific educational preparation of an advanced psychiatric nursing provider enabled the creation of the CNS role at Rutgers University in 1956 as a Masters-prepared nurse [50]. Peplau's designation of educational preparation being the Masters (minimum) level has persisted and has been a key component of the expectations for the CNS role globally [20].

When countries identify that they have CNSs in the healthcare provider team, there is a mix of practice locations that primarily include hospital or community-based providers. Clinical Nurse Specialists (CNSs) in hospital settings are most often focused on medical–surgical care of the adult, including critical care [35]. Clinical Nurse Specialist (CNS) providers on a global level are identified in rural communities where their role is to reduce transmission of disease and work with the local population to improve health overall.

Nurse Practitioner

The first Nurse Practitioner program globally is reported to have been created by Dr. Loretta Ford and a physician colleague in 1965 as a response to the shortage of primary care physicians. The need for a Nurse Practitioner was a direct response to "... the expansion of coverage by Medicare and Medicaid to include low-income women, children, the elderly, and people with disabilities" [40]. The role was not initially conceived as a Masters-level preparation and was a post-baccalaureate certificate [3]. It was not until 1967 that the first proposed Masters preparation was created at Boston College and by 1989 "...Ninety percent of NP programs are either master's degree programs or post-master's degree programs" [3].

Role Confusion and Clarification

The National Association of Clinical Nurse Specialists [36] provided an updated definition of what a clinical nurse specialist is, in an effort to clarify the role and distinguish it from a Nurse Practitioner. A CNS is an "...Advanced Practice Registered Nurse (APRN) [designation in the United States] prepared by a master's, or doctoral, or post-graduate certificate level CNS program. CNSs diagnose, prescribe, and treat patients and specialty populations across the continuum of care. The CNS improves outcomes by providing direct patient care, leading evidence-based practice, optimizing organizational systems, and advancing nursing practice" [36]. The key distinguishing component of this definition is the improvement of patient care outcomes through the optimization of healthcare systems. This component is unique to the CNS role as an advanced practice nurse and what is so valued by the global community with "...the ultimate goal [being] to optimize patient care and individualize care delivery to attain health for men, women, children, and the family in the context of their communities..." [32].

There continues to be a lack of clarity within the public and the healthcare team, however, as to how the CNS differs from the role of the Nurse Practitioner. This is in spite of the fact that the definitions as presented above are very different. The Joint Dialogue Group [23] in the United States (US) defined a Nurse Practitioner as someone whose "...care includes health promotion, disease prevention, health education, and counseling as well as the diagnosis and management of acute and chronic diseases. Certified nurse practitioners are prepared to practice as primary care CNPs and acute care CNPs, which have separate national consensus-based competencies and separate certification processes" [23]. This definition is clearly focused on care of the individual primarily within the primary care or acute care environments. The CNS, however, is focused on both individual complex care and the systems/operational improvement overall. The roles are complementary and, as defined, should rely on each other within the clinical setting.

This confusion extends to the global perspective as well with inconsistent titling and variations in scope of practice in various countries [14]. The variety of titles for APNs globally is quite expansive and not easily tracked due to differences in the scope of practice and range of care being provided also being very different in each country [26].

The Global Demographics of Persons Served by APNs

In order to understand the need for APNs, there needs to be a general understanding of the current global trends in demographics, population growth and distribution, the incidence of non-communicable diseases (chronic illnesses), and how geopolitical and environmental forces impact the ability of the healthcare providers to address the health needs of the population [58].

The World Health Organization (2019) Department of Economic and Social Affairs identified that the burden of an aging populace globally will have a potentially negative impact on healthcare systems everywhere (WHO 2019). It is predicted that the population of those older than 65 will at least double in most countries and will have an explosive growth in others. Examples show that developed countries such as those in Europe and North America will have the lowest rate of growth at an expected 48% increase from 2019 numbers with underdeveloped countries such as Central and Southern Asia expected to have an increase of 226% by 2050 ([27]; WHO 2019). Ladd et al. [27] identified that non-industrialized nations will comprise 80% of this growth. Data from 2019 showed that this segment of the population comprised only 6% of the total population but trajectories and predictions based on past data shows an exponential increase to approximately 16% of the global population by 2050 (WHO 2019).

Along with aging comes the increase in non-communicable diseases (NCDs) such as cardiac health, cancer, diabetes, and chronic obstructive pulmonary diseases [64]. Approximately 73% of the deaths caused by NCDs were in low- and middle-income countries meaning that their healthcare system is unable to provide chronic disease care and education to their population which may be scattered across vast geography and not easily accessed [64]. The APN, in particular the CNS, is known to be a strong advocate and provider of chronic disease education in communities. Their role is ever more important in the provision of healthcare to the aging population. Nurse Practitioners (NPs) of course, provide direct primary care to individuals. Both roles are imperative and need to be supported into the future.

Healthcare systems in lower-income countries that are already struggling to keep up with the demands at this time will be overburdened by 2050 [64]. Plans and strategies need to be put in place now to address this expected population increase with its concomitant increased burden on the healthcare system. This is where APNs come into play. By being more available, costing less, having skills in consultation and collaboration while developing policy and education, and having equal or better health outcomes to physicians, the APN can fill the gaps in healthcare and establish efficiencies that will increase the ability of healthcare workers to meet the coming demand.

Rural to urban migration is an additional consideration. Although the possibility exists for urban to rural migration, it is not the primary direction that people tend to move. There are many reasons why people move from rural to urban areas. These include the following: economics—poor standard of living and far fewer job opportunities in a rural environment as compared to an urban area, a low standard of living, insecurities or wars, natural disasters, and political factors such as oppression or instability in local government [7]. The movement from rural to urban again presents stressors to the healthcare system as the population increases in the urban setting. By having CNSs and NPs who can reach out the rural population, this may assist in reducing the migration to urban settings. Provision of education on health matters, learning about increased sanitation and cleanliness of water supplies, methods of making farming an accessible and realistic occupation, all can mean increased job opportunities in the rural areas and potentially mitigate the migration to urban settings. Advanced Practice Nurses (APNs) can have a significant impact on these elements. Wars, conflicts and political instability are more difficult to mitigate.

Consideration needs to be given to current fertility and birth rates. The global average of births has been on a steady decline over the last 75 years (United Nations [UN] 2023). Women in the 1960's reached a birthrate of 5.3 births per person. In 2023 this number had dropped to 2.2 births per person. Reasons behind this decline include the availability of contraceptives, higher education in general for women, higher costs for care of a child, and a reduction in infant mortality (UN 2023). All of these are good things for the health of women and children globally but it also means a reduction in the number of children being born. This is of concern with the elderly population on the rise in that there will be fewer healthcare providers into the future simply because of a decline in population. There will be a push to increase the need for healthcare providers who can be at the point of care where and when needed but with population trends moving as they are, there will be fewer people able to meet those needs.

Global Trends in Legislation and Policy Actions Regarding Advanced Practice Nursing and Autonomy

Barbara Safriet [42] began the discussion regarding the regulation of the advanced practice nurse based on case law and administrative rules from both the United States and Canada. Her seminal work as a lawyer assisted lawmakers at the time regarding how to approach the regulation of the APN role. Her work was foundational and continues to be relevant to the current regulations and legislative actions that allow APNs to function autonomously.

Legislation and Policy

The World Health Organization (WHO) [65] identified that there is growing evidence that communities are satisfied with the "…efficacy, efficiency, quality and satisfaction of nurse-provided care" (p. 71). Studies conducted looking at the outcomes of care, patient satisfaction, costs of care, and the evolving role of the APN have generally stated positive outcomes, however the sample sizes have been small [1, 5, 26]. In spite of these findings, the APN roles still face significant barriers to being fully implemented in a manner that allows for autonomous practice without oversight or management by a physician.

Brownwood and LaFortune [5] conducted a study for the Organization for Economic Cooperation and Development (OECD) which looked at how the APN role had been helped or hindered as a result of the pandemic. Five countries (Australia, Canada, France, Italy, and the US) were the focus of the study and it was noted that the following factors hindered APN role development: no position created, administrative issues, insufficient patient referral from physicians, insufficient income, and insufficient training [5]. Indications are that the following were affecting APN development: (1) opposition from the medical and nursing community, (2) policy restrictions on APN practice, (3) poor APN and administrative relations, (4) lack of understanding of the APN role, (5) issues related to regulation, and (6) limited educational opportunities [5, 43, 56].

Counter to the above, factors that facilitated the development and expansion of APN roles were, (1) high levels of autonomy/independent practice and (2) positive

APRN–physician relations [43]. Another factor that supports the development of the APN roles is clear statements of APN function, regulation, and legislative action that support and define the roles. This is where policy specifically plays a role.

The ICN defined that APN roles needed to have the following regulatory mechanisms clearly defined in policy or legislative action: the right to diagnose, inclusive of the following authorizations—ability to prescribe medication, prescribe treatment, refer clients to other professionals when needed, and the ability to admit patients to hospital when needed [20]. Title protection in the form of legislation outlining who can use the titles of Clinical Nurse Specialist, Nurse Practitioner, or Advanced Practice Nurse is also essential in managing those who are practicing as APNs [21].

Regulatory models have already been well-established in many countries such as Australia, Belgium, Canada, the United States, Finland, France, Ireland, Japan, Poland, the United Kingdom, and the Czech Republic [14]. Chile, New Zealand, and Mexico are in the advanced stages of APN implementation [14, 28–30]. Of note is that there are developing roles for APNs (specifically CNSs) in China, Turkey, Thailand, Japan, and Nigeria [14, 18]. While there is still much to do in order to assure public access and safety when dealing with APN roles, there are many models that can be used to frame the needed work in countries that have not yet begun the processes of regulatory clarity.

Current State of Regulatory Changes for APN Practice

The United States

The APRN Consensus Model [23] was developed in an effort to clarify the expectations on a national level for APN licensure/title protection, accreditation of educational programs, certification requirements as validation of entry level competence, and core requirements for education of the roles (LACE) [16, 17]. These guidelines are provided to all state licensure boards in the United States (US) to assist with ensuring that laws and regulations relative to APRNs are evaluated for safe practice [37]. The NCSBN is not, in itself, a regulatory body. It is an advisory group comprised of representatives from each state who assist each state with regulatory consistency across the nation. Each state, however, has its own specific legislative process to assure how and what an APN can or cannot do within the scope of practice for that state [17]. Unfortunately, this leads to inconsistencies with autonomous practice and full practice authority due to the influences of physician group lobbyists and their sway with the legislative members in each state.

The APRN Consensus Model [23] was an ambitious undertaking. The joint dialogue group was made up of representatives from each of the four APN roles in the United States, representatives of certification examination groups, the NCSBN, accrediting agencies and educational organizations. The document took 4 years to bring to fruition and was expected to be fully implemented by 2015. It continues to be in variable levels of implementation across the 50 states and territories [16, 17].

The NCSBN provides a map of the states and territories and an evaluation of whether each state has implemented the consensus model based on identifying whether or not the state has incorporated into regulation the seven criteria outlined in the model. The link below is provided for you to review of the status of each state's implementation: https://www.ncsbn.org/nursing-regulation/practice/aprn/aprn-consensus-implementation-status.page

Global Policy Changes

The International Council of Nurses [20, 22] is the global body that provides information regarding the current state of regulation in each country and also guidance to countries on how best to move forward should they choose to implement the APN roles. The focus of the guidance is to identify how APNs should be educated, regulated, and how to develop practice standards or competencies [22]. Unfortunately, there continue to be inconsistent applications of the ICN guidelines around the world. This inconsistency means that there are varying levels of recognition and/or advancement of APN roles across the globe. The inconsistency ranges from countries with no formal recognition of APN roles at all to countries with well-established advanced practice roles [11, 14, 18, 22].

Once a country determines that APN roles should be incorporated as a component of the healthcare team, there needs to be strong development of legislation and policy, a robust regulatory framework, and standardized practices that ensure quality of care [22]. The formal nursing organization in each country needs to follow the guidance provided by the ICN so that a robust development of APN practice can ensue. Much work still needs to be done.

The Social Determinants of Health, Sustainable Development Goals, and Implications of Universal Healthcare

The social determinants of health (SDOH) were identified as important factors in the health and well-being of individuals on a global scale [57]. Factors such as education, social support, economic stability, environmental issues, homelessness or housing instability, lack of access to healthcare are just a few of the factors that play a part in the overall health of the global community [31]. As such they were integrated into the United Nations Sustainable Development Goals and a plan was established for improvement in all 17 goals and 169 indicators for attainment by 2030 [45, 59].

Support for the Social Determinants of Health (SDOH) and the Sustainable Development Goals (SDGs) goes all the way back to the development of nursing itself [12]. Florence Nightingale [39] identified that many times the health of an individual depended not on the how the disease presented or the symptoms but instead on what we now identify as the SDOH "…the need for fresh air, warmth, a home, a proper diet and other affecting events in the person's life" [39].

The Social Determinants of Health (SDOH) [62, 63] and the Sustainable Development Goals (SDGs) [51] are intricately tied together through a plan for transformation of the world into a more equitable, and healthy environment. Health and well-being for all at all ages and the determinants of health are at the heart of the United Nations 2030 Agenda for Sustainable Development [51].

While the obvious choice for nursing and APN interaction and support is Sustainable Development Goal 3 (Attaining Universal Healthcare for all), that is not the only SDG that nursing can and does impact. Nursing also has an influence over SDGs 4, 5, 6, 8, 10, and 17 [49]. Although some of these may seem tangential, there is a direct link back to nursing in each case. The need for nursing to engage in the support and implementation of all of the SDGs is imperative.

The United Nations Sustainable Development Goal (SDG) 3 is focused on the attainment of universal healthcare on a global level. Additionally, it is also focused on the need to optimize the nursing and healthcare workforce [60]. This will mean that there need to be nurses participating in the development of policy to support attainment of universal healthcare in each country, a focus on public health and preventative programs, growth in the scope of practice for nurses, and sufficient care providers to meet the need for individualized healthcare. The CNS is well-positioned to provide support for both policy and public health initiatives. The NP, on the other hand, is well positioned to address the need for direct care providers in sufficient numbers to meet the needs of the public. Again, by working together, the two advanced practice roles can assist in meeting the needs of the general population.

Sustainable Development Goals (SDGs) 4 and 5 are connected through ensuring quality education and gender equality for women. As nursing is primarily a female-dominated profession, on a global level it provides an opportunity for higher education with at least a diploma and higher earning potential for women and girls who seek to learn and grow [49, 52–54].

One of nursing's key roles is the focus on preventative health education. Sustainable Development Goal (SDG) 6, which focuses on basic sanitation and achieving clean drinking water in every community with the associated health promotion, relies heavily on the active role of nurses. Advanced Practice Nurses (APNs) can provide education regarding how to assess water safety and potability of water for human consumption [49]. By educating the community and advocating for clean water, the CNS/APN is likely to achieve higher health metrics and lower disease/illness issues.

As identified earlier under SDGs 4 and 5, nursing is one of the professions that women contribute to significantly. This is also tied to SDG 8 (decent work and economic growth). Nursing contributes significantly to the global economy by creating jobs and opportunities for women in particular [49]. The APN roles carry this to a higher level and increase the overall salary and spending power in the community. All of this increases the global economy.

Nursing in general, but the advanced practice roles in particular, stand out when considering attainment of SDGs 10 and 17. These two SDGs focus on reducing inequalities within and between countries and collaborating to improve health outcomes and improvements to the healthcare system [49]. The role of collaborator and focused attention to healthcare systems is the purview of the CNS as defined in many countries. The SDGs are an opportunity for the CNS to shine in the international field and the NP to shine in provision of individual/primary care in areas that are deficient in primary care physicians.

The World Health Organization (WHO) and the International Council of Nurses (ICN) worked together to create a comprehensive report on the state of nursing in 2025 [65]. The data showed that the nursing workforce had increased since the last assessment (2021–2023) and that a further increase was projected to occur over the next and final 5 years of the initiative supporting the sustainable development goals. This growth in the nursing population is good, however, the concern is that the growth still may not meet the needs of the global community as the population ages and youth decrease in number. Additionally, if the APN is not allowed to function to the full scope of their education and abilities the SDGs will not be achievable. It is imperative that APNs are given the ability to function autonomously if the SDGs are to be attained and the SDOH are improved on a global level for all.

The Impact of Technology, Telehealth, and Digital Health Tools

A number of technologies have been developed and embraced recently due to the global pandemic [5, 46]. Care is able to be provided without having to have the patient/family/community travel to the healthcare centers. This means that the costs of care are reduced and care is more accessible to all, regardless of where they live. Alternatively, the care providers may travel and connect with systems that can track and trend the healthcare of numerous patients. In either case the movement directly to wi-fi-enabled technology rather than the traditional infrastructure means that the time and costs associated with laying cables, lines for telephone etc., are not needed. Placement of towers for both phone and internet access is much more feasible from a cost/benefit perspective and also opens the door to the use of many different technologies in the care of patients, families, and communities [6]. These technologies have become commonplace and are facilitating quality care and direct follow-up with patients to manage non-communicable diseases, extending lifespan well into the future [6].

The World Health Organization [58] articulated a vision that by 2030 unbiased universal healthcare would be available to all and that care would be non-discriminatory. Accomplishing this will require a thorough look at effective policies at regional, national, and global levels with an understanding that there needs to be sufficient financial investment to bring this vision to life [58]. Primary ways in which technology has been used by APNs is telehealth modalities, digital health tools such as the “Simple” app created by the non-profit organization Resolve to Save Lives [6], and the burgeoning area of Artificial Intelligence as applied to healthcare [24, 44, 48].

Telehealth

Use of telehealth came into being in a healthcare setting well before the pandemic but there was not widespread use in nursing [44]. Its use grew exponentially when the global pandemic occurred and meant that healthcare could not be provided in person due to the risks associated with transmission of the COVID-19 virus [13]. Telehealth was a tool that had low adoption rates prior to the pandemic when it was perceived to be inconvenient, too technical to learn, too time consuming, and generally "not as good as" face to face interactions with a patient and their family. A tool that had been underutilized, however, became the backbone of health services during the pandemic despite barriers to use and low health literacy [15].

Advanced Practice Nurses use telehealth modalities with great effect. Advanced Practice Nurses (APNs) use the technology to communicate, perform remote assessments to determine best means of treatment, consult with the patient and their family, and provide health education and guidance to both individual patients and to communities [8]. Telehealth interactions were found to have lower costs, high levels of patient safety, and comparable quality to in person assessments [8]. As the SDG 3 identifies the access to universal healthcare is an imperative [51]. The use of telehealth modalities and the implementation of policy and regulation that allow the APN to use this technology makes the potential of achieving SDG 3 more realistic.

Digital Health Technology

Digital health technology includes a variety of applications that we are using each and every day [38]. These tools include such things as remote healthcare monitors (blood pressure), apps on our smartphones, devices we wear such as step counters, heart rate monitors, and diabetes glucose level monitors [38]. Again, the advent of the global pandemic meant a significant increase in the use of these tools and ability of healthcare providers to monitor their patients from a distance.

The fact that these tools are spreading broadly and are accepted by most means that the transfer of information and interconnectedness is happening on a global level. This has great potential to accelerate progress in provision of healthcare and develop new global communities based on commonalities, healthcare knowledge, and understanding [61]. The digital bridge to healthcare will be essential to ensuring that "…1 billion more people benefit from universal health coverage, that 1 billion more people are better protected from health emergencies, and that 1 billion more people enjoy better health and well-being (WHO's triple billion targets, [61]). The APN plays a significant part in the full implementation and follow-up on the data that is collected for personal health issues, taking that data and looking at the global trajectories, and ensuring the health of both the individual and the community.

The goal articulated in the World Health Organization Thirteenth General Programme of Work, 2019–2023 [61] was to support the acceleration and adoption of digital health programs that could potentially detect another pandemic on the rise. The purpose was to collect and use health data in order to support the SDGs and the triple billion targets as articulated by WHO [61]. Sustainable Development Goal 3 is intended to be a well-rounded effort at increasing the efficiency of existing systems with a focus on health promotion and disease prevention on a global level. Digital health tools in the hands of APNs can assure a positive outcome [41].

The WHO [61] recognized that the full implementation of their 2019–2023 plan may encounter some barriers, especially in low- and middle-income countries. To that end, they created a plan with four priorities that countries could use to bring digital health tools into play. They acknowledged that: (1) each national health system needed to commit to integration of the technology, (2) an integrated strategy will be needed to successfully implement digital tools, (3) there needed to be a statement from the governing body that digital technologies for health should be used appropriately, and (4) each health agency needed to recognize the major barriers that least-developed countries face when trying to implement digital health technologies. If countries follow the pathway set by WHO [61], they stand a better chance of appropriate interlinking of the healthcare systems and the APN providing patient care.

Artificial Intelligence (AI)

Artificial Intelligence (AI) is not a new phenomenon with research into the new tool being conducted as far back as the 1950s [9]. It has seen a bold growth pattern in the recent 5 years with significant resources being put into its development and revenues showing reciprocal growth. Between 2018 (10.0 billion dollars in revenue) and 2025 (projected revenue at 126 billion), the potential profit grew exponentially [19]. This makes AI both the most lucrative and potentially the most difficult trend to corral when profits are high and expected to continue to climb. This raises some issues with potential breaches in ethical comportment that are not easily resolved. In spite of the ethical issues, healthcare providers should expect an increased use of AI as time moves forward and the systems mature. Healthcare providers need to understand the potential complicated issues and guard against the possibility of data being misused or shared inappropriately [47].

Kilpatrick et al. [25] identified a number of areas where research is currently lacking on the impact of AI on advanced practice nurses. As AI becomes more reliable, in both seeking information to support practice and in potentially recommending a diagnosis or treatment plan, it will need to be integrated as a tool in the world of the APN. This area is changing almost literally on a daily basis. Currently, AI tools are not infallible and require that the healthcare provider is aware that the system may provide information that is inaccurate. The APN needs to understand enough about what they looking for in order to know when the information is incorrect or potentially harmful.

Some specific concerns are related to bias in the algorithm that provides answers to diagnostic questions. Data that is input to the AI determines its algorithm and racist, biased, or harmful ideas that have been put into the system through the internet could influence AI's decision-making [4]. Data is used to train AI. If all of that data comes from one group of people to the exclusion of others, the AI may not work well. This in turn could lead to unfair treatment or outcomes. The healthcare provider, again, needs to understand this issue and ensure that decisions made in diagnosis and treatment take potential biases into consideration [4].

The possibilities are amazing when taken at face value and the thought of very personal plans of care for patients that integrate SDOH information, genetic patterns, and more "...will allow AI to predict risks, customize treatment, and enhance health outcomes" Sharma et al. [48]. The development and refinement of such things, as sensors that can be worn to measure blood glucose or blood pressure and can transmit that information in real time to a healthcare provider when issues arise, is going to change how we deliver healthcare as APNs [24, 48, 55].

All of this is going to need careful attention and the development of new and forward-thinking policies to govern the use of AI in healthcare settings [44]. Regardless of the need to establish policies, it is clear that AI is not going away and can be very supportive of the care process. As AI matures and becomes more accurate, the systems will be able to provide plans for preventative care, detect diseases earlier in the trajectory, and increase efficiency of care by streamlining clinical workflows [10]. All of these changes are going to mean that patient outcomes will improve. Chatbots in healthcare are already assisting patients to find the right resources [2]. When AI is fully integrated into the APN workflow, the possibilities are endless.

Conclusion: Future Outlook and Challenges

The world of the APN is changing rapidly on a global basis. With the potential that the roles bring, it is possible to envision a future that is healthier, overcome barriers such as distance, lack of resources, and inefficient workflow and policies. Policies need to be developed that support the ongoing growth of the APN roles and allows them to flourish on an international level. The work of the ICN is assistive in this and the guidelines provided can clearly support and expand the role of the APN. Challenges continue to exist though when other professions see the APN role as a threat and work to limit the scope of practice inappropriately.

The APN can work toward the reduction of both communicable and non-communicable diseases. Their skillset of clinical practice, collaboration, knowledge of policies and how they need to change, and interpersonal effectiveness with the client, all support the health of the client and their community. Areas that are challenging but can be managed by the APN include the aging population, reductions in birthrate, and issues surrounding maternal and neonatal health.

As identified, the APN has a significant role to play in the SDOH and attainment of the SDGs. Advanced Practice Nurses (APNs) working together to achieve these goals both internal to their region or country and internationally will mean healthier outcomes for all on a global level.

Technology will play an important role in all of these actions as telehealth, digital health technology, and AI can support the provision of care to low- and middle-income countries. The APN needs to be a part of the future as technology becomes more accurate and can provide suggested plans of care for specific individuals or communities. The potential is boundless but not without its challenges as identified previously.

Future outlook is clearly positive for the APN on a global level. The outcomes of care can be better and will be with the support of the APN and their expansion of role and provision of safe, effective, and efficient systems of care; bring to the future a positive perspective and a better understanding of what all the APN roles can accomplish.

References

1. Abraham CM, Norful AA, Stone PW, Poghosyan L. Cost effectiveness of advanced practice nurses compared to physician led care for chronic diseases: a systematic review. Nurs Econ. 2019;37(6):293–305. https://pmc.ncbi.nlm.nih.gov/articles/PMC8491992/
2. Al Khatib I, Ndiaye M. Examining the role of AI in changing the role of nurses in patient care: systematic review. JMIR Nurs. 2025;19(8). https://doi.org/10.2196/63335.
3. American Association of Nurse Practitioners. Historical timeline. n.d. https://www.aanp.org/about/about-the-american-association-of-nurse-practitioners-aanp/historical-timeline
4. British Columbia College of Nurses and Midwives. Using artificial intelligence in practice. 2025. https://www.bccnm.ca/NP/learning/artificial-intelligence/Pages/Default.aspx
5. Brownwood I, Lafortune G. Advanced practice nursing in primary care in OECD countries: recent developments and persisting implementation challenges, OECD Health Working Papers, No. 165. Paris: OECD Publishing; 2024. https://doi.org/10.1787/8e10af16-en.
6. Burka D, Gupta R, Moran AE, et al. Keep it simple: designing a user-centred digital information system to support chronic disease management in low/middle-income countries. BMJ Health Care Inform. 2023;30. https://doi.org/10.1136/bmjhci-2022-100641.
7. Chukwuemeka ES. Rural-urban migration: meaning, causes and effects. Bscholarly; 2021. https://bscholarly.com/rural-urban-migration/#Causes_of_Rural-urban_Migration
8. Costa I, Silva Costa A, Garbuio DC, et al. Telehealth in patient care by advanced practice nurses: a systematic review. Acta Paul Enferm. 2025;38(12). https://doi.org/10.37689/acta-ape/2025ar0003141i.
9. Coursera. The history of AI: a timeline of artificial intelligence. 2025. https://www.coursera.org/articles/history-of-ai?msockid=0a6849b72e8069b52f56466e2fa86806&isNewUser=true
10. Dailah HG, Koriri M, Sabei A, Kriry T, Zakri M. Artificial intelligence in nursing: technological benefits to nurse's mental health and patient care quality. Healthc Basel. 2024;12(24):2555. https://doi.org/10.3390/healthcare12242555.
11. Delamaire M, Lafortune G. Nurses in advanced roles: a description and evaluation of experiences in 12 developed countries, OECD Health Working Paper No. 54 [Internet]. Paris: Organization for Economic Cooperation and Development; 2010. https://doi.org/10.1787/5kmbrcfms5g7-en.
12. Dossey BM, Rosa WE, Beck DM. Nursing and the Sustainable Development Goals: from nightingale to now. Am J Nurs. 2019;119(5):44–9. https://doi.org/10.1097/01.NAJ.0000557912.35398.8f.
13. Ezeamii VC, Okobi OE, Wambai-Sani H, Perera GS, Zaynieva S, Okonkwo CC, Ohaiba MM, William-Enemali PC, Obodo OR, Obiefuna NG. Revolutionizing healthcare: how telemedicine is improving patient outcomes and expanding access to care. Cureus. 2024;16(7). https://doi.org/10.7759/cureus.63881.

14. Fulton JS, Holly VW, editors. Clinical nurse specialist role and practice: an international perspective. Springer: Cham; 2021.
15. Garber K, Chike-Harris K, Vetter MJ, Kobeissi M, Heidesch T, Arends R, Teall AM, Rutledge C. Telehealth policy and the advanced practice nurse. J Nurse Pract. 2023;19. https://www.npjournal.org/article/S1555-4155(23)00157-5/fulltext
16. Goudreau KA. Updates on the implications for practice: the consensus model for advanced practice registered nurse regulation. In: Goudreau KA, Smolenski MC, editors. Health policy and advanced practice nursing: impact and implications. 4th ed. New York: Springer; in press-a. 2026.
17. Goudreau KA. State level implementation of the APRN consensus model: progress to date. In: Goudreau KA, Smolenski MC, editors. Health policy and advanced practice nursing: impact and implications. 4th ed. New York: Springer; in press-b. 2026.
18. Holly V, Fulton JS, Goudreau KA. International clinical nurse specialist practice. In: Fulton JS, Goudreau KA, Swartzell KL, editors. Foundations of clinical nurse specialist practice. 4th ed. New York: Springer; in press. 2027.
19. Howarth J. 50 new artificial intelligence statistics. 2025. https://explodingtopics.com/blog/ai-statistics
20. International Council of Nurses [ICN]. Guidelines on advanced practice nursing. 2020. URL: chrome extension://efaidnbmnnnibpcajpcglclefindmkaj/https://www.icn.ch/system/files/documents/2020-04/ICN_APN%20Report_EN_WEB.pdf
21. International Council of Nurses [ICN]. What is an advanced practice nurse? 2022. https://internationalapn.org/what-is-an-apn/#:~:text=%E2%80%9CA%20Nurse%20Practitioner%2FAdvanced%20Practice%20Nurse%20is%20a%20registered,country%20in%20which%20s%2Fhe%20is%20credentialed%20to%20practice
22. International Council of Nurses. International Nurses Day 2025: Caring for nurses strengthens economies. (Lead authors: David Stewart & Gillian Moore; Contributors: Dr Gill Adynski, Erica Burton, Howard Catton, Helen Donovan, Hoi Shan Fokeladeh, Christine Hancock, Karine Lavoie, Colin Parish; Editor: Lindsey Williamson). International Council of Nurses. 2025. ISBN: 978-92-95124-48-6. https://www.icn.ch/sites/default/files/2025-04/ICN_IND2025_report_EN_A4_FINAL_0.pdf.
23. Joint Dialogue Group. Consensus model for APRN regulation. 2008. Available at URL: https://www.ncsbn.org/public-files/Consensus_Model_for_APRN_Regulation_July_2008.pdf
24. Kamei T. Telenursing and artificial intelligence for oncology nursing. Asia Pac J Oncol Nurs. 2022;9(12). https://doi.org/10.1016/j.apjon.2022.100119.
25. Kilpatrick K, Savard I, Audet LA, Costanzo G, Khan M, Atallah R, Jabbour M, Zhou W, Wheeler K, Ladd E, Gray DC, Henderson C, Spies LA, McGrath H, Rogers MA. Global perspective of advanced practice nursing research: a review of systematic reviews. PLoS One. 2024;19(7):e0305008. https://doi.org/10.1371/journal.pone.0305008. PMID: 38954675; PMCID: PMC11218965.
26. Kilpatrick K, Tewah R, Tchouaket E, Jokiniemi K, Bouabdillah N, Biron A, Emed J, Martel B, Atallah R, Jabbour M, Bryant-Lukosius D. Describing clinical nurse specialist practice: a mixed-methods study. Clin Nurse Spec. 2024;38(6):280–91. https://doi.org/10.1097/NUR.0000000000000856. PMID: 39437208.
27. Ladd E, Miller M, Wheeler K, Wainaina S, Aguire F, McGrath H, Lee S, Nashwan A, Neary A, Core K. A global SWOT analysis of advanced practice nursing: policy, regulation, and practice. Research Square. 2020. https://doi.org/10.21203/rs.3.rs-113320/v1.
28. Levine N. What does a nurse practitioner do? New York: Cedars-Sinai; 2019. https://www.cedars-sinai.org/blog/nursepractitioners.html#:~:text=Broadly%20speaking%2C%20NPs%20are%20trained,even%20from%20hospital%20to%20hospital
29. Lopes-Junior LC. Advanced practice nursing and the expansion of the role of nurses in primary health Care in the Americas. Sage Open Nurs. 2021. https://doi.org/10.1177/23779608211019491.

30. Maier C, Aiken LH. Task shifting from physicians to nurses in 39 countries: a cross-country comparative study. Eur J Pub Health. 2016;26(6):927–34. https://doi.org/10.1093/eurpub/ckw098.
31. Marmot M, Wilkinson R, editors. Social determinants of health, 2nd ed. Int J Epidemiol. 2006;35(4). https://doi.org/10.1093/ije/dyl121.
32. Matthews JH, Whitehead PB, Ward C, Kyner M, Crowder T. Florence nightingale: visionary for the role of clinical nurse specialist. Online J Issues Nurs. 2020;25(2):Manuscript 1. https://doi.org/10.3912/OJIN.Vol25No02Man01.
33. McClelland M, McCoy MA, Burson R. Clinical nurse specialists: then, now and the future of the profession. Clin Nurse Spec. 2013;27(2):96–102. https://doi.org/10.1097/NUR.0b013e3182819154.
34. National Association of Clinical Nurse Specialists. Happy birthday and thank you Hildegard! 2021. URL: https://nacns.org/nursing-news/happy-birthday-and-thank-you-hildegard/
35. National Association of Clinical Nurse Specialists [NACNS]. Leading the next generation: Insights from the NACNS 2022 census; 2022. https://NACNS-2022-Census-Results-Infographic.pdf.
36. National Association of Clinical Nurse Specialists. CNS definition gets an update to foster understanding and visibility. NACNS; 2024. URL: https://nacns.org/2024/03/cns-definition-gets-an-update-to-foster-understanding-and-visibility/
37. National Council of State Boards of Nursing. Nursing regulation: APRN consensus model. 2025. https://www.ncsbn.org/nursing-regulation/practice/aprn.page
38. National Institute for Health and Care Research [NIHR]. NIHR evidence: what is digital health technology and what can it do for me? 2022. https://doi.org/10.3310/nihrevidence_53447.
39. Nightingale F. Notes on Nursing: What it is and what it is not. Harrison and Sons, London. 1859. ISBN: 0-397-55007-3.
40. Ohio Association of Advanced Practice Nurses. History of NPs in the United States. OAAPN. 2021. URL: https://oaapn.org/2021/06/history-of-nps-in-the-united-states/#:~:text=The%20first%20NP%20program%20was%20founded%20by%20Loretta,women%2C%20children%2C%20the%20elderly%2C%20and%20people%20with%20disabilities
41. Registered Nurses Association of Ontario. Best practice guidelines: clinical practice in a digital health environment. 2024. https://rnao.ca/bpg/guidelines/clinical-practice-digital-health-environment
42. Safriet BJ. Closing the gap between can and may in health-care providers' scopes of practice: primer for policymakers. Yale J Regul. 2002;19(2):301–34.
43. Schirle L, Norful AA, Rudner N, Poghosyan L. Organizational facilitators and barriers to optimal APRN practice: an integrative review. Health Care Manag Rev. 2020;45(4):311–20. https://doi.org/10.1097/HMR.0000000000000229.
44. Schlachta-Fairchild L, Varghese SB, Deickman A, Castelli D. Telehealth and telenursing are live: APN policy and practice implications. J Nurse Pract. 2010;6(2):98–106.
45. Schmets G, Rajan D, Kadandale S. Strategizing national health in the 21st century: a handbook. Geneva: World Health Organization; 2016. https://www.who.int/publications/i/item/9789241549745.
46. Schultz M. Telehealth and remote patient monitoring innovations in nursing practice: state of the science. Online J Issues Nurs. 2023:2023. https://doi.org/10.3912/OJIN.Vol28No02ST01.
47. Seh AH, Zarour M, Alenezi M, Sarkar AK, Agrawal A, Kumar R, Khan RA. Healthcare data breaches: insights and implications. Healthcare (Basel). 2020;8(2):133. https://doi.org/10.3390/healthcare8020133.
48. Sharma K, Ramawat VK, Kant R, Bhatt S, Nain N. The role of artificial intelligence in nursing: advancements, challenges, and future directions. Tuijin Jishu/J Propuls Technol. 2024;45(3). https://doi.org/10.52783/tjjpt.v45.i03.7378.

49. Taminato M, Fernandes H, Barbosa DA. Nursing and the Sustainable Development Goals (SDGs): an essential commitment. Braz J Nurs [Rev Bras Enferm]. 2023;76(6). https://doi.org/10.1590/0034-7167.2023760601.
50. Thompson CJ. Hildegard Peplau: the creator of the CNS role. Nursing Education Expert. 2023. URL: https://nursingeducationexpert.com/patho,EBP,education,nursing,podcast,blog/creator-of-the-cns-role/
51. United Nations [UN]. Sustainable Development Goals: Goal 3 – Good health and well being. Health - United Nations Sustainable Development. 2015.
52. United Nations Department of Economic and Social Affairs. Transforming our world: the 2030 agenda for sustainable development. New York: United Nations; 2015. https://sdgs.un.org/2030agenda
53. United Nations Department of Economic and Social Affairs. The 17 goals. 2022. Available from: https://sdgs.un.org/goals
54. United Nations Population Division. World Population Prospects: fertility rate, total (births per woman). Statistical databases and publications from national statistical offices, National statistical offices; Demographic Statistics, Eurostat (ESTAT). 2023. https://data.worldbank.org/indicator/SP.DYN.TFRT.IN
55. Walton AML, Nikpor JA, Randolph SD. Population health in a global society: preparing nurses for the future. Public Health Nurs. 2022;39(5):1098–106. https://doi.org/10.1111/phn.13081.
56. Wheeler KJ, Miller M, Pulcini J, Gray D, Ladd E, Rayens MK. Advanced practice nursing roles, regulation, education, and practice: a global study. Ann Glob Health. 2022;88(1): 42, 1–21. https://doi.org/10.5334/aogh.3698.
57. Wilkinson R, Marmot M, editors. Social determinants of health: the solid facts. 2nd ed. Geneva: World Health Organization; 2003.
58. World Health Organization. Global strategy on human resources for health: workforce 2030. Geneva: World Health Organization; 2016. https://iris.who.int/bitstream/handle/10665/250368/9789241511131-eng.pdf?sequence=1
59. World Health Organization. A regional guide to the development of nursing specialist practice. Cairo: WHO Regional Office for the Eastern Mediterranean; 2020. Licence: CC BY-NC-SA3.0 IGO. https://WHOEMNUR432E-eng.pdf.
60. World Health Organization. Global strategic directions for nursing and midwifery: 2021–2025. Geneva: World Health Organization; 2021. Licence: CC BY-NC-SA 3.0 IGO.
61. World Health Organization. Global strategy on digital health 2020–2025. Geneva: World Health Organization; 2021. Licence: CC BY-NC-SA 3.0 IGO.
62. World Health Organization. Social determinants of health. Geneva: World Health Organization; 2022. https://apps.who.int/gb/ebwha/pdf_files/EB152/B152_22-en.pdf
63. World Health Organization. Social determinants of health: progress of the world report on social determinants of health equity. 2023. https://apps.who.int/gb/ebwha/pdf_files/EB154/B154_21-en.pdf
64. World Health Organization. Noncommunicable diseases. Geneva: World Health Organization; 2024. https://www.who.int/news-room/fact-sheets/detail/noncommunicable-diseases
65. World Health Organization. State of the World's nursing: investing in education, jobs, leadership and service delivery. WHO. 2025. URL: www.who.int/publications/i/item/9789240110236

Conclusion

Jackie Rowles

As a nurse, we have the opportunity to heal the heart, mind, soul, and body of our patients, their families, and ourselves. They may forget your name, but they will never forget how you made them feel.

—Maya Angelos, American Poet and daughter of a nurse. May 2013

Nursing is a calling. It is the giving of oneself to care for others, to help move patients closer to optimal health given the patient's health challenges. It is not a profession for those faint of heart, or who do not value humanity. Our profession is exhausting, challenging, largely unappreciated, undervalued, unseen, and flooded with artificial barriers to practice. Yet the nursing profession has survived and thrived since its recognition in the mid-nineteenth century under the influence of Florence Nightingale. For more than 170 years, nursing has progressed in education, practice authority, recognition and respect, having to continually prove itself worthy of recognition and respect along the way. Nurses are the largest healthcare workforce globally [1]. According to the International Council of Nurses (ICN) and the World Health Organization (WHO), there are currently over 30 million nurses around the world, however the number of global Advanced Practice Nurses (APN) remains unknown [1, 2]. As an APN example, current data from the US reports 461,000 Nurse Practitioners, 90,000 Clinical Nurse Specialists, 62,000 Certified Registered Nurse Anesthetists and 14,000 Certified Nurse Midwives [3–6].

The WHO reported that 62% of the 194 countries who provided data for the 2025 State of the World's Nursing Report indicated the presence of advanced practice nurses in their country, an increase of 11% over the 2020 report [7]. Data collection on the numbers and types of APNs is difficult given the various names assigned to the role, lack of official education, recognition, registration or titling of the role, variation in scope of practice, lack of data collection combined with challenges of

J. Rowles (✉)
School of Nurse Anesthesia, Harris College and Nursing and Health Sciences,
Texas Christian University, Fort Worth, TX, USA
e-mail: j.rowles@tcu.edu

A. Kapu et al. (eds.), *A Global View on Clinical Autonomy for Advanced Practice Nurses*, Advanced Practice in Nursing,
https://doi.org/10.1007/978-3-032-21458-4_21

where to obtain data on nursing practice and practice authority. However, the lack of official data does not mean that advanced practice nursing care is not being provided.

A global nursing shortage, with a predicted shortage of 4.5 million nurses by 2030, remains a major concern for the future of healthcare [7]. Additionally, there is much discussion concerning a global shortage of physicians [8] and other healthcare workers. The WHO reports a deficit of 11 million healthcare workers by 2030 [9]. The greatest shortage will occur in low and lower–middle income countries, although all countries have been identified as having difficulties with healthcare workforce educational capacity, geographic placement, retention, and performance [9]. A lack of investment into the education of healthcare workers is a major precursor of the shortage. Further, the WHO reports that 67% of the global workforce are women. Gender bias has resulted in nursing subsisting as an almost invisible, unrecognized, and undervalued profession. Gender equity and equality is a key factor in strengthening health systems and workforce retention [7, 10]. Further, nursing faces an age-old hierarchical bias by being placed on a lower level of the healthcare pyramid than medicine [11]. Despite these hierarchies, all APNs are educated to provide clinically autonomous care via a team approach or in solo as dictated by timing, workforce deployment inequities, or unavailability of a physician.

The United Nations (UN) confirms we are in an era of longer life span, yet the ability to meet 2025 targets for healthcare Sustainable Development Goals (SDGs) is poor [12]. Governments are facing a healthcare crisis, with grave concerns about how they will finance and ensure equitable healthcare availability for their citizens. The logical, and economic, choice demands an increased role for advanced practice nurses. In fact, the WHO has called for increased, and more advanced roles for nurses [7]. Advanced Practice Nurses (APNs) are trained in medical models. The research evidence from multiple studies of APN roles have concluded APNs are high-quality care providers with a patient outcome profile comparable to physicians [13–16]. Development of APN roles, or expansion of the roles, are a logical, timely, and sustainable way to bridge the workforce gap. Why? Because nurses are tried and true, trusted members of the healthcare team who offer a cost-effective care option for provision of care [17]. For example, in the US, nurses have been voted by the public as the most honest and ethical profession in the Gallup Poll each year since 1999 (when nursing was added to the list) with the exception of 9/11 when firefighters were awarded top place [18]. Formalized APN education incurs less cost and provides a more rapid entry to practice than medical education. APNs are held to advanced standards of practice in their specialty area [19–21]. Patients have reported increased satisfaction rates with APN care, citing reduced wait times, increased appointment more one-on-one time, better communication, provision of holistic care, and effective outcomes [13, 22, 23]. Moreover, nurses are effective team members, having been educated in collaborative models with an emphasis on building trust, cooperation, and engaging the patient as an active member of the healthcare team.

As noted in this book, an Advanced Practice Nurse (APN) commonly refers one of four recognized advanced practice specialties: Nurse Practitioner, Nurse Midwife,

Nurse Anesthetist, and Clinical Nurse Specialist. The history of evolution of each APN role and responsibilities has been detailed in chapters “Clinical Autonomy for Nurse Practitioners”, “Clinical Autonomy in Midwifery”, “Clinical Autonomy for Nurse Anesthetists Globally” and “Clinical Autonomy for Clinical Nurse Specialists (CNSs)”. Undoubtedly, these readings have demonstrated that “advanced practice” has been in effect long before its proper definition and recognition.

This book is timely and necessary. Discussions are brought forth into the light that have often been held in secret and in the dark. Throughout the journey that resulted in the final writing of this book, the authors and editors have searched extensively for the evidence needed to verify existence and contribution of APNs around the world. We have addressed global APN roles, regulation, stages of authority, contributions of clinical autonomy in practice, global differences/challenges, and specifically how strengthening an APN’s clinical autonomy expands high quality, safe, access to care—especially in low-resource settings.

Thus, from beginning to end, this book demonstrates the past, current, and future contributions to accessible, high-quality, and equitable healthcare delivery by advanced practice nurses throughout the world. Moreover, it attempts to calm the murky waters through a thought-provoking discussion of what clinical autonomy is and is not. The authors seek to make sense of the ongoing challenges to clinical autonomy despite the vast amount of evidence supporting improved access to timely care, patient outcomes, patient satisfaction, and economic benefit.

Some may view this discussion and this book as controversial but that is neither our aim, nor was meant to be our approach. This book assesses the current state of APN global practice and contribution to universal health. We examined the current global status and considered future requirements of overburdened, and undermanned healthcare systems. Governments are currently struggling to meet, and prepare for, the weight of increasingly complex and costly healthcare demands of their citizens.

The future of global health is tumultuous at best given the lack of manpower [9] and the burden that increased life expectancy has placed on every country’s global healthcare system. Adding in the current nursing shortage and future need for nurses [7], citizens are left wondering who will care for them in their time of need. As previous stated, our profession faces many challenges, leaving nurses feeling undervalued, underpaid, burned out, and disrespected.

The ICN reports member countries have difficulty in retaining nurses [7]. Low salaries, long work hours, staffing shortages, lack of respect have all been offered as reasons nurses leave the profession—with a staggering 18% of nurses leaving within their first year of practice [24]. The Institute of Medicine’s (USA), 2010 report, *The Future of Nursing,* called for removal of barriers to practice so nurses may function to the full extent of their education and training, citing the role of nurses as key to the provision of future healthcare needs of the public [25]. The WHO recently called for increasing the role of nurses in the delivery of healthcare in order that we may improve the global reach of care and make a positive impact toward realization of the UN’s SDG targets [7]. Advanced Practice Nurses (APNs) whose practice allows for use of their education, skills, competencies, critical thinking and experience have improved job satisfaction and are more likely to stay in the workforce [26, 27].

A lack of an understanding of the education, skills, competencies, and benefits of APN clinical autonomy often results in artificial and unnecessary barriers to practice. Nurses are trained in team-based healthcare, but in order to lead future healthcare to the optimal benefit that our public deserve, nurses must be given unencumbered education, recognition, and respect to practice to the full extent of their role. In tandem with the rest of the medical care team, nurses can ensure the provision of high-quality care to patients in all communities.

Disbursement of healthcare services must be considered in all countries and across all economic and geographic borders. Nurses are the lifeblood of patient care and are also the lifeline in rural, underserved, low economic communities, as well largely populated urban communities struggling to recruit and maintain an optimal healthcare workforce. In addition to high quality, safe and cost-effective care, equity matters.

The future of accessible, timely, and high-quality healthcare demands recognition of all advanced practice nurses, and the removal of artificial barriers to practice. Advanced Practice Nursing is not in competition with medicine. Advanced Practice Nurses (APNs) are complementary to medicine and serve to transform the reach of quality access and care to positively impact universal health.

Research has demonstrated that access to care is not the be all, end all. Rather, access to quality care is the key. A 2018 study highlighted preventable deaths in 137 low and lower–middle income countries. Death statistics were higher in those who sought care (5 million) than those who did not (3.6 million), concluding the preventable deaths were due to an inferior quality of care [28]. This is a travesty and an area where APNs can make a difference. Nurses have the willingness and capacity to take on higher education and increased care duties. Nurses have proven to be accountable, valued members of the healthcare team. Expansion of nursing roles and practice after successful education, mentoring or proctoring is a not a gamble, it is an opportunity for the healthcare system to flex its workforce to meet its ever-changing needs.

Clinical autonomy should not be an objection but a celebration of how the APN education, skills, training, and critical thinking ability lead to timely, high-quality healthcare. Research supports both the use and empowerment of APNs globally to meet our world's unprecedented healthcare challenges. These include aging populations, increasingly chronic disease processes, pandemics, increasing health disparities, and healthcare manpower shortages [29].

Advanced Practice Nurses (APNs) are educated first as generalist nurses, taught to see and assess the big picture, be an effective team member, and ensure patient-centered care. These foundational concepts motivated an entire profession's desire to do more. The APN aspired to be more, to give more to effect change for the patient, the health system, communities, and the world.

Simply put, APNs are underutilized. We are experts in our area of practice yet often overlooked in our ability to provide high-quality care, often in remote locations, and in a way that is proven to increase patient satisfaction, reduce cost, and bridge manpower needs. We are not interested in a struggle over practice authority. We understand the healthcare team is stronger together and we embrace teamwork, acknowledging that more can be achieved together as a united group of healthcare professionals committed to enhancing universal health for all.

The future is bright. Advanced Practice Nurses are committed to achievement of the United Nation's healthcare-related SDGs, strengthening global healthcare systems through timely, high-quality, and equitable care. We have demonstrated impact in addressing workforce gaps and reducing inequities worldwide. We can do more. That is, if our governments and health systems recognize our value and partner with us. Clinical autonomy enables APNs to practice to the full extent of our education, skills and competencies resulting in expansion of care, improved outcomes, narrowing of manpower gaps, strengthening of economies, and accelerating progress toward universal health. We are stronger together.

References

1. World Health Organization. Global health workforce statistics database. https://www.who.int/data/gho/data/themes/topics/health-workforce. Accessed 20 Jan 2026.
2. International Council of Nurses. Recover to rebuild: investing in the nursing workforce for health system effectiveness. 2023. https://www.icn.ch/news/icn-report-says-shortage-nurses-global-health-emergency. Accessed 20 Jan 2026.
3. American Association of Nurse Practitioners. 2025. https://www.aanp.org/news-feed/a--behind-the-scenes-look-at-the-2025-nurse-practitioner-count. Accessed 19 Jan 2026.
4. National Association of Clinical Nurse Specialists. 2025. https://nacns.org/2025/. Accessed 19 Jan 2026.
5. National Board for Certification and Recertification of Nurse Anesthetists. https://www.nbcrna.com/about-us/history. Accessed 19 Jan 2026.
6. American Midwifery Certification Board. https://www.amcbmidwife.org/. Accessed 19 Jan 2026.
7. World Health Organization & International Council of Nurses. State of the world's nursing 2025: investing in education, jobs, leadership and service delivery. Geneva: World Health Organization; 2025. https://www.who.int/publications/i/item/9789240110236. Accessed 18 Jan 2026.
8. Lawson E. The global primary care crisis. Br J Gen Pract. 2022;73(726):3. https://doi.org/10.3399/bjgp23X731469. PMID: 36543556; PMCID: PMC9799366.
9. World Health Organization. https://www.who.int/health-topics/health-workforce#tab=tab_1. Accessed 18 Jan 2026.
10. World Health Organization. https://www.who.int/activities/value-gender-and-equity-in-the-global-health-workforce. Accessed 17 Jan 2026.
11. Bueter A, Jukola S. Multi-professional healthcare teams, medical dominance, and institutional epistemic injustice. Med Health Care Phil. 2025;28:219–32. https://doi.org/10.1007/s11019-025-10252-z.
12. The United Nations. https://www.un.org/en/desa/we-live-longer-ever-many-health-related-sdg-targets-are-track-ahead-2030-deadline. Accessed 18 Jan 2026.

13. Htay M, Whitehead D. The effectiveness of the role of advanced nurse practitioners compared to physician-led or usual care: a systematic review. Int J Nurs Stud Adv. 2021;3:100034. https://doi.org/10.1016/j.ijnsa.2021.100034. PMID: 38746729; PMCID: PMC11080477.
14. Lewis SR, Nicholson A, Smith AF, Alderson P. Physician anaesthetists versus non-physician providers of anaesthesia for surgical patients. Cochrane Database of Syst Rev. 2014;(7):Art. No.: CD010357. https://doi.org/10.1002/14651858.CD010357.pub2.
15. Dulisse B, Cromwell J. No harm found when nurse anesthetists work without supervision by physicians. Health Aff (Millwood). 2010;29(8):1469–75. https://doi.org/10.1377/hlthaff.2008.0966.
16. Barnett M, Balkissoon C, Sandhu J. The level of quality care nurse practitioners provide compared with their physician colleagues in the primary care setting: a systematic review. J Am Assoc Nurse Pract. 2022;34(3):457–64. https://doi.org/10.1097/JXX.0000000000000660. Erratum in: J Am Assoc Nurse Pract. 2022 Apr 1;34(4):696. http://doi.org/10.1097/JXX.0000000000000718. PMID: 34678807.
17. Cintina I, Hogan PF, Schroeder C, Simonson BE, Quraishi JA. Cost effectiveness of anesthesia providers and implications of scope of practice in a Medicare population. Nurs Econ. 2018;36(2):67–73.
18. https://news.gallup.com/poll/700736/nurses-continue-lead-honesty-ethics-ratings.aspx. Accessed 22 Jan 2026.
19. International Council of Nurses. Guidelines on Advanced Practice Nursing. 2020. Geneva, Switzerland. https://www.icn.ch/system/files/documents/2020-04/ICN_APN%20Report_EN_WEB.pdf. Accessed 17 Jan 2026.
20. International Council of Nurses, Guidelines on Advanced Practice Nursing: Nurse Anesthetist. 2021. Geneva, Switzerland. https://www.icn.ch/resources/publications-and-reports/guidelines-advanced-practice-nursing-nurse-anesthetists-2021. Accessed 18 Jan 2026.
21. International Federation of Nurse Anesthetists. IFNA Standards. https://ifna.site/etusivu/practice/ifna-standards/Education. Accessed 15 Jan 2026.
22. Mahmood HR, Hossain L, Sayeed A, Azrin F, Mallick T, Hayder T, Ahmed A, Jabeen S, Tonmon TT, Rahman MM, Akm MH, Siddique MAB, Zaman S, Rahman A, Murshid HB, Nadia N, Mahmud M, Alim MA, Hoque DME, Hasan ASM, El Arifeen S, Rahman AE, Rasghuvanshi VS. Effect of involvement of midwives in maternal care on patient and provider satisfaction in secondary-level public health facilities in Bangladesh: a comparative quasi-experimental study. J Glob Health. 2025;15:04183. https://doi.org/10.7189/jogh.15.04183. PMID: 40611805; PMCID: PMC12231468.
23. Eriksson I, Lindblad M, Möller U, Gillsjö C. Holistic health care: Patients' experiences of health care provided by an Advanced Practice Nurse. Int J Nurs Pract. 2018;24(1):e12603. https://doi.org/10.1111/ijn.12603. Epub 2017 Oct 25. PMID: 29071766; PMCID: PMC5813192.
24. American Nurses Association. Why nurses quit and leave the profession. May 2023 https://www.nursingworld.org/content-hub/resources/nursing-leadership/why-nurses-quit/. Accessed 19 Jan 2026.
25. Institute of Medicine (US) Committee on the Robert Wood Johnson Foundation Initiative on the Future of Nursing, at the Institute of Medicine. The Future of nursing: leading change, advancing health. Washington, DC: National Academies Press; 2011. https://doi.org/10.17226/12956. Available from: https://www.ncbi.nlm.nih.gov/books/NBK209880/. Accessed 19 Jan 2026.
26. Duignan M, Drennan J, Mc Carthy VJC. Work characteristics, job satisfaction and intention to leave: a cross-sectional survey of advanced nurse practitioners. Contemp Nurse. 2024;60(4):382–94. https://doi.org/10.1080/10376178.2024.2327353.
27. Kim DK, Scott P, Poghosyan L, Martsolf GR. Burnout, job satisfaction, and turnover intention among primary care nurse practitioners with their own patient panels. Nurs Outlook. 2024;72(4):102190. https://doi.org/10.1016/j.outlook.2024.102190. ISSN 0029-6554.

28. Kruk ME, Gage AD, Joseph NT, Danaei G, García-Saisó S, Salomon JA. Mortality due to low-quality health systems in the universal health coverage era: a systematic analysis of amenable deaths in 137 countries. Lancet. 2018;392(10160):2203–12. https://doi.org/10.1016/S0140-6736(18)31668-4. Epub 2018 Sep 5. Erratum in: Lancet. 2018 Nov 17;392(10160):2170. https://doi.org/10.1016/S0140-6736(18)32337-7. PMID: 30195398; PMCID: PMC6238021.
29. Mackavey C, Henderson C, Morris G. Empowering advanced practice nurses: a review of addressing global health needs. Ann Glob Health. 2025;91(1):45. https://doi.org/10.5334/aogh.4723. PMID: 40821623; PMCID: PMC12352385.

GPSR Compliance

The European Union's (EU) General Product Safety Regulation (GPSR) is a set of rules that requires consumer products to be safe and our obligations to ensure this.

If you have any concerns about our products, you can contact us on ProductSafety@springernature.com

In case Publisher is established outside the EU, the EU authorized representative is:

Springer Nature Customer Service Center GmbH
Europaplatz 3
69115 Heidelberg, Germany

Batch number: 10399441

Printed by Printforce, the Netherlands